GREAT DOCTORS
OF THE
NINETEENTH CENTURY

GREAT DOCTORS
OF THE
NINETEENTH CENTURY

By

SIR WILLIAM HALE-WHITE

Essay Index Reprint Series

originally published by

EDWARD ARNOLD & CO.

 BOOKS FOR LIBRARIES PRESS

FREEPORT, NEW YORK

First Published 1935
Reprinted 1970

STANDARD BOOK NUMBER:

8369-1575-5

LIBRARY OF CONGRESS CATALOG CARD NUMBER:

74-108639

·PRINTED IN THE UNITED STATES OF AMERICA

PREFACE

I am glad to have been asked to write this book, for doing so has enabled me to pass pleasantly many hours of the leisure which follows retirement from practice.

In the nineteenth century some doctors, e.g. Keats, became famous in literature or art; many, e.g. T. H. Huxley, became famous in sciences other than that of medicine—these are not here considered. The book is confined to the life and work of the more eminent of those in these islands, who, in this century, attained great distinction in medicine, using this word in its usual comprehensive sense.

Not all who might be included are here, because the book is written to a prearranged size. Some of those omitted belong more to the eighteenth or twentieth centuries than to the nineteenth.

Other selectors would have chosen other lists, but I can only hope that the reader will consider that the seventeen men herein delineated do fairly represent the development of medicine in this country during the last century. They fit in well, for, from the birth of Jenner to that of Ross is a hundred and eight years, and from the discovery of the efficiency of vaccination to that of the transmission of malaria is a hundred and one years.

In each article there are brief accounts of those who were associated with the subject of it, consequently many more doctors than seventeen are described. The index gives references to them.

W. H.-W.

CONTENTS

GREAT DOCTORS OF THE
NINETEENTH CENTURY

EDWARD JENNER

No other country doctor has reached the fame acquired by Edward Jenner. His ancestors were a Gloucestershire family of antiquity and distinction; his father, the Rev. Stephen Jenner, who owned much land in the county, was Vicar of Berkeley; he married the daughter of the Rev. Henry Head, who had been Vicar of the same place.

Half-way between Bristol and Gloucester, a country lane turns west from the main road. After going about two miles along it you reach Berkeley, once a town, now a characteristic English village, peaceful, unspoiled by motor traffic and still just as it was two centuries ago. Westward, across the fields, lies the Severn. Adjacent to the east end of the village is Berkeley Castle, the seat of the Earls of Berkeley, a formidable example of a thirteenth-century stronghold; in it Edward II was murdered. Between the village and the castle is the fine old church, close to which is the ancient vicarage where Edward, Stephen's third son and youngest child, was born, May 17, 1749. Stephen died in 1754. He had formerly been tutor to an Earl of Berkeley, and, as will be seen later, there was always close friendship between the Berkeleys and the Jenners.

Little Edward was brought up with " affectionate care and judicious guidance " by his elder brother, the Rev. Stephen Jenner, who sent him, at the age of eight, to school at Wotton-under-Edge, where he was taught by Mr. Clissold and was under the medical care of Dr. Capell, and later to one kept by the Rev. Dr. Washbourn, at Cirencester. From childhood he was a naturalist; he made a collection of nests of the dormouse before he was eight and collected fossils when at Cirencester. Leaving there he went to the Ludlows, practitioners at Sodbury, near Bristol, as an apprentice for six years; in 1770 he came to London and for two years lived in the house of John Hunter as a pupil. The master was forty-two, the pupil twenty-one years old. Nothing could have been more fortunate than this association of these two, they became fast friends. Dr. Drewitt has told us of the widespread interest in natural history during the second half of the eighteenth century. We have no evidence how far this influenced Jenner, but Hunter's enthusiasm must have strengthened Jenner's fondness for it. On Hunter's recommendation he was appointed to examine and prepare the specimens of natural history brought back by Captain Cook, in 1771, and was offered the post of naturalist to the expedition which sailed in 1772; this he declined.

After Jenner left London many letters passed between them until Hunter's death in 1793. Unfortunately, all Jenner's have been destroyed, but Hunter's have been preserved, and from them we learn that these two men kept up an extraordinary correspondence. Hunter was always much interested in the hibernation of animals and their temperature, and Jenner made many observations for him, especially on bats and hedgehogs. There are many allusions to these animals. In one letter Hunter thus disposes of Jenner's disappointment in love:

I own I was glad when I heard you was [about to be] married to a woman of fortune; but let her go, never mind her. I shall employ you with hedgehogs, for I do not know how far I may trust mine. I want you to get a hedgehog at the beginning of winter and weigh him; put him in your garden, and let him have some leaves, hay or straw to cover himself with which he will do; then weigh him in the spring and see what he has lost. Secondly, I want you to kill one at the beginning of the winter to see how fat he is, and another in the spring to see what he has lost of his fat. Thirdly, when the weather is very cold, and about the month of January I wish you would make a hole in one of their bellies and put the thermometer down into the pelvis and see the height of the mercury.

Probably no other disappointed lover has been bid to seek solace in hedgehogs. One letter asks for a large porpoise for love or money. Another begins: "I received yours with the eel," another thus: "What are you doing? How do the hedgehogs go on?" We get a glimpse of Hunter's menagerie when he writes to say an eagle ate one of his hedgehogs; in a later letter he says he will willingly give three guineas for a bustard—Jenner sent one; there is a long letter about colour vision and indeed nine-tenths of the letters are taken up with

requests for specimens of animals and fossils or for experiments
to be made in natural history. That Jenner had in him the
soul of a naturalist is shown by the fact that one of Hunter's
letters begins: "I do not know anyone I would sooner write
to than you: I do not know anybody I am so much obliged
to." We see further proof of Jenner's capacity as a naturalist
when we find Hunter writing to him to suggest that he should
come to London and that they should teach natural history.

Jenner was incited by Hunter to study the natural history
and habits of the cuckoo, this he did so successfully that he
completely solved the riddle. His observations were made, in
1787, at his aunt's farm, about four or five miles from his own
home in Berkeley. His nephew, Henry, helped him. The
note-book in which were jotted down some of the facts is in
the library of the Royal College of Physicians of London.
He sent a paper on the subject to the Royal Society the same
year, but the Council was evidently sceptical, for he was
asked to make more observations and to send the paper again
next year, when it was read in March 1788. Cuckoos do not
build a nest. Jenner dissected female cuckoos and found each
one capable of laying more than twenty eggs. She flies round
and deposits an egg in some other bird's nest, or lays it outside
and then pushes it in. The kind of bird whose nest is to receive
the cuckoo's egg varies in different parts of the country, and as
a rule the cuckoo lays an egg which closely resembles in form
and colour the egg of the bird who built the nest. Jenner
observed the laying of cuckoos' eggs in hedge-sparrows' nests:
this is exceptional in that the cuckoo's egg bears no resemblance
to the greeny-blue eggs of the host. The hedge-sparrows, or
other birds, whose nests have been visited by the cuckoo, actually
sometimes turn out their own eggs but not those of the cuckoo
which they hatch; at other times they hatch their own and
the cuckoo's. Jenner watched a nest containing two newly-
hatched cuckoos, a newly-hatched hedge-sparrow and an un-
hatched hedge-sparrow's egg. The cuckoos began to fight;
the contest lasted for over twenty-four hours, when the stronger
had turned out the weaker cuckoo, the hedge-sparrow and the
egg. This is how Jenner describes the performance:

The mode of accomplishing this is very curious. The little animal, with
the assistance of its rump and wings, contrived to get the bird (the young hedge-

3

sparrow) upon its back, and making a lodgement for the burden by elevating its elbows, clambered backward with it up the side of the nest till it reached the top, where, resting for a moment, it threw off its load with a jerk.

He then describes a special groove on the young cuckoo's back which renders the performance possible, as the bird grows older the groove disappears. The adult hedge-sparrow feeds and brings up the cuckoo. Many naturalists would not believe this extraordinary story, but, as Professor Alfred Newton says, these observations have been corroborated by others in the most minute detail. Recently photography has completely confirmed them. Shortly after the cuckoo paper Jenner was elected a Fellow of the Royal Society.

He also observed and wrote to Hunter about other things. He proved that migratory birds return to the same place in successive summers, that the supposed hibernation of birds does not exist, and that the robin not the lark is the first bird to sing at dawn. He said that earthworms prepare materials for the vegetable kingdom by breaking stiff clods to pieces and he dissected animals dead of hydatids and of distemper. Both correspondents were evidently fond of pictures, for Hunter offers to lend some of his to Jenner, who got much pleasure out of art; he sang, played the violin, belonged to a musical society, and wrote light verse—the poem to a Robin is best known, that on the Signs of Rain shows what an excellent country-man he was, nearly forty signs of coming rain are given in it.

In 1773, returning to Berkeley, he lived with his elder brother Stephen, and at once started to practise his profession, in which he took the same interest as he did in other branches of natural history. He was thoroughly happy, riding through the beautiful country and filling up his spare time by answering Hunter's demands for specimens and observations, and preparing specimens for his own museum of Natural History and Comparative Anatomy.

If a patient was very ill he would stay in the house a few days, doing his practice from it. In the winter it was hard work. Jenner fortunately had physical strength and endurance. Describing a drive over the Cotswolds in a snow blizzard he says:

There was no possibility of keeping the snow from drifting under my hat, so that half of my face and my neck were for a long while wrapt in ice. . . . When I came to the house I was unable to dismount without assistance. I was almost senseless, but I had just recollection to prevent the servants bringing

4

me to the fire. I was carried into the stable first and from thence was gradually introduced into a warmer atmosphere.

He rapidly made a great reputation. A patient in the Infirmary at Gloucester required an immediate operation for strangulated hernia, neither of the surgeons was available, so Jenner, at Berkeley, sixteen miles off, was summoned; he went and performed the operation successfully, although an attack of vomiting forced a large volume of intestines out through the wound. The patient lived for twenty years. Jenner was an investigator by nature. Being disappointed by the uncertainty of the action of tartar emetic, which he attributed to imperfection in preparation, he made experiments to improve this, and wrote to Hunter about them. Hunter replied "I am puffing off your tartar as the tartar of all tartars. . . . Let it be called Jenner's Tartar Emetic." He published Jenner's letter.

The annual fair at Berkeley in 1783 was unusually exciting, for, to amuse the folk, Jenner showed them a hydrogen balloon which had only been invented that year. He filled it with hydrogen in the great hall of Berkeley Castle. When taken outside it rose "magestically," went over the hills to come down at Symonds Hall. At a large dinner party a question arose as to the hottest part of a flame, Jenner putting his finger in the centre showed this to be cooler than the outside. This so impressed a guest that he offered Jenner an appointment in India with an annuity of £2,000. In this year his nephew, Henry Jenner, son of Henry, Jenner's brother, came as an apprentice. He seems not to have been suited for practice, for six years later his uncle writes of him as "a simple, inoffensive lad . . . so very *fifteenish* that a poor mortal on the bed of sickness will hardly look up to him with that eye of confidence and hope that might be safely placed in him."

In 1788 Jenner married Miss Catharine Kingscote, member of a well-known family. They went to live in The Chantry, a pleasant old-fashioned house in Berkeley near the church; in the garden the quaint arbour, described in glowing terms by Fosbroke, in which Jenner used to write can be seen to-day much as it was in his lifetime. The house is described as containing "every kind of apartment which the eye of philosophy could desire." Their eldest son Edward was born the following year and John Hunter stood godfather.

The busy naturalist doctor, who kept a tame eagle and delighted in landscape gardening, was as much liked by his medical brethren as he was by the people of Gloucestershire. He was instrumental in founding a medical society called the Medico-Convivial, which usually met at The Fleece Inn, Rodborough. He also belonged to another called the Convivio-Medical, which met at the Ship at Alveston. Among his many occupations he found time to be a morbid anatomist, and Dr. Parry tells us he was an excellent one—a rare accomplishment in those days. He read a paper before the first Society on the Association of Coronary Disease with Angina Pectoris, saying that he had made two autopsies on patients dead of this disease —in one the coronary arteries were thickened, in the other ossified, as he, in a letter to Dr. Parry of Bath, thus describes,

I was making a transverse section of the heart pretty near to its base, when my knife struck against something so hard and gritty as to notch it. I well remember looking up at the ceiling, which was old and crumbling, conceiving that some of the plaster had fallen down. But on further scrutiny the real cause appeared; the coronaries had become bony canals.

and he suggests that the symptoms are due to this. A large literature has sprung up on this subject, but to Jenner is due the credit of being the first to point out the association of cardiac pain with diseased coronary arteries. Dr. Parry, a great friend of Jenner's, incorporated his views in a book he wrote on Angina Pectoris. Hunter's health became bad, he arrived at Bath and Jenner went to see him and came to the conclusion he had angina pectoris; he did not tell him but wrote to Heberden for advice whether he should be told. Jenner says he knows of no remedy and if Hunter were told he would be deprived of hope. He died from angina pectoris in 1793, and Sir Everard Home wrote to Jenner to tell him that the coronary arteries were ossified.

Before the same Society he read two other original papers, one on the serious heart disease which may complicate rheumatic fever, and the other on ophthalmia. All these papers are unhappily lost, but the mere fact that a busy country doctor could find opportunity to write them shows Jenner to have been a singular man. Before the other Society he often talked about the popular belief that cow-pox protected against small-pox, the other members were well aware of the belief, which they regarded as merely an old woman's tale and they used to threaten Jenner with expulsion if he persisted in boring them with such rubbish.

The winter after Hunter's death was unfortunate for Jenner as several members of his family were ill with either typhus or typhoid. In 1792, that is to say when he was 43, the fatigues of an ever increasing practice had become so great that he resolved to practise solely as a physician, and accordingly he obtained the M.D. degree of the University of St. Andrews. He had been a general practitioner for twenty years, during which, in addition to his clinical and pathological professional work, he had carried out observations on the migration of birds, on the cuckoo, and on geology; he had dissected numberless animals, had experimented with hydrogen balloons and had conducted innumerable investigations for Hunter on hedgehogs and a host of other animals.

Jenner was a favourite both at the medical discussions of the two local medical societies and at the dinner which followed; when he was ill several of his colleagues gladly helped to look after him, when he stayed for days at a patient's home the household were sorry at his departure, educated people loved his conversation, he used to encourage those whom he liked to ride twenty or thirty miles with him on his rounds and he would talk to them all the way; when he left a patient's house often some of the family would ask permission to ride home with him even if it was midnight.

What figure of a man was this unique country practitioner? His friend Gardner describes him thus:

His height was rather under the middle size, his person was robust but active and well formed. In dress he was particularly neat. . . . He was dressed in a blue coat and yellow buttons, buckskins and well polished jockey boots with handsome silver spurs and he carried a smart whip with a silver handle. His hair, after the fashion of the times, was done up in a club and he wore a broad-brimmed hat.

Everything we know of him indicates that he was usually cheerful and sociable, very occasionally he was depressed, and we find him complaining that he was an example of the sin of indolence. Many busy people, being aware how much there is to do in the world, at times blame themselves for this.

I have tried shortly to picture Jenner the naturalist, pathologist, and country doctor, but now we come to that part of his work which has made him one of the greatest benefactors to the human race. Before his great discovery small-pox was an awful scourge; in 1572 a special medal was struck to commemorate Queen Elizabeth's recovery from it; in the latter half of the eighteenth century it killed 40,000 people in this country every year: many who got well were disfigured for life. Three-fourths of the blind owed their loss of sight to small-pox. It was quite common for a man to prefer to marry a woman marked by it, for then he was less likely to be a widower. Jenner not only showed how to prevent this frightful malady so well that most doctors to-day have never seen a case of small-pox, but, from his discovery followed the principle of vaccination which, for example, in the late war saved whole regiments of soldiers from typhoid fever.

Ever since the dawn of history every man, woman and child had passed through life, with small-pox close by, ready without warning to kill or cruelly disfigure. In desperation, in the eighteenth century the practice of inoculation was tried, the word being used for the first time in a pathological sense. Healthy people voluntarily acquired small-pox which they trusted would be mild, as but a small dose of exudate from a patient having small-pox was injected under the skin, because a mild attack of small-pox rendered them immune from further attacks. This shows the terrible dread of small-pox, for there was always a considerable chance that the inoculated disease might be severe, indeed it was sometimes fatal. Still in many countries people willingly ran this risk. But every successfully inoculated person really suffered from small-pox and often transmitted the disease to others: the result was, in some countries, an appalling increase in the number of cases of small-pox. Often the total mortality from small-pox was higher after the introduction of inoculation than before. In France the practice was condemned by the Faculty of Medicine and was prohibited by royal authority in 1763. The Royal College of Physicians of London declared its approbation of inoculation, but, for some incomprehensible reason, omitted to state that those inoculated should be isolated until they ceased to be able to infect others. Inoculation was later made illegal in England. When Jenner began to think about small-pox there was therefore no real preventive in the field. He certainly had no reason to be well inclined to inoculation. His friend Fosbroke writes,

At a very early period of the life of Dr. Jenner the foundation was probably laid for his subsequent investigations as to a Preventive of Small-Pox by the following circumstances. He was a fine ruddy boy, and at eight years of age was, with many others, put under a preparatory process for Inoculation with the Small-Pox, by the late Mr. Holbrow of Wootton Underedge. This preparation lasted six weeks. He was bled to ascertain whether his blood was fine; was purged repeatedly, till he became emaciated and feeble; was kept on very low diet, small in quantity and dosed with a diet-drink to sweeten the blood. After this barbarism of human-veterinary practice he was removed to one of the then usual inoculation stables, and haltered up with others in a terrible state of disease, although none died. By good fortune the doctor escaped with a mild exhibition of the disease.

It is said that this torture affected his health for several years.

A chance remark by a milkmaid ultimately led to the control of small-pox throughout the world. The story of the discovery of vaccination is this. The maid came to the house of Mrs. Ludlow of Sodbury when Jenner, then a youth, was living in it as an apprentice. The word small-pox was mentioned in her presence; he heard her say, " I cannot take that disease, for I have had cow-pox." He pondered on this remark for years, he talked about it to Hunter, who mentioned it in his lectures and characteristically said to Jenner, " Don't think, but try; be patient, be accurate." We have seen that he so often talked of it at one of his medical clubs that his fellow members got bored with it. Still he communed within himself and observed and experimented whenever opportunity arose. Then in 1780, riding with Gardner between Gloucester and Bristol, as the two were passing Newport, Jenner made an historic communication to his friend, telling him of all his experiments and observations and his hopes of extinguishing small-pox, winding up by saying,

Gardner, I have entrusted a most important matter to you, which I firmly believe will prove of essential benefit to the human race. I know you, and should not wish what I have said to be brought into conversation; for should anything untoward turn up in my experiments, I should be made, particularly by my medical brethren, the subject of ridicule—for I am the mark they all shoot at.

This remark had reference to the chaff he underwent at the Convivio-Medical Club; no discoverer was ever more willing than Jenner to share his discoveries with others.

Observations and experiments continued. In 1788 he went to London and showed a drawing of cow-pox on the hands of a milker to Sir Everard Home and others. Cline told Dr. Adams about Jenner's investigations. Haygarth got to hear of them and wrote, "Your account of the cow-pox is indeed very marvellous; being so strange a history, and so contradictory to all past observations on the subject, very clear and full evidence will be required to make it credible."

Back again in Berkeley, his original work continued, and, on May 14, 1796, the famous experiment was made, so famous that for many years an annual festival to commemorate it was held in Berlin on the fourteenth of May. Jenner thus describes it in a letter to Gardner:

A boy named Phipps was inoculated in the arm from a pustule on the hand of a young woman who was infected by her master's cows. Having never seen the disease but in its casual way before, that is, when communicated from the cow to the hand of the milker, I was astonished at the close resemblance of the pustules in some of their stages, to the variolous pustules. But now listen to the most delightful part of my story. The boy has since been inoculated for the small-pox which, as I ventured to predict, produced no effect. I shall now pursue my experiments with redoubled ardour.

Believe me, yours very sincerely,
EDWARD JENNER.

BERKELEY, *July* 19, 1796.

From this date till the spring of 1798 his researches were discontinued because no cases of cow-pox appeared in the dairies; then it appeared again, he repeated his experiments and wrote a paper on the subject. He discussed this with his friends near Berkeley, Mr. Westfaling, Dr. Worthington, Mr. Paytherus and Mr. Hicks, who approved of it. He suggested sending it to the Royal Society, but, acting on the advice of Dr. Worthington, it was published, as a quarto pamphlet of seventy-five pages, at the end of June 1798, and dedicated to his friend Dr. Parry of Bath. The title of this immortal pamphlet is *An Inquiry into The Causes and Effects of The Variolae Vaccinae, A Disease discovered in some of the Western Counties of England particularly Gloucestershire and known by the name of The Cow Pox.* It is usually referred to as The Inquiry. The author begins with a description of "grease," a disease of horses shown by inflammation of the heel, which swells and discharges. Should the groom who attends to the horse get some discharge on his hands and then, without washing them, milk a cow, he will infect the cow whose illness is cow-pox. The symptoms in this animal are pustules, which later discharge, on the nipples, and general illness. If a dairymaid milk such a cow, her hands will very likely be infected. She then has cow-pox, her symptoms are vesicles, which may form pustules and break down to become ulcers, most frequent on the hands, swelling of the axillary glands and general malaise lasting from one to four days. After Jenner's description of this he writes, "but what renders the cow-pox virus so extremely singular is that the person who has been thus affected is, for ever after, secure from the infection of the small-pox; neither exposure to the variolous effluvia, nor the insertion of the matter into the skin, producing this distemper." Then follows an account of many cases to support this statement. I cannot, for want of space, quote more than two. A woman had cow-pox in 1765, in 1792 she nursed a child with small-pox without catching it, Jenner thereupon inoculated her with small-pox, but without any result. A girl at the age of 9 years had had cow-pox; when she was 62 Jenner inoculated her with small-pox, the only results were very slight transitory signs of illness. He reminds us that it is well known among dairy farmers that most of those who have had small-pox are protected from cow-pox and with the few that get it, the disease is exceedingly mild; he quotes cases to illustrate this. He tells us that in a village a large number of persons were inoculated against small-pox, eight had had cow-pox, in not one of the eight did the inoculation succeed. Examples are given to show that the infection of human beings by the discharge from the heel of a horse with grease confers considerable immunity against small-pox, Jenner calls attention to the popular belief that farriers are, generally speaking, free from small-pox, but he believes that to confer complete immunity the virus from the horse must pass through the cow. Experiments are described in which cow-pox was successfully transferred, by inoculation, from one human being to another, and it is shown that the person to whom it is transferred is completely immune against small-pox inoculation even if the cow-pox has been transferred from one human being to another through a considerable series.

At the end of the cases he asserts " That cow-pox protects the human constitution from the infection of small-pox." Cow-pox never kills human beings, nor are there any disfiguring scars in those artificially inoculated, hence vaccination with it is far superior to inoculation by small-pox.

The following year he published another pamphlet entitled *Further Observations*, also dedicated to Dr. Parry. He did so because some observers reported they had not obtained his results. This he showed was for two reasons. Firstly, they had failed to recognize that pustules and vesicles, which are not due to true cow-pox, may be present on cows' udders; these are spurious cow-pox and have no preventive influence against small-pox, only true cow-pox has this. Secondly, for the matter from the cow to be protective against small-pox, it must be taken from the vesicle before it bursts, if taken after the vesicle has burst, it may produce a serious illness following injection (which is what we should expect, but Jenner knew nothing of septic micro-organisms) which does not protect. He gives further reasons for thinking that grease causes cow-pox but admits that this is not completely proved. The rest of the pamphlet is occupied with many extraordinarily interesting cases. A child 20 hours old·was vaccinated, subsequently it was inoculated with small-pox without any effect.

In 1800 he issued a third pamphlet called *A Continuation of Facts and Observations*. By then he says over 6,000 people had been vaccinated, far the greater number had been subsequently inoculated with small-pox without any effect. His neighbour, Dr. Marshall, had vaccinated 423, of whom 211 were afterwards inoculated with small-pox, but everyone resisted it. As vaccination spread, it was early found that a recently vaccinated person was incapable of giving cow-pox to others by propinquity. Some in Gloucestershire were vaccinated with cow-pox lymph from cows in London, the result was as good as with lymph from cows in the neighbourhood. The important discovery was made that, if a patient be vaccinated soon after exposure to small-pox, he will fail to contract this disease; for example, two children were in contact, often in bed, with their father for five days, during which he had the small-pox eruption on him, they were then vaccinated and did not get small-pox. Another similar case is given. Dr.

Marshall inadvertently took vaccine matter on a lancet previously charged with small-pox matter. He, thinking he was only going to vaccinate, used this lancet for this purpose on a woman and four children, none had any signs of small-pox, but all had genuine cow-pox. Later they were all inoculated again with small-pox matter and were found to be immune. Jenner, with perfect propriety, concludes thus:

May I not with perfect confidence congratulate my country and society at large on their beholding, in the mild form of the cow-pox, an antidote that is capable of extirpating from the earth a disease which is every hour devouring its victims; a disease that has ever been considered the severest scourge of the human race!

The *Inquiry* went through several editions and was translated into many languages. The rapidity with which knowledge of it spread is remarkable, German and Latin editions appeared in 1799, French and Italian in 1800. Jenner and his wife were in London from April 24 till July 14, 1798, partly to see the *Inquiry* through the press—it appeared late in June—and partly to arouse interest in vaccination, for this was the name given to the inoculation of cow-pox, and, from it, the word vaccine is derived. He returned to Berkeley, having failed to persuade Londoners to be vaccinated, with the exception that Cline, always on the look out for any scientific advance, had vaccinated a boy with cow-pox material given by Jenner and had found him subsequently immune to small-pox inoculation. Cline became enthusiastic in the cause, wrote to Jenner, advised him to leave the country and take a house in Grosvenor Square, prophesying he would become famous and make £10,000 a year. After the *Inquiry* had been read, Cline was backed up by Sir W. Farquhar and others, but Jenner refused, writing, " Shall I, who even in the morning of my days sought the lowly and sequestered paths of life, the valley, and not the mountain; shall I, now my evening is fast approaching, hold myself up as an object for fortune and for fame ? " He goes on to ask how would either add to his happiness, he has all he wants where he is. " And as for fame what is it ? A gilded butt, for ever pierced with the arrows of malignancy." A letter characteristic of the true country-loving philosopher that he was.

The publication of the *Inquiry* made him very busy, for many wrote to him. Some to help him, for example there is a long letter from Lord St. Asaph in strong support of the opinion that grease leads to cow-pox, some to congratulate him, some writers gave him their favourable experience, some criticized severely. All, especially the last, meant an enormous correspondence. Those who quoted results which were supposed to tell against vaccination either did not understand the matter, or had used wrong material, as has been mentioned already. Jenner encountered fewer opponents than most discoverers, who are usually pestered by ignoramuses, fools, knaves and cranks, still he suffered from attacks, for he writes that brickbats and hostile weapons are flying around him and he is beset by snarling fellows. He was fortunate in his lay support; his neighbour, Mr. Hicks, was the first gentleman to have his children vaccinated, Lady Ducie and the Countess of Berkeley quickly followed, and he had good professional support from the beginning, e.g. Cline, Lettsom, Abernethy and many others declared their faith in vaccination.

Things were not going well for vaccination in London because two doctors, Pearson and Woodville, were talking and writing about it, and practising it extensively, without having grasped the features of true cow-pox. They were using matter from vesicles—occasionally those of small-pox—which were not those of true cow-pox, often with serious results to the patient and great damage to the reputation of vaccination. This brought Jenner to London in March 1799, where he stayed nearly three months. His presence did good. Mr. Ring got up a testimonial signed by over seventy of the best-known physicians and surgeons in London, stating their belief in the efficiency of vaccination from true cow-pox.

Jenner had hardly got back to Berkeley when he received a letter from Pearson saying that he had formed an Institution or Vaccine Board for vaccinating the poor and asked Jenner to be a corresponding member. This was an insult, for Jenner, the discoverer of vaccination, who had never been consulted about the formation of the Institution, was now offered a subordinate position, the letter actually said the subscription due from Jenner would be a guinea annually, but if he liked he could be exempt from paying. Having a generous nature he would have treated the letter with contempt, had it not been that, knowing Pearson's incompetence, he was fearful of the results to the cause of vaccination, especially as Pearson had secured the Duke of York as patron and Lord Egremont, who had always been interested in Jenner's work, as one of the officers. He came back to London, the Duke asked to see Jenner who had told his friend, Lord Egremont, of the harm the proposed Institution would do. The result was that both the Duke and Lord Egremont withdrew and the Institution collapsed. During this stay in London, Jenner, introduced by Lord Berkeley, presented a copy of the *Inquiry* to the King, he was also received by the Prince of Wales, the Duke of Clarence and the Queen, he saw hosts of people of note both in his profession and outside it, he attended meetings, wherever he went he explained vaccination and he vaccinated many children. Lady Rous, one of his ardent admirers, sent some vaccine lymph to her sister Mrs. Gooch at Hadleigh, whose husband wrote to say that the whole town had been vaccinated without a single mishap. On his way back to Berkeley in June, he stayed a day in Oxford, where he met many distinguished persons and received a testimonial in favour of vaccination. Within two years of the publication of the *Inquiry* there was a full flood-tide in favour of Jenner and vaccination.

The rapid and ubiquitous spread of vaccination was remarkable. Less than a year after the appearance of the *Inquiry*, De Carro, of Vienna, was using vaccine lymph. He began by vaccinating his own two children and the son of a doctor; under his enthusiastic advocacy the practice spread to Switzerland, Germany, Poland, Italy and Constantinople and from thence to Bombay and India. Dr. Scott, of Bombay, at once vaccinated his own children and family, soon after every European family in the city and upwards of 3,000 children had been vaccinated. The request was made that vaccine lymph should be sent by every courier. The swift spread of vaccination in India, and from there to the Far East, was helped by the religious veneration of the Hindus for the cow. Jenner, not knowing that vaccination had reached India so quickly, was wishful to send a mission to India to spread vaccination; he offered to subscribe 1,000 guineas for the purpose, the project dropped when he learned that it was not necessary.

In December 1799 Princess Louisa of Prussia wrote asking Jenner to send lymph to Berlin, which he did. Next year the use of it began in Spain, where vaccination spread rapidly; in this year when the *Inquiry* was translated into French, three editions were sold in seven months, and vaccination was widely used. A most singular mission sailed from Portsmouth in 1800 under the sanction of the British Government. Its object was to convey the benefits of vaccination to the inhabitants of the Mediterranean countries; Gibraltar, Mahon, Malta, Sicily, Naples, Egypt and other places were visited, thousands of people were vaccinated. The new preventive was introduced into the Navy and Army, and the naval doctors gave Jenner a gold medal.

The United States quickly adopted vaccination. Jefferson and many of his relations were vaccinated, so were the native Indians. Jenner sent them his book. The chiefs held a meeting to thank him, and in their reply said:

We shall not fail to teach our children to speak the name of Jenner; and to thank the Great Spirit for bestowing upon him so much wisdom and so much benevolence. We send with this a belt and a string of Wampum in token of our acceptance of your precious gift; and we beseech the Great Spirit to take care of you in this world and in the land of Spirits.

Then follow the native signatures and marks.

The Government of Spain fitted out an expedition to carry the practice to all Spanish dependencies throughout the world. It was under the care of Dr. Balmis, and set sail from Corunna on November 30, 1803. There were on board twenty-two children who had never had small-pox, selected for the preservation of the vaccine fluid, by transmitting it successfully from one to another during the voyage. In three years the expedition returned to Spain, having circumnavigated the globe and successfully introduced vaccination to Central America, South America, and many other places.

It spread to the most remote parts of Russia and China; in this last country a book about it was published. The number vaccinated must have been several millions, for Dr. Sacco and two assistants vaccinated 1,300,000 persons in Italy in eight years. At Palermo it was not unusual to see on the mornings of the public inoculation at the hospital, a procession of men, women and children, conducted through the streets by a priest carrying a cross, on their way to be inoculated. In Geneva a priest exhorted the members of his congregation to be vaccinated and had a physician present to do it for them after the service. An English clergyman preached a sermon advocating it, and, whenever he baptized a child, gave the parents a tract urging vaccination. The Dowager Empress of Russia recommended it fervently, decreeing that the first child in Russia to be vaccinated should be called Vaccinoff; it was a girl, and provision was settled on her for life. The Empress sent Jenner a diamond ring. A letter from Dr. Davids, of Rotterdam, is addressed to the "Benefactor of Mankind, Dr. Jenner."

Such great fame taxed the discoverer sorely. His correspondence was prodigious. Letters came from everywhere asking for lymph, for advice, telling him of results, praising him, criticizing him. Journeys to London were frequent. No time remained for earning his living by his practice, yet he was put to considerable expense. His neighbours in Gloucestershire saw this, they showed their admiration and affection by a present of silver plate, they talked of a subscription. But, in the opinion of many influential persons, the benefit conferred upon the world by Jenner was so great that his proper recompense was a national matter, accordingly he came to town in December 1801 and in January 1802 had a satisfactory interview with Addington, the Prime Minister. On March 17, 1802, "The humble Petition of Edward Jenner, Doctor of Physic," was presented to the House of Commons. This admirable, temperate document, given in full by Baron in his *Life of Jenner,* indicates the importance of the discovery, the fact that its author has given it to the world freely and without recompense and that he has suffered considerable financial loss thereby. The petition was referred to a strong committee which examined many witnesses of great distinction, both medical and lay. It was pointed out that if Jenner had kept the discovery secret he could have made £10,000 a year by it. The committee reported to the House on June 2, 1802, entirely favourably to Jenner on all grounds, and recommended that a grant of not less than £10,000 should be made to him. It was moved that a grant of this amount be made, an amendment was proposed that it be £20,000. The division was between those who supported this sum and those who supported £10,000. Those supporting the lesser sum won by 59 votes to 56.

As the beneficent results of vaccination became certain, Jenner was honoured by medical societies everywhere. In 1802, at a meeting in Paris and also at one in Breslau, his portrait was surrounded by a garland of flowers; he was elected a corresponding member of the American Academy of Arts and Sciences; several English societies honoured him, but what gave him "the greatest satisfaction" was that the Physical Society arranged a debate on vaccination at Guy's Hospital, and invited Jenner, who attended all four evenings on which the debate lasted. This was the first time he had an opportunity of addressing a London audience on the subject. "On entering the theatre he was constantly received with universal and rapturous applause; and as no discussion was ever of greater importance or of deeper interest, none, probably, ever attracted in a higher degree the attention of professional and scientific men." The Society conferred a special order of merit upon him.

He returned to the country in the autumn. In December he received a letter from London saying that it was proposed to found a Jennerian Institute, he replied that he would abide by the advice of his friend Lettsom as to whether he should take part. In January 1803 a large meeting, at which the Lord Mayor presided, was held at the London Tavern. It was decided to found a Jennerian Institute for the extermination of small-pox and for the furtherance of vaccination. The King and Queen were patrons, the supporters formed a galaxy of persons of note, Jenner was President. An office was taken in Salisbury Square and thirteen vaccinating stations were opened in London; thousands were vaccinated, but, alas, the committee appointed the wrong man as "resident inoculator and medical secretary." He was thoroughly unsatisfactory, was about to be dismissed when he resigned, but the Institute never recovered; gradually its activities ceased.

His friends now thought that the rare distinction of the Parliamentary grant already sanctioned would so enhance his reputation that he would make a handsome income if he settled in London; consequently he tried this plan, practising at 14, Hertford Street, Mayfair—on the house there is now a tablet to him—but it was a failure. In the first place the grant was not paid for at least two years and £1,000 was deducted for expenses. Most persons seemed to consider that as he had the grant he was the servant of the public, thus he was inundated with letters and callers; so many were able to vaccinate that few came to Jenner for this, although he was called upon to vaccinate numbers of patients gratuitously. Therefore, after giving practice in London a fair trial, he relinquished it, returned to Berkeley and again became the village doctor, coming to London very rarely. But the experiment had been extremely costly, and consequently his supporters brought before Parliament the question of a further grant. The Government called upon the Royal College of Physicians to report upon the subject of vaccination. This body examined the matter most carefully and judiciously, and on April 10, 1807, presented a report signed by Sir Lucas Pepys, the president. It strongly recommended the practice of vaccination, the truth of which "seems to be established as firmly as the nature of such a question admits," and the College considered that the public may look forward to the end of the ravages, if not the existence, of small-pox. As a result of this report the Chancellor of the Exchequer proposed a grant of £10,000. Mr. Edward Morris, the member for Newport in Cornwall, moved an amendment to make it £20,000. The amendment was carried by a majority of thirteen, with, for Jenner, the fortunate condition attached that the grant was to be free of fees. India sent him a present of over £7,000.

He now lived at his house, The Chantry, in Berkeley, doing the ordinary work of a country practitioner. In the garden was the arbour in which he used to vaccinate the poor gratuitously. Sometimes he visited Cheltenham or Bath; occasionally he had the opportunity of seeing celebrated visitors to his neighbourhood. He delighted in walks and rides; he visited Matthew Baillie who had retired to Duntisbourne; he was as eager as ever in the study of nature. There exists a charming note by him describing how moths feed upon the night-blowing primrose. It was now that he did most of his work on the migration of birds, but his enormous correspondence must have occupied much of his time. In no wise was he puffed up with his fame, he remained a simple unostentatious man, a friend of his neighbours whom he liked to meet at dinner. He gave freely of that most valuable of all commodities, his time; he was assiduous as a magistrate; he would listen to all callers, rich or poor, at whatever time they came to him. He was particularly cordial to all his fellow-practitioners, and especially liked talking with the younger of them. His kindness to the needy was continual. Phipps became very ill, and, as he lived in a miserable place, Jenner built him a comfortable cottage, himself stocking the garden with shrubs and flowers. One of the villagers showed considerable musical ability, whereupon Jenner took him to a music meeting at Gloucester. Indeed, as far as we can gather, he led the happy life of the perfect country doctor.

Nevertheless, in the last twenty years of his life, which he spent almost entirely in the seclusion of a country village, his fame continued to spread and honours fell thick upon him from all over the world. The list of diplomas, honours and addresses awarded to him numbered, according to Baron, forty-seven and of these more than half were received after his final return to the country. Several medals were struck to commemorate his discovery. The freedom of the City of London was presented to him in a box valued at a hundred guineas. He was also made a freeman of Edinburgh, Glasgow, Dublin, Liverpool and Kirkcaldy. He received an honorary degree from the University of Oxford, he was made Physician Extraordinary to the King. One of the greater of his distinctions was that he was unanimously elected a Corresponding Member of the National Institute of France, and later on he was made one of its Foreign Associates. Addresses, resolutions, letters from societies and from distinguished people, not included in the above forty-seven, all thanking the discoverer of vaccination, were innumerable.

Such was the gratitude of mankind to him that he attained an influence throughout the world probably never before or since acquired by a private individual. Dr. Wickham and Mr. Williams were detained in Geneva by Napoleon. All efforts to obtain their release had been fruitless. Jenner wrote to Napoleon asking that they should be set free, and they were, Napoleon saying: "Jenner! Ah, we can refuse nothing to that man." On another occasion he liberated two other Englishmen on Jenner's request. The Emperor of Austria also set free an Englishman when asked by Jenner, and on his intercession the King of Spain gave a prisoner his liberty. Those who travelled abroad were able to dispense with passports if they took a certificate by Jenner, for it was respected everywhere. Here is an example:

> I hereby certify that Mr. A., the young gentleman who is the bearer of this, and who is about to sail from the port of Bristol on board the *Adventure*, Captain Vezey, for the island of Madeira, has no other object in view than the recovery of his health.
>
> EDWARD JENNER,
> Member of the N.I. of France.
>
> BERKELEY, GLOUCESTERSHIRE, *July* 1, 1810.

In his letter to the young man's father Jenner says that if the boy is captured the certificate will secure his release.

His wife died of phthisis at Cheltenham on September 13, 1815. After this Jenner retired from public life, he bought The Chantry and hardly ever left Berkeley, but continued to work at vaccination correspondence, his practice and nature studies. In August 1820 he had a cerebral hæmorrhage, from which he recovered, although he was never quite himself again; on January 25, 1823, he was found insensible from a second attack and he died the following day. He is buried in Berkeley Church, next to his wife; on the wall of the church is a large tablet to commemorate him and there is a statue in Gloucester Cathedral.

Since his death statues of him have been put up in many countries, the London statue is in Kensington Gardens. His portrait was painted by Lawrence, Northcote, Hobday and J. R. Smith. That by Hobday is now at the Royal Society of Medicine, that by Northcote is in the National Portrait Gallery. Collections of things of interest about him have been made, the best is in the Wellcome Historical Medical Museum in London. Institutes have been named after him. On the centenary of his death a special meeting was held at the Royal Society of Medicine in London, a wreath was placed at the foot of his statue in Gloucester Cathedral and an "In Memoriam" notice appeared in *The Times*. The centenary was also celebrated at the Académie de Médecine in Paris by an address from Professor Chauffard.

SIR ASTLEY PASTON COOPER

Early in the nineteenth century it used to be said that the two best-known men in London were George the Fourth and Sir Astley Cooper. His ancestors and numerous relations had lived in Norfolk for many generations. With them, as was usual in those days, large families were common. His great-great-grandmother, Cassandra, had twenty-one children; he was one of ten, of whom three at least died of consumption. The Coopers, like several other Norfolk families, were well educated, well off, took their place in county society and inter-married with members of it.

His paternal grandfather, Samuel Cooper, a surgeon in Norwich, was a man of considerable literary attainments. He had two sons: the elder, Samuel, was the father of Astley; the younger, William, became surgeon to Guy's Hospital. Samuel was a wrangler and a Doctor of Divinity; he held several livings, the last being the important one of Great Yarmouth. He was an authoritative man, inclined to lay down the law both in his life and in his writings, which consisted mostly of sermons. He married Miss Bransby, a woman of property: "in her person were remarkably exhibited the close affinity between cultivated talents and virtuous affection." She was the authoress of many novels, popular in their day; they were of a religious character, written in the form of letters supposed to pass between the different characters.

Astley Paston Cooper, her fourth son, was born on August 23, 1768, at Brooke Hall, where the family were then living; it is about seven miles from Norwich. At that time ladies in East Anglia, who could afford it, put their children out to nurse; young Astley's foster-mother was Mrs. Lowe, a farmer's wife. About eleven years later his foster-brother, young Lowe, had his femoral artery severed by a wheel going over his thigh. His parents tried to stop the bleeding by pressure on the wound. Astley, hearing of the accident, rushed round, found blood flowing out and stopped it by tying a handkerchief tightly round the thigh above the wound. He used to say that this incident made him think he would like to be a surgeon.

Astley was an idle young fellow, the teaching of his father, mother and a Mr. Larke, the village schoolmaster who taught him mathematics, made little impression, but he was greatly daring, loving to be in all sorts of mischief. Riding a horse, he set it to jump a sleeping cow, but the cow got up inopportunely throwing Astley and breaking his collar-bone. He fell from the roof of the church several times, he was nearly drowned, he tumbled from the top of a hay-stack, he dressed up as the devil to frighten an old woman. These and many like activities seem to have been due to mere mischief, people liked the idler, admiring his fearlessness but they marvelled that he never killed himself. At the age of twelve he moved to Yarmouth with his parents. His uncle, William Cooper, who came to stay with them occasionally, took a liking to the lad which led to his taking him as a pupil, to learn surgery, at Guy's Hospital. He was only sixteen, so it may be that the wish to see London operated more strongly than the desire to be surgeon.

St. Thomas's and Guy's Hospitals were then on opposite sides of St. Thomas's Street, in the borough of Southwark. The students at each were free to attend both. William Cooper became surgeon to Guy's Hospital in 1783. He did not trouble much about private practice, but attended the hospital daily, superintending carefully the work of his dressers and taking a personal interest in each. One of them having made an apt classical quotation about a patient, William Cooper was so pleased that, next day, he presented the dresser with a handsome edition of the author of the quotation. His nephew said he had too much feeling to be a surgeon—in those days anæsthetics had not been discovered—and to illustrate this related that William on one occasion was going to amputate a man's leg; the patient, arriving in the operating theatre, saw its display of instruments, lost his courage and rushed from the hospital. William Cooper made no attempt to recover him; he merely remarked, "By God! I am glad he is gone."

Why young Astley did not live with his uncle is unknown. He lived instead at St. Mary Axe with Henry Cline, who favoured the French revolution, was a devoted friend of Horne

Tooke and who held opinions on religion and politics so completely opposed to those of Astley's parents that we can only suppose they knew nothing about them, but did know Cline to be an able man, surgeon to St. Thomas's Hospital and lecturer on anatomy there. It was a good thing for Astley because it widened his horizon, enabled him to meet people who would not be allowed in the rectory at Yarmouth, and gave him, in Cline, a kind friend whose influence in Paris made it possible for him to study there in 1792. Cline, who did a large practice, was respected by his fellow-surgeons, for he became President of their College, also by his pupils, who subscribed to obtain a bust of him by Chantrey.

Guy's Hospital Physical Society was founded in 1771, its members being drawn chiefly from Guy's and St. Thomas's. It was famous; Jenner gave his first account in London of vaccination before it, Hunter read a paper on ligature of the popliteal artery for aneurism. Crowded meetings were held; in fact, it was *the* Society to join. Therefore, in October 1784, Astley, on the nomination of his uncle, became a member. During the winter session 1784–5 this young, handsome, finely-built, popular medical student did little work, his amiable qualities quickly gave him the companionship of equally idle youths, he continued much the same practical jokes as had amused him at home, and his inattention to his profession is shown by the number of times he was fined for non-attendance at the Physical Society or for leaving meetings before they were over. He thus describes his first six months:

The conversation of these men (i.e. those living at Mr. Cline's) improved me : the indolence of L—— and his gold-laced waistcoats, made him our laughing stock, C—— promised too much to be always right, J—— was always a gentleman. I was very idle, quick, lively, a favourite with the family, especially with Mr. Cline's mother, a highly informed reading woman, and with her I spent many hours.

Towards the end of this session he transferred from his uncle to Cline, whose pupil he became. Probably, as William Cooper was a strict disciplinarian, the nephew did not enjoy working with him.

He was now completely under Cline, his idleness ceased, and he was enthusiastically led into the path of the science of anatomy as taught by John Hunter. Thanks to Cline he worked diligently at it. The demonstrator was John Haighton, an original and able man in many directions, but irritable, opinionated and argumentative, consequently students did not care to ask his help in their dissections, preferring to ask their popular fellow-student to assist them. Haighton, realizing that he would not get promotion in the anatomical department, resigned his post there in 1789 to lecture on physiology, and also on midwifery. He was a good lecturer, an admirable operator in obstetrics, his distinction in mathematics and astronomy obtained for him his F.R.S. He died in 1823.

In those days, there was no summer session at the medical school, therefore Astley went home at the end of his second winter session, during which he had made for himself a good position in the dissecting-room; he had begun to go round the wards and take notes under the direction of Cline; he had attended the Physical Society; indeed, the contrast between the stern student of the second session and the idler of the first is extraordinary. Even his mother was astonished. She writes: " You seem to have improved every moment of your time, and to have soared not only beyond our expectations, but to the utmost height of our wishes."

During his summer vacation in 1786 he made the acquaintance of a medical student named Holland who, liking Astley, came also to live with Cline for the winter session 1786-7. The dissecting-room was so full that these two enthusiasts took home their parts to dissect quietly in their room. They ligatured the femoral and humeral arteries of a dog, later they killed it and injected the arteries in order to study the anastomoses. Astley worked hard at anatomy and surgery, and found time to attend John Hunter's demonstrations and the Physical Society where he took part in the debates. Towards the end of the session he caught typhus fever and was nursed by the Clines, afterwards going home to convalesce.

In the autumn of 1787 he went to Edinburgh for seven months. He took a room at six shillings and sixpence a week, arranging for a daily dinner for a shilling; having presented his numerous introductions, he started study at the University. On December 1 he was elected a member of the celebrated Royal Society of Medicine at Edinburgh; he attended the meetings regularly and took part in many debates, during one of which he heard a reply which amused him greatly. An Irishman declared that cancer did not occur in women who had borne children; in disproof a Scotchman cited a woman who had twice borne twins and yet had cancer. The Irishman instantly replied, " Ah, by my soul, don't you know that's an exception—where's the wonder in cancer following gemini—it always does." The ease with which Astley acquired the esteem and affection of his fellows is shown by his election to the presidency of one of the student societies soon after his arrival. His was a very practical mind, perhaps he thought it was too much so, for he joined the Speculative Society and read a paper before it in which he maintained the Berkelian Theory of matter; he was teller for the noes in a debate on " Is a man a free agent."

The chief part of his time was spent on anatomy and surgery; he used to say that he learnt a great deal in Edinburgh, especially the art of arranging his thoughts systematically, particularly when they were applied to the elucidation of a patient's illness; also it was an advantage to his education to mix freely with many people celebrated for their learning. He admits he enjoyed this seven months, but remarks that distance enhances the character of men beyond their deserts. The summer of 1788 was passed partly in a tour through the Highlands with a servant and two horses; he returned to Cline's house in the autumn.

Fortunately he discovered a new pupil here named Colman. The two used to attend Hunter's lectures, they dissected, experimented and argued together. Between them there grew a close friendship which lasted fifty years. Edward Colman was four years older than Astley. Before he came to London he had been, for seven years, a surgeon's apprentice at Gravesend, to Mr. Kite, who was much interested in asphyxia, hence Colman's anxiety to understand it. His scientific work on the subject was rewarded by the medal of the Humane Society and his book on it brought him much reputation. He practised as a surgeon until he became Professor at the Veterinary College in 1793; his famous book on the foot of the horse was published in 1799. His chief claim to our gratitude is his unceasing insistence upon the need for the proper ventilation of stables. The Army, which was saved thousands of pounds annually by following his advice, made him Veterinary Surgeon-General to the British Cavalry. He became an F.R.S. and is

justly regarded as one of the founders of the science of Veterinary
Medicine.

In 1789 Astley Cooper was appointed demonstrator of
Anatomy at St. Thomas's, in place of Haighton who had
resigned the post. For the next two years the young demonstrator
studied and taught with such success that in 1791, although
his pupilage had not expired, Cline offered him a part share
in the lectures, saying he should have £120 a year, to be
increased £20 annually, until he gave half the lectures when
the fees from them should be divided equally. He gladly
accepted what was an extremely complimentary offer to one so
young, but Cline had foreseen his future greatness. His first
step was to persuade Cline, which he did with difficulty, that
anatomy lectures should be separated from those on surgery,
an alteration which greatly enhanced the value of the lectures.
Astley took those on surgery, giving them in the evening. He
began by trying to imitate Hunter's lectures. This was a
mistake, for, although he had learnt much from Hunter and
admired him greatly, Cooper's mind was practical not philosophic. Few students came; then he changed his method by
lecturing on individual patients and the students flocked to him.

Cline had a friend, a Mr. Cock, a wealthy Hamburg merchant, to whose country house at Tottenham he often took
Astley on Sundays, with the result that in about 1789 he became
engaged to Miss Cock. The wedding was fixed for November
21, 1791; Mr. Cock, however, died the same day. In December a christening took place, Astley and Miss Cock attended
and, after it was over, were married, thus the wedding was
quite private; the married couple went straight to their house
in Jefferies' Square, which Mr. Cock had bought and furnished
for them. In the evening Astley, as usual, delivered his lectures
at the hospital. His wife brought him a fortune of £14,000,
consequently he was left free to study and to teach without
financial anxiety.

Lecturing and demonstrating forbade an immediate honeymoon, and when it came, in June 1792, it was unlike most,
for Astley and his wife went to Paris, then in revolutionary
turmoil. He wished to see surgery in the Parisian hospitals
and also the revolution, for he was, at this time, a thorough
democrat like Cline, through whose help it was made possible

for him to go. When there he wore his democratic badge. He visited hospitals but learned little or nothing, for all work was disorganized; he was, however, of use in looking after the wounded. He attended meetings of the National Assembly and several times heard Danton, Marat and Robespierre. The difficulties of life for visitors were very great, they often had to remain shut up for days, the horrors were bad for Mrs. Cooper, who was with child, so in August they decided to come home. There was, however, much trouble about passports, consequently they did not reach London till the end of September.

By October Astley was in professional harness again. He took much pains with his lectures, constantly attending the wards with Cline in order to obtain clinical material for them. His reputation as a lecturer led to his appointment as lecturer on Anatomy at the Surgeons' Hall for the three years 1793–5, his duty being to dissect in public the bodies of criminals executed at the Old Bailey. He continued his dissecting at St. Thomas's, spending much time, when not teaching, in dissecting on his own account. A day's work is summarized thus: " I went to the hospital before breakfast to dissect for lecture. I demonstrated to the students before lecture. I injected their subjects. I lectured from two o'clock till half-past three. In the evening, three times a week, I lectured on surgery. I attended the interesting cases in the hospital making notes of them." Until 1795 he made no attempt to earn anything by practice, although he would see a few poor patients gratuitously. A daughter was born to him; she died at the age of twenty months. A little girl of the same age was taken as an adopted child; she ultimately became Mrs. Parmenter.

The well-known democrat, Thelwall, who had always been a friend of Astley's, took out tickets for some of the lectures at the schools of St. Thomas's and Guy's, although he had no intention of becoming a doctor. He joined the Physical Society, taking a considerable part in its management; he became a bit of a nuisance, for he would read papers on metaphysical and semi-political subjects and these often led to prolonged discussion; one on vitality was discussed for five or six meetings. Subsequently, he read one on " The Origin of Mental Action explained on the System of Materialism." The discussion of this occupied five meetings. This was more than the Society could stand, so Dr. Relph moved and Dr. Saunders seconded that, as the paper had no bearing on medicine, discussion on it should cease. This was carried by 39 votes to 19. Thelwall resigned, Astley saw less of him, and from this time gradually moved in thought more from the left to the right, retaining however the friendship of Thelwall.

In 1797, Cline having left 12 St. Mary Axe, Astley moved there from his house in Jefferies' Square, he was partly influenced by the fact that the St. Mary Axe house had a large warehouse attached to it which could be used as a dissecting-room. In the same year he invited Mr. J. C. Saunders, who had been a student under him for two years, to live with him in order to dissect for comparative anatomy lectures and make preparations. Saunders accepted and afterwards became Demonstrator of Anatomy at St. Thomas's. That some help was wanted is shown by the statement that Astley kept many " snakes, vipers and frogs " for his studies, and they sometimes got loose to the annoyance of his neighbours.

A little while before his move he had a strange adventure. A duel was to be fought between Mr. Gawler and Lord Valentia. Hamburg was the place selected; Astley was asked to go as surgeon; he readily agreed as he wished to see his wife's relations in Hamburg. Lord Valentia was hit just below the collar-bone; the bullet ran round the second rib. Mr. Gawler thought he had killed his enemy and therefore fled with his companions. Lord Valentia recovered and became a friend of his surgeon, Astley, who was so seasick on the return journey that he never afterwards took a longer voyage than between Dover and Calais.

Astley Cooper was a great believer in the value of discussion. He frequently spoke at the Physical Society where, about this time, a great debate took place between him and Abernethy. He formed a private medical society confined to the staffs of St. Thomas's and Guy's. The members discussed cases, kept records of them and published a volume of *Medical Researches and Records*. Two essays in it show Astley's industry and thoroughness. He belonged to the Edinburgh Club founded in London in 1800 from those who had studied in Edinburgh. The members met in each other's houses to discuss interesting cases, and often distinguished foreigners were present.

We have now reached the most important year of Astley Cooper's life, namely 1800. He was 32. For many years past he had shown indefatigible perseverance; he was an excellent anatomist and surgeon; he had devoted all his spare time to anatomical and physiological researches; he was a renowned teacher, a good writer, and he was liked by crowds of people. In this year his uncle, William Cooper, resigned his post of surgeon to Guy's Hospital. There were four candidates of whom Astley was by far the best qualified, but the treasurer of Guy's Hospital feared he might damage the reputation of the hospital by appointing a revolutionary democrat. He had several interviews with Astley, who said his political opinions should never prevent his doing his hospital work as well as he could, that he had for some time been gradually getting less democratic and had resolved to have nothing more to do with politics, but to devote himself to surgery. This satisfied Mr. Harrison, the treasurer, who recommended him to the Govenors for the appointment, which he received in October 1800.

Two or three months earlier Travers had come to live with Astley as a pupil; he describes his master as then being the most handsome and intellectual-looking man he ever met; his portrait by Lawrence confirms Travers, who goes on to say that his energy was untiring; he was a good companion, with a sense of humour; he took little time over his meals, drank water with his dinner and two glasses of port after it; he always maintained he could digest anything except sawdust; he needed no recreation from his professional pursuits; he did not think much of books, for he believed the best way of acquiring knowledge was to look for yourself.

Young Travers was soon taught this, for within twenty-four hours of his arrival as a pupil he was, although he had never seen a corpse, taken to help Astley make a post-mortem examination as he was anxious to have the stomach for his museum. Astley, like Hunter, had his own private museum and dissecting-room; in it he collected pathological specimens and animals from which he taught himself comparative anatomy. He arranged with the keeper of the menagerie at the Tower, with dog dealers, with bird stuffers, and with fishmongers at Billingsgate to send carcases. A dead elephant arrived; nohow could it be got into the museum, so it was dissected in the yard, carpets being hung over the railings to intercept the public gaze of those in St. Mary Axe. His enthusiastic industry for dissecting, if possible, increased when in 1806 he went to live in Broad Street. Here two dissecting-rooms over the stables were fitted up with sinks, tables and a proper water supply. He obtained his pathological supplies from the post-mortem rooms and operating theatres of Guy's and St. Thomas's, from numbers of doctor friends and from his own practice, in which he was most successful in obtaining autopsies. He left careful directions for a post-mortem examination on himself and had one performed on his infant daughter. He engaged assistants to help him, a man to make plaster casts, and an artist to make drawings. His chief assistant, Mr. Lewis, accompanied him in his carriage, when Astley dictated notes to him. He and Hey, of Leeds, had a difference of opinion about the anatomy of hernia. Astley ordered a dead body to be taken to his private dissecting-room and invited Hey from Leeds. The two met one afternoon, dissected and studied preparations by candle-light till between two and three in the morning, finally concluding that Astley's view was correct. He spared no expense—he paid thirteen guineas for the body of a man who had been operated on twenty-four years before. Every morning, at six, he began dissecting in his private room, the specimen was left when he went to breakfast, so that he could return to it if he had time during the day. All this was done, not in the spirit of the mere collector, but first to add to his own know-ledge, secondly to provide specimens for illustration of his lectures and for the museums of the Borough Hospitals.

Breakfast over, his wife saw him no more till dinner, a small rapid meal, after which he swallowed his glasses of port, slept for ten minutes, then generally went to see private patients, to lecture at the hospital, or to dissect, only a few evenings being spent in the drawing-room. His enormous practice came slowly, in his ninth year at it he made £1,100, ultimately it was worth £15,000, but one year he made, including hospital fees, £21,000. The practice of a successful doctor is often largely run by a capable servant, so it was here, the servant being Charles Osbalderson, generally known as Charles, who was keenly alive to his master's interests and his own. He boasted that for twenty-six years he never lost a patient for his master whom it was possible to retain. He would tear off in a post chaise to fetch him wherever he was. He was said to make £600 a year by showing in patients out of their turn. Astley Cooper would slip out by a back door at the end of a morning's work, pick up his carriage and rush off to Guy's, leaving Charles to deal with the waiting patients, which he did very tactfully. There was a rumour that he sometimes saw them himself, pretending to be his master: the probable explanation of this tale is that Astley had had Charles's son educated as a doctor, he practised close by and may have sometimes acted for Astley.

It would be tedious to mention the numerous aristocratic and wealthy people who consulted him, but exception may be made of Lord Liverpool whom Astley had treated, and who liked him, and, therefore, recommended that he should be sent to Brighton in 1821 to advise about a sebaceous cyst on the King's head, which became inflamed from time to time. The patient wished for its immediate removal, but Astley told him he must come to London for other surgeons to be consulted. They were, and it was agreed to remove the cyst, Astley suggested Sir Everard Home, the Serjeant Surgeon, but the King, on the advice of Lord Liverpool, chose Astley, who asked for Cline to help him. The King naturally demurred, for he hated Cline's politics, but he gave way, so the popular pupil, helped by his old teacher, removed the tumour. Erysipelas was then dreaded by all operating surgeons, and George the Fourth was just the kind of man to get it; fortunately all went well. Astley was made a baronet, with permission for succession to his nephew, whom he had adopted in 1800 to be a companion to his adopted daughter. Before leaving this short account of his practice, it should be added that his object was not money-making; he was accustomed to set aside times for the seeing of gratuitous patients; after the Peninsular War he insisted on not taking fees from those who had been engaged in it.

Busy as he was, he nevertheless took his part in medical affairs. In the early nineteenth century there was much dissatisfaction with the management of the Medical Society of London, Dr. Saunders, physician to Guy's Hospital, in March 1805 refused to serve on its Council. Many members resigned from it and founded the Medical and Chirurgical Society—

now called the Royal Society of Medicine. Saunders was its first President and Astley Cooper held the post of treasurer to the new Society, subscribed fifty pounds towards obtaining a charter, attended its dinners and its ordinary meetings. He contributed ten papers to the *Transactions* of the Society.

We have seen Astley studying Comparative Anatomy first hand, and he frequently used his knowledge of it in his hospital lectures, consequently it was natural that when, in 1813, he and Abernethy were appointed Professors at the College of Surgeons, he should have been allotted Comparative Anatomy and Abernethy surgery, although Cooper would have much preferred surgery. The strain of preparing the lectures was intense, for he was teaching in the wards and lecture theatre of the hospital and his practice was large. Sometimes he only got four hours' sleep, he began dissecting specimens to illustrate the lectures at four or five in the morning, they went by " coach loads " to the college and the lecture theatre. His nephew Henry Cooper and Mr. Parmenter were sent to stay a fortnight in a hotel at Weymouth, to collect marine animals from the fishermen. The lectures appear to have been extremely interesting, the only objection to them was due to the number of exhibits. Clift says : " This was an overpowering discourse and highly perfumed ; the preparations being chiefly recent and half dried and varnished." Astley resigned the Professorship in 1815.

This year he moved to the West End, taking a house in New Street, because he was clearly overworked, he was taking no exercise, was getting stout and was liable to attacks of giddiness. At his new address he hoped to shed many of the patients who visited Broad Street, he would be nearer those who lived in the West End and he would be able to ride in the park. Mrs. Cooper disliked London and was usually at their country house at Gadesbridge, therefore in 1817 his surgeon nephew Bransby Cooper and his wife went to live in the house in New Street with their uncle, staying there till 1827, when Astley retired. Life went on in New Street pretty much as before, he had a dissecting-room both here and at Gadesbridge, usually rising at half-past five or six to work in it ; he employed an artist named Canton to make drawings, an untidy, idle fellow, nevertheless an excellent draughtsman, who was later artist to Guy's Hospital, and did the beautiful coloured drawings in Bright's *Medical Reports*. The disposition of the rooms was such that Charles could not obtain so much money from patients as formerly; occasionally patients complained to the master of the extortions of the servant, who was immediately summoned into the consulting-room, where he received, in the patient's presence, a severe scolding from his angry master who threatened him with dismissal, which did not take place because Charles had made himself indispensable. A sense of duty and a love of clinical surgery were probably the reasons why Astley continued to see patients, for he certainly did not need the money and did not allow them to interfere with anything of professional interest to him; for example, Mr. Read, the inventor of the stomach pump, called on him to show his invention; Astley took him in to breakfast, after which he talked with him for over two hours, leaving a large room full of patients to take care of themselves, which meant that several, after hours of waiting, would have to take their chance another day. The famous wax modeller, Joseph Towne, when in his teens called on Astley to show a beautiful wax skeleton he had made. Astley saw him, instantly recognized the skeleton to be a work of genius, gave the youth an introduction to the Treasurer of Guy's, further, fearing to lose him, made him promise not to show the model to anyone till after his interview with the Treasurer, who secured him to work for Guy's Hospital for the rest of his life, with the result that the hospital museum has one of the best collections of wax models in the world.

His interests and his friends were almost entirely professional; his mind does not appear to have needed any change but from surgery to dissecting and then back to surgery. He was hospitable, often having doctors and students to dine with him; he belonged to several medical clubs, the two best were the Athletæ and the Pow Wow. The first was mostly composed of doctors, e.g. Babington, Lettsom, Relph, but there were a few outside the profession, e.g. Boswell the biographer. The club began by meeting at some bowling green, then it met at Dr. Lettsom's in Camberwell, after this at Dr. Babington's in Tottenham. There was always a dinner with, during the summer, some form of outdoor exercise—during the winter, chess. The Pow Wow, founded by John Hunter, was a rather exclusive, expensive dining club. He was also a member of the Askesian, a scientific club founded in 1796.

Except for his giddy attacks his health remained good, but they gradually became more frequent. Whenever he could, he went to his country house, Gadesbridge, Hemel Hempstead. He amused himself by farming but lost money over it; his chief pleasure was having friends to stay—Babington, Marcet, Colman were often guests; he did not, however, rest in the country; he was up between five and six to dissect before breakfast, and, if the weather prevented his going out, he was in his dissecting-room for many hours in the day. Babington and he left on Monday mornings by post chaise at four-thirty in order to begin their work in London punctually. What with journeys to Hemel Hempstead and his practice Astley spent a good part of his time in post-chaises. It was his habit to bribe the post-boys to go as fast as possible; he had no serious accidents from this, if a breakdown occurred, he would never get out to help, always preferring to sit still until matters were put right.

A century or more ago medical instruction was a private affair. Several distinguished teachers taught by lectures and dissection on the human body at institutions unconnected with hospitals, and even when the teaching was connected with a hospital it was also regarded as a private speculation on the part of the teacher who took the fees and when he retired sold or gave the goodwill to his successor. Astley ultimately paid Cline £1,000 for the right to lecture jointly with him, he contributed another £1,000 towards rebuilding the lecture theatre at St. Thomas's, and the fine museum there, used to illustrate lectures, was almost entirely of his making. Towards the end of 1824 his attacks of giddiness became more frequent and he was short of breath; he determined therefore to give up lecturing entirely. He had before this got Aston Key to give some of the surgical, and Bransby Cooper some of the anatomical lectures, it being generally understood that, being his nominees, they would succeed him in these lectureships at St. Thomas's in which he had invested his money. The Governors of this hospital, to his intense chagrin, appointed Mr. South, and would not let Astley withdraw his resignation from a lectureship he had held more than thirty years. Looking back it seems as though the Governors ought to have told Astley that they did not intend to follow the usual custom.

The Treasurer of Guy's Hospital, being indignant at the slight put upon the distinguished surgeon to Guy's Hospital, immediately began in 1825 to build a medical school of his own. Key and Bransby Cooper were appointed respectively to the lectureships of surgery and anatomy. This ended the association of teaching at Guy's and St. Thomas's, known till then as the United Borough Hospitals, the popular United Hospitals Dining Club composed entirely of men educated either at Guy's or St. Thomas's still exists as a memory of bygone days. Astley Cooper's fame attracted many of the St. Thomas's students to Guy's, and the new school at Guy's flourished exceedingly from the very first. He occasionally lectured, always to huge audiences, but his health soon compelled him to desist and also caused him, towards the end of this year, to resign his surgeoncy to Guy's Hospital, to which he was appointed Consulting Surgeon.

Much happened to him in 1827; his patient the Duke of York died after a long illness in January, later his old friend Cline died at the age of 76; in the summer he lost his wife; lastly in September he retired from practice, going to live entirely at Gadesbridge. Country life was so boring to him that before the year was out he returned to town to practise. At first he took lodgings, then a house in Dover Street, then one in Conduit Street. In this year he was elected President of the College of Surgeons and, as such, was connected with the founding of King's College. Next year, in July, he married Miss C. Jones, in the same month he was appointed Serjeant Surgeon to the King. He passed much of his leisure revising his books for the press and also in dissecting, which occupation was his absorbing passion. He had been on the Council of the Royal Society; in 1830 he became Vice-President. During the autumn he made a long tour on the Continent, and next year another through Cornwall.

Honours poured on him. To mention some, he was made a member of the Institute of France, an officer of the Legion of Honour, a fellow of the Royal Society of Göttingen, and distinctions came from the Netherlands, Russia, Heidelberg, New Orleans, Palermo and Mexico. He received the degree of D.C.L. from Oxford in 1834. Two years later he was for the second time President of the Royal College of Surgeons and was awarded the Grand Cross of the Guelphic Order. In 1835 he was made an Honorary Fellow of the Royal College of Surgeons in Edinburgh; when he visited this city in 1837 the College gave a banquet in his honour, the University made him an LL.D. and he became a Freeman of the City. Later he was nominated as a candidate for the Lord Rectorship of the University of Glasgow: the Duke of Wellington was successful.

He indulged his liking for travel during the last few years, always seeing the hospitals of the towns he visited. His passion for dissecting continued, he records a visit to Dupuytren, who provided bodies for him to dissect while in Paris. At Cromer he dissected fish. His diary says: " Sunday, Sept 25.—Rose early and dissected eels; went to church "; this entry is similar to many. The heart of a porpoise was forwarded by him to Wilkinson King, the Curator of the Guy's Museum, to which he constantly contributed, for his great desire was to make it as complete as possible.

Towards the end of 1840 his breathlessness was severe, he could not visit a patient unless the stairs were few; later he was unable to lie down. Drs. Bright and Chambers attended him from January 22, 1841, previous to which he had refused to see a doctor. On February 10, he said, " My dear sirs, I am fully convinced of your excellent judgement and of your devotion to me, but your wishes are not to be fulfilled. God's will be done ! God bless you both ! . . . You must excuse me, but I shall take no more medicine." Death took place on February 12. He had expressed a wish that a post-mortem examination should be made, with special reference to a cured inguinal hernia, a cured umbilical hernia, suspected phthisis in his youth, and an inability to sleep on his left side. The examination was made at 9 p.m., thirty-two hours after death, by Mr. Hilton in the presence of Dr. Chambers, Dr. Bright, Mr. Key and Mr. Cock. The cured hernias were confirmed, cured phthisis, as shown by a depressed scar with a calcareous centre, was found at the upper part of the right lung, the kidneys were granular, the heart hypertrophied. A detailed account is published in the Guy's Hospital Reports for April 1841, according to Sir Astley's desire. It is a noteworthy coincidence that the same number contains a description of three interesting cases communicated by him. By his own wish he was buried in the crypt of Guy's Hospital Chapel. In his will he left capital to provide a triennial prize of £300 for the best essay on a nominated subject, saying that the first six subjects were to be the thymus, the spleen, the thyroid, the suprarenals, the blood in inflammation and the coagulation of the blood. The endowment failed to attract good essays, for an individual writer never knew who was competing against him. The terms of the bequest were subsequently altered with the consent of the Charity Commissioners.

Sir Thomas Lawrence painted an admirable portrait of him, from this Cousins made a beautiful mezzotint; there is a good bust by Towne in the Guy's Hospital Library, one at the Royal College of Surgeons, and a statue by Baily in St. Paul's Cathedral.

Sir Astley Cooper was neither an original thinker nor a discoverer, yet, incontestably, he was a really great surgeon. He was never content with the second best; he did an operation, gave a lecture, wrote a book, prepared a specimen as well as in him lay. Then there was his indefatigable industry. He spoke and wrote well, he was a magnificent teacher, proud of his profession and loyal to its members. His handsome, commanding figure compelled admiration.

His own opinion of himself was that he had a flair for correct diagnosis (this was true) but " never was a good operator where delicacy was required." Probably this merely meant that he was so good as to be aware of his shortcomings, for he undoubtedly was a fine operator.

The elegance of his operations, without the slightest affectation, all ease, all kindness to the patient, and equally solicitous that nothing should be hidden from the observation of his pupils, rapid in execution, masterly in manner, no hurry, no disorder, the most trifling minutiæ attended to, the dressings generally applied by his own hand. . . . Sir Astley's operations appeared like the graceful efforts of an artist.

His surgical colleagues at Guy's could hardly be got to operate unless he was present to help them out of their difficulties. He tied the abdominal aorta just above its bifurcation for an aneurism of the common iliac, which had begun to leak blood, so it is not surprising that the patient died, but the operation was perfect. In 1824 he amputated at the hip joint, the first time the operation had been performed. The whole operation, with the dressing, took half an hour. The patient, who bore it with extraordinary fortitude, said "that it was the hardest day's work he had ever gone through," to which Sir Astley replied that it was almost the hardest he had ever had. Our admiration is increased when we remember he had not anæsthetics, antisepsis nor asepsis to help him.

His fame was European, and distinguished foreigners often came round his wards or to see him operate. Students flocked to him—when he retired he used to say that 8,000 students had come under his sway—Dr. Pettigrew tells us they "followed him in troops." Tuesdays and Fridays were the days he went round the wards, and, as his carriage drove up quickly, he was out in a moment, skipping up the steps like a bright schoolboy, surrounded by a crowd of pupils; rushing up the staircase, pupils pushing and scrambling to get near, he went round the wards, the audience hanging on every word he said. The visit over he crossed quickly to the theatre at St. Thomas's to lecture on anatomy, the surgical lectures being in the evening. The students tore to secure the best places; by the time he arrived they were sitting on the stairs and passage, fully 300 being in the theatre. When he came in he was greeted with tremendous applause, but, for the hour the lecture lasted, you could hear nothing but his silvery voice and the scratching of the students' note-taking pens. There was no oratory, he spoke in a conversational style, every statement was clear and he mostly told only of that which he knew from personal observation. His exceptional success as a teacher is beyond doubt. Among the pen scratchers sat John Keats, likewise scratching, his notes of Cooper's lectures may be seen in the Keats Museum, Hampstead. It is a severe test to judge any lectures by a student's notebook, but these appear interesting and likely to be useful to the learner. Keats entered as a student at Guy's in October 1815, just when Cooper was as busy as could be. He was not dresser to Cooper, but to Mr. Lucas; it is therefore greatly to Astley Cooper's credit that he took an interest in golden-haired little Keats, only just over five feet high. That he did we know from South who writes "George Cooper told me that whilst at Guy's Hospital, where he was dresser to Astley Cooper for eighteen months, he lived in St. Thomas's Street, at a tallow chandlers, named Markham, where John Keats the poet lived with him, having been placed under his charge by Astley Cooper." In both his surgery and physiology lectures (see Lecture 10 in Keats's notebook) Astley alludes to the Polish General Kosciuszko, who had a pike wound of his sciatic nerve. Quite likely this was the first Keats heard of him, if so we owe the sonnet on him published in the *Examiner*, February 16, 1817, indirectly to Astley Cooper.

The popularity of Astley Cooper's lectures is shown by the fact that the first article in the first number of the *Lancet*, which appeared October 5, 1823, is a lecture by him. The reporter was Thomas Wakley, the editor, who attended the lecture, made longhand notes and from them composed the lecture as though it had been taken down verbatim. Cooper, who was naturally very angry, called on Wakley to protest, for his permission had not been asked, nor had he seen a proof. Wakley talked him round to consent that other lectures should appear after he had seen a proof, and several did. The *Lancet* later became so scurrilous that Astley Cooper, in public, used very strong language about it and afterwards ceased to have anything to do with it.

He wrote many papers and books and he wrote well. Perhaps he is best remembered to-day for his papers on ligation of arteries, which he had studied in many animals; further he knew his anatomy so well as to understand the paths of collateral circulation. Before he ligatured the aorta he had shown that in dogs the collateral circulation was efficient. The popliteal artery had been ligatured by Hunter, but Cooper was the first to put a ligature round the common carotid. He lost his first case, the wound suppurated; his second was completely successful, the patient lived thirteen years subsequently; both patients suffered from aneurism. It had been the common opinion that such an operation was unjustifiable, because damage to the brain must follow. Cooper, by observing cases in which the common carotid was obstructed by disease and by ligaturing the artery in dogs, convinced himself that this fear was groundless. On the day of operation on the second patient he ligatured the external iliac artery in another patient who survived for eighteen years.

He obtained his F.R.S. and was awarded the Copley medal on account of two papers presented to the Royal Society. The earlier, read February 6, 1800, was entitled " Observations on the Effects which take place from Destruction of the Membrana Tympani of the Ear." It was then thought that absence of this membrane always entailed deafness, he showed this was not so ; he noticed that the muscles of the external ear grew active in the deaf, who could therefore slightly move the external ear. In the second communication, read June 21, 1801, he records that the examination of twenty more persons confirmed his previous conclusion. He also tells us that if an aperture in the membrane is small no effect on hearing ensues, if the whole membrane and the small bones are removed almost total deafness follows, but after a time considerable hearing returns. It is necessary to have air both sides of a membrane for it to vibrate ; if the Eustachian tube is blocked, deafness results, because there is no air on the inner side of the membrane, so it cannot vibrate. He punctured the membrane in several of these cases, thus admitting air to the inner side of the membrane, with the result that hearing was restored.

Astley Cooper's determination never to be content with the second best is well shown in his books on hernia, on fractures and dislocations, on diseases of the breast, on the testis and on the thymus. The first was prepared because of the many lives lost owing to strangulated hernia, he describes clearly the anatomy, the treatment and the details of operation. It is a magnificent large atlas folio, beautifully printed and with dozens of fine line engravings. All his books contain not only perfectly clear descriptions in excellent English, but they are works of art, the coloured plates in the book on the breast are particularly fine. It is no wonder he lost £1,000 by that on hernia, although every copy was sold. The one on fractures and dislocations is dedicated to his friends the students of St. Thomas's and Guy's, for he says it is written for their use. The *Anatomy of the Thymus Gland* was published in 1832, which shows he was working hard at the age of 64. The preface indicates admirably how he had in him the instinctive desire of a great teacher to diffuse knowledge. He writes: " As the preparations which form the foundation of these observations on the structure of the thymus gland are carefully preserved, it will, at all times, afford me great pleasure to exhibit them to those of my professional brethren, whether domestic or foreign, who are zealous in the science of anatomy."

41

SIR CHARLES BELL

The family to which Bell belonged had existed for several centuries in and around Glasgow. His grandfather, John Bell, minister in the parish of Gladsmuir in Haddington, wrote two manuscripts on witchcraft from which Sir Walter Scott thus quotes in his letters on *Demonology and Witchcraft*: " anno 1697, a time when persons of more goodness and esteem than most of their calumniators were defamed for witches, and which was occasioned mostly by the forwardness and absurd credulity of divers otherwise worthy ministers of the gospel, and some topping professors in and about the city of Glasgow." John, whom we see from this to have been an enlightened man, died at the age of thirty-two, leaving several children, one of whom, William, the father of Charles, was a minister in the Episcopal Church of Scotland; domestic affairs did not trouble him, for his chief delight was to sit surrounded by his books. In 1757, being then fifty-three years old, he married, as his second wife, Margaret Morice, the daughter of an Episcopal clergyman. William died in 1779. His wife and her six children were left in very poor circumstances. George, the fourth son, tells us that his schooling, which required only five shillings a quarter, could not be continued after he was eleven years old. Nevertheless the lives of three of her children, John, George and Charles, are to be found in the *Dictionary of National Biography*, and Robert, the eldest, became a Writer to the Signet.

There is liable to be confusion about the Edinburgh surgeons named Bell. Benjamin Bell, appointed surgeon to the Royal Infirmary, Edinburgh, in 1772, was distinguished both by his practice and his writings; his sons George and Joseph were surgeons and so was Joseph's son, Benjamin.

This family was not the same as that of Charles Bell, whose brother John, born in 1763, became a member of the Royal College of Surgeons, Edinburgh, and, in 1790, established himself in that city as a successful extra-mural lecturer on surgery.

He attacked the teaching of Benjamin Bell. Among his pupils was his brother Charles, who helped him with his book, the *Anatomy of the Human Body*. The family ability in art is shown in John's *Engravings of the Bones, Muscles and Joints* and in his *Observations in Italy*; his *Discourses on the Nature and Cure of Wounds* was an admirable work. For twenty years he was the leading operating surgeon in Edinburgh. Unfortunately much of his time and energy was spent in a bitter controversy with the unscrupulous Dr. Gregory, which led to his exclusion from the post of surgeon to the Royal Infirmary.

George Joseph Bell, born at Fountain Bridge near Edinburgh, in 1770, was the favourite brother of Charles; it is to him that the *Letters of Sir Charles Bell*, published in 1870, are addressed. In 1822 he was elected Professor of Scots Law in the University of Edinburgh, the motion, seconded by Sir Walter Scott, who was a friend of the Bell family, being carried unanimously. Some of his books—all on legal subjects— passed through several editions and are still quoted as authorita- tive. He served on Legal Commissions and left behind him the reputation of being one of the many eminent Scottish jurists.

Charles, the fourth son and youngest of the family, was born in November 1774, five years before his father's death. Thus it came about that he was entirely dependent on his mother for his upbringing. Although he went to the High School of Edinburgh, where during the last years of the century Walter Scott, Francis Jeffrey, Henry Brougham and Cockburn were pupils, he did not consider that he learnt much there, for opposite the statement in Pettigrew's *Medical Portrait Gallery* that he was educated at this school, he wrote: " Nonsense ! I received no education but from my mother, neither reading, writing, cyphering, nor anything else." Her children adored her. Charles says: " For twenty years of my life I had but one wish—to gratify my mother." She was well educated, of a sweet disposition, devoted to her children, using every endeavour to bring them up as well as her poverty allowed. The two younger boys, who loved her dearly, were her especial care. Charles writes: " I know no more of the motions of the earth, moon and stars, than her little contrivance then taught me as a boy. I recollect the room and the spot where she formed a ball, and passed a stocking wire thro' it to show me the poles and the revolution of the seasons." There was something wrong either with the Edinburgh High School or with Charles Bell, for his two years' attendance there were "torture and humiliation." Adams, loved by all good scholars, was to him a stupid tyrant. The bright spot of his schooldays was his friendship with David Allan the painter, who recognized Charles's genius for and pleasure in drawing. Allan, who had studied long in Italy, became Master of the Academy in Edinburgh; he is sometimes called the "Hogarth of Scotland"; he was a lively, cheerful old fellow, just the kind of man to attract the boy, whom he used to hail with "Ha ! brother Brush, let's see what you have been doing." The beauty of Charles's draughtsmanship probably owes much to Allan.

Charles Bell decided to become a surgeon and studied at Edinburgh under Black, Gregory and Alexander Munro, the anatomist, whose lectures he attended and of whom he always spoke with respect. His artistic ability led him, while still a student, to publish in 1798 his *System of Dissections*. This well-printed folio, dedicated to Dr. Daniel Rutherford, Professor of Botany in the University of Edinburgh, contains descriptions of how to inject a body, how to make anatomical preparations and how to dissect each part of the body, all in accurate detail. Great as is the praise due to it for the letterpress, still greater is that which must be given to it for its thirty large plates, all of which are beautiful works of art, a real joy to the eye. Many would say that no finer anatomical plates have ever been published. They are obviously the work of a considerable artist, even the red of the arteries and the yellow of the veins are harmonious. This book, which must have been expensive, was at once recognized as something out of the common and a second edition was called for within a year. Modern anatomy books are poor affairs compared with it. Equally fine engravings from drawings by him illustrate his brother John's lectures and a book on anatomy by himself and John.

In 1799 he was elected a member of the Royal College of Surgeons, Edinburgh, and about this time he made excellent wax models of anatomical and pathological conditions. He had a class of ninety pupils to whom he lectured and he taught himself to be a highly skilful operator.

We have seen that his turbulent brother John was engaged

44

in fierce controversy with Dr. Gregory, the result was that early in the nineteenth century both brothers were excluded from the Royal Infirmary, consequently Charles, seeing no chance of a career in Edinburgh, determined, after consultation with brother George with whom he lived, to seek his fortune in London, for these two brothers, devoted to one another, had both made up their minds to reach a distinguished position in their respective professions and both did. Charles's years in Edinburgh had brought him many friends among celebrated people such as Brougham, Cockburn, Jeffrey, Walter Scott and Sydney Smith: he took with him a letter to Horner from Jeffrey, who wrote:

Nothing but emigration to London. My good friend Charles Bell is about to follow your cursed example. He has almost determined to fly and take shelter in the great asylum. I have a very great affection and esteem for him, and can, moreover, assure you that you will find him very modest, intelligent, honourable, grateful and gentle.

He reached the great asylum at the end of November 1804, having had to walk from Huntingdon because the coach did not go forward from there on Saturday evening and Sunday morning.

It must be unique for a young doctor's passport into the higher medical circles to be his reputation as an artist, but so it was with Bell, for his fame as the draughtsman of the plates in his *System of Dissections* had preceded him. Within a day or two of his arrival Astley Cooper called and finding Bell out, left an invitation to dinner, Sir Joseph Banks asked him to breakfast, he dined with Matthew Baillie and Dr. Adams. Within a week Astley Cooper had suggested he should live with him, which he did not do, preferring to be in his own lodgings. Before the end of the year 1804 he had made the acquaintance of most of the prominent people in his profession. Lynn laughingly said they were afraid young Bell was going to knock them all out and become Professor of Anatomy at the Royal Academy, for his book had been seen on Sir Joseph Banks's table. Some three months later Abernethy, who had become a great friend of Bell, told him that the Academy must appoint him their professor. He describes in one of his letters to George how he went to the St. Bartholomew's dinner:

Sir C. Blicke paid me every possible honour and civility, and at dinner placed me in the centre of the surgeons of the hospital, between himself and Sir J.

Earle. The situation was so particular that the Lord Mayor, the president, drank to me individually among a hundred at dinner. Great honours for Charlie, who sat pining that he had not an eligible permanent situation among them.

His friend Lynn, the surgeon to the Westminster Hospital, had from the first given him work by asking his assistance at operations. Dr. Maton, the court physician, had also aided him, but it was the want of a permanent situation that troubled Charlie, for somehow he must earn his living. During his first six months in London he had a pleasant time. Longman offered him £300 for two volumes introductory to surgery, he got to know West the painter, whom he found to be a stiff, reserved man, and he spent much time enjoyably visiting art galleries. He speaks of the bad drawing and bad colouring of English artists, says he could pour ridicule upon them for their ignorance of anatomy, but, like a canny Scot, he concludes that this would not be wise. He drew and modelled a good deal, sometimes for his amusement, sometimes for his friends; he went to the opera, which he thoroughly enjoyed, for he had considerable musical taste; he read the classics. Still, all this led to nothing; Lynn was constantly trying to cheer him up, but, as his money gradually ran out, in July 1805 George came from Edinburgh to stay with him at his rooms in Fludyer Street, in order to discuss what should be done. The brothers had much conversation, Charles suggested returning to Edinburgh, but George opposed this; finally it was decided to take a house in which Charles should lecture to artists and medical students, and from which he could practise his profession. The two brothers, after much wandering, fixed on an old house in Leicester Street, Leicester Square, which had been inhabited by Speaker Onslow. It was in a bad state of repair, the roof caused much trouble; the first night that Charles went into it the floor gave way under him; the surveyor said he would sooner have nine children laid to his charge than this house over his head. Further it was haunted by the subject of *The Pathetic Ballad of the Invisible Girl* which made students chary of living in it. Charles, who did it up as well as he could afford, moved into it in October 1805, departing from Fludyer Street with £12 in his pocket.

When he left Edinburgh he brought with him the manuscript of a new book, which he finished soon after his arrival

in London. With difficulty a publisher was found; his friend
Horner helped to correct the proof and early in 1806 the book
appeared under the title of *An Essay on the Anatomy of Expression
in Painting*, a quarto volume of only 186 pages. The second
enlarged edition was published in 1824 with the title altered to
Essays on the Anatomy and Philosophy of Expression. It is fuller
than the first, for it contains much about the nerves, a subject
which Bell had studied so profitably in the interval. A later
edition has additions he made after a long holiday in Italy.
This famous book is of great interest to anatomists, but was
written for artists. Its theme can be gathered from the preface
which tells us that anatomy stands related to the art of design
as the grammar of that language in which this art addresses us.
The expressions, attitudes and movements of the human frame
are the characters of this language. All lesser embellishments
and minuteness of representation are foreign to the painter's
main subject, he should copy what he sees merely as the means
of communicating his thoughts and presenting the creations
of his fancy; until he has acquired a poet's eye for nature, and
can seize all the effects produced upon the body by the operations of the mind he has not raised himself above the mechanism
of his art, nor does he rank with the poet. Bell is at great
pains to maintain that the mind does not directly cause the
appearances associated with the emotions, but indirectly through
the heart—hence pallor—or through the lungs—hence the implication of many respiratory muscles, for example in fear and
terror. He gives an anatomical account of the muscles concerned with all the many human expressions such as fear and
joy, and he points out that many artists have erred ridiculously
by trying to depict upon the faces of lions and horses expressions
which can be attained by human beings, but which the muscles
of these animals are incapable of producing. We see that he
had educated himself well in literature by the quotations he
gives from English and other writings to show how admirably
inspired authors depict the emotions in words. To quote only
one example of the interesting matter of the book. The statue
of David with his sling is wrong, for, to convey the idea of
resolution and energy, he is biting his lip, but this is a motion
intended to suppress an angry emotion; on the other hand the
dying gladiator is correct, for he is seeking support for his arm,

not to rest or prevent himself from falling, but to give a fixed point for his labouring muscles of respiration. Fortunately for Charles, Jeffrey, his friend, wrote, not a caustic, but a just and kindly review in the *Edinburgh Review*, in which he said that hitherto there had been no such book for artists, that the author knew his subject thoroughly and had a better taste in painting and sculpture than many artists, and he skilfully induced his readers to read the book by quoting many long passages. It was extremely well received by everybody and has become a standard classic. Flaxman and Fuseli covered the author with compliments; the Nabob of Arcot had a copy bound in red morocco and satin; the Queen had a copy which she read for two hours, on hearing which Bell irreverently exclaimed, " Oh happiness in the extreme ! that I should ever write anything fit to be dirtied by her snuffy fingers." Bell's book made him famous, but did not lead to the Professorship of Anatomy at the Royal Academy, which is, perhaps, a good thing, for his mind might have been diverted from the great discoveries he was about to make.

He was now in the happy position of being a celebrated man, friends with the chief doctors and artists, whenever he felt lonely he could always associate with distinguished Scotsmen such as Brougham, Sidney Smith and Horner. He went about dreaming dreams, " the prevailing cast of my mind was to gain celebrity and independence by science "; nothing gave him anxiety but the fear he could not meet the expense of his tumbledown house. To begin with there were two resident pupils, soon another came; by February 1805 his surgical pupils had brought £82, his lectures to painters £25 (there were seven painters working under him, each had a little table where he drew skulls and skeletons), and on the tenth of the month he received his first fee in consultation; the struggle was severe, but by hard work he succeeded. Two months later he wrote, " After breakfast to see a patient at Brompton Row, come home and study for my lecture; after lecture visit three patients; dine near six; prepare for my evening lecture; in the evening probably Brompton again." He had a Russian baron as a patient, his pupils were very fond of him, his wax models kept him busy. Sidney Smith wrote of them, " I could not have conceived that anything could be so perfect and beautiful as his wax models. I saw one to-day which was quite the Apollo Belvedere of Morbid Anatomy." He dines with the Abernethys, and accompanies them afterwards to Vauxhall. A pleasant week-end is spent with Tom Campbell, the poet, at his country house at Sydenham. The two "wander over the forest: not a soul to be seen in all Norwood." Tom, sitting on a felled tree, repeats delightful extracts. Charles certainly was happy and cheerful. After he had been in the Leicester Street house a little more than a year he tells George that lecturing, which used to be his bane, is now his delight, that Fuseli has called on him and overwhelmed him with compliments. " I am merriest in my own house, and I find no gloom ever encroaching on me, no melancholy. I am satisfied with London and with myself, my reception and my expectations. I have got a great deal of money from my pupils, from my class, from Longmans, from my patients." John Richardson, the lawyer friend of Walter Scott, Cockburn, the Bells and Campbell, writes to George, saying that he has been playing chess with Charles who is in excellent spirits, his class has trebled and he has made a great reputation as an anatomist.

In July 1807 George, who had married Barbara Shaw, visited Charles, and, in a letter to his wife, says he found Charles strong, hearty and in admirable spirits, his pupils adored him, his housekeeper looked after him like a kind old nurse who had brought him up from childhood, his museum was becoming famous. Many of Charles's letters show the happiness that beauty gave him, he writes of the Elgin marbles, celebrated pictures, good literature, plays, the opera, music and the joy to be derived from the country. The letters to George dated May 21 and November 26 give the first hint of his work on the nervous system. "I have done a more interesting nova anatomia cerebri humani than it is possible to conceive. I lectured it yesterday. I prosecuted it last night till one o'clock, and I am sure that it will be well received." In his next letter he says, "I really think this new Anatomy of the Brain will strike more than the discovery of the Lymphatics being absorbents." The remaining letters of 1807 and those of 1808, 1809 and 1810 show that his mind was burning with his new discovery which will be described in detail later. He thought of announcing it to the world by lectures, and by papers to the Royal Society, he sent his writings on it for criticism to George, to Jeffrey and others.

His busy life continued, he volunteered to go to Haslar to look after the wounded home from Corunna, coming back to London with some " noble specimens of injured bones." He gives an account of the fire at Drury Lane which shows the artist in him, makes etchings and paintings of gunshot wounds, paints and then dissects a dead lioness, buys etchings of the best masters and hangs them around him. The letters to George written in 1809 are all cheerful. " My little red book says now £900 : D's fee will make it £1,000." His reputation, scientific position, and writings are progressing. In December an attack of scarlet fever caught from his friend John Shaw compels him to rest from his labours. Up to now, in addition to the books already mentioned, he had in 1802 published a quarto *The Anatomy of the Brain explained in a Series of Engravings*. There are twelve beautiful plates from his drawings, many are coloured. I doubt whether any medical illustration has ever excelled plate twelve showing the arteries and sinuses at the base of the skull. In 1803 *A Series of Engravings explaining the Course of the Nerves* appeared. These nine quarto plates were very fine. He wrote a large book, *A System of Operative Surgery founded on the Basis of Anatomy*. The first volume is dated 1807, the second 1809. The dedication is to his friend William Lynn, senior surgeon to the Westminster Hospital. Bell says: " This work I profess to be original. . . . I have described no operation I have not performed, from bleeding in the arm to lithotomy with the knife alone; from tying the umbilical cord to the operation of Cæsarian section." Both letterpress and plates are excellent. In 1810 he left Longmans who had published all these books and Murray published for him *Letters Concerning Diseases of the Urethra*. The advertisement in it shows him at work, for we learn that Mr. Charles Bell's lectures on anatomy and surgery are given at 10 and 11 Leicester Street. A first course is five guineas. The dissecting-rooms are open from 8 a.m. to 10 p.m. Either Mr. Bell or Mr. Roberton is in constant attendance. His books were read, for several editions of them appeared. He was thirty-six years old; truly he had worked hard.

Next year he married, on June 3, Marion, the second daughter of Charles Shaw of Ayr, and the two started housekeeping at 34 Soho Square. Her elder sister, Barbara, had married George Bell. The dreaded critic Jeffrey, always true to his friends, wrote, " You will be delivered from the persecution of my admonitions, as it would be a piece of unpardonable presumption to lecture a man who has a wife to lecture him at home."

More than forty years before this time William Hunter had founded the famous Great Windmill Street School of Medicine, it was now owned by the surgeon James Wilson; with the aid of his wife's dowry, Bell bought a part interest in it. Doing this filled him with joy. Wilson had in the School a fine museum, Bell added his own collection and wrote to his brother of "the happiness of this life of exertion, modelling, writing and putting this great museum in order." He woke his wife in the middle of the night by calling out, " Oh, May, it will be a noble museum." His lectures drew large audiences. Nevertheless, he was still worried by his finances, for he spent much on the museum, but his reputation was increasing fast. In 1813 he, by invitation, became a member of the Royal College of Surgeons of England, and the year after he was elected surgeon to the Middlesex Hospital, where he worked diligently seeing patients and teaching; his fame attracted foreigners to the hospital and many distinguished patients to his consulting-rooms; they came partly because of his skill, but also because everyone liked him personally.

One of the many traits in Bell which charmed people was his enthusiasm. When on June 22, 1815, the news of the Battle of Waterloo reached London, Charles exclaimed to his doctor brother-in-law, John Shaw, " Johnnie ! how can we let this pass ? Here is such an occasion of seeing gunshot wounds." Off they went, reaching Brussels on the 30th without any passports, if these were demanded they exhibited a fearsome array of dreadful surgical instruments, and were at once allowed to proceed. Bell operated in Brussels from early morn till late evening, finding, as have others in like circumstances, that he could do with little sleep. He made many water-colour sketches of the surgical conditions he saw, some of these were deposited in Edinburgh, in University College, London, and at Netley. The first letter he wrote to his brother George from Brussels had an important result, for Lockhart tells us that George showed it to Sir Walter Scott, who said " it set him on fire." It did this with good purpose, for on July 27 Sir Walter started for the battlefield at Waterloo, from whence he went to Paris, returning to Abbotsford in September.

On coming back to London, Bell settled down for some years to the routine work of a busy teacher and surgeon. When patients were few he was easily cast down, being " quite in the blue devils," when they were many he was elated, and contemplated a house in the country; he was much pleased because a Frenchman wrote that he operated " quickly and with grace, without affectation." So many foreigners came to see his hospital work that he took lessons in French and was soon able to talk to them fluently. Love of the country called him into it whenever possible, he would drive to Box Hill and sleep there, returning the next morning; on these excursions he always amused himself by sketching. There was so much in his make-up to remind us of Izaak Walton that it is surprising he did not take to angling till the autumn of this year. He quickly became a devoted disciple; a few years later he writes, " I often go a-fishing and without it I know I could not exist;" no better description of the joys of fishing is to be found than that which he gives in a letter to George written in 1824; unfortunately it is too long to quote. But behind all this, as his letters show, he led a second life, constantly pondering on the nervous system, and the first of his many papers on this subject communicated to the Royal Society was read on July 12, 1821.

In July 1824 he was appointed Professor of Anatomy and Surgery to the English Royal College of Surgeons; the lectures he consequently gave were an immense success, theatre crowded to suffocation and as many turned away as got in. This year he sold his collection in the Windmill Street Museum to the Edinburgh College of Surgeons, and published the second edition of the *Anatomy of Expression*, dedicating it to George. He contributed an article on " Animal Mechanics " to the publications of the Society for the Diffusion of Useful Knowledge, Brougham writes to him from Lancaster about it, saying, " I cannot refrain from telling you the prodigious success your admirable treatise has among us on this circuit—judges, lawyers, wranglers, metaphysicians and theologians, men who are devoid of science, saint, savage and sage, all unite in its praise and in gratitude to you."

From now until he left London twelve years later he was in the thick of things. His friend Brougham obtained his active help in the foundation of the London University; he served on committees, gave a general inaugural lecture and also one in the medical department, but there was so much bickering and squabbling that he and Horner in disgust resigned from all connection with the University. He served on the Council of the Royal College of Surgeons; he was active in forming a medical school attached to the Middlesex Hospital, " a complete little thing—theatre, museum, clinical classroom and dissecting-room." He lectured there, but he did not receive one guinea for his lectures, " On the contrary I have subscribed £50 as one of the hospital surgeons, £30 as a lecturer. Nevertheless, the main object will be gained—the preserving the hospital respectable." In a letter to his brother he mentions that he is just going to dine with Horne, next sunday with Lord Lans-downe, on friday at John Murray's, meeting there many dis-tinguished people, which made him feel as if he had been gazing all night at skyrockets. Cuvier was the chief guest at one of Bell's dinner-parties. A Royal Society Medal was awarded to him; in 1831 he received the Guelphic Order of Knighthood, and, in 1833, Bell and Astley Cooper were awarded the M.D. of Göttingen. He gave evidence before a House of Commons Committee on the Medical Bill, and an address at Edinburgh, when the British Association met there in 1834. Private practice, hospital practice, lectures, writing, especially his publications on the nervous system, all combined to make him a very busy man, but whenever a day off was possible he went fishing, his longer holidays were also devoted to it.

Three of his publications during the later half of his London period should be mentioned.

The Rev. Francis Henry, 8th Earl of Bridgewater (1756–1829), left £8,000 for the best work on " The Goodness of God as manifested in the Creation." This sum was divided among eight authors selected by the Archbishop of Canterbury, the Bishop of London and the President of the Royal Society. One of the eight was Sir Charles Bell, who received £1,000, taking for his subject *The Hand, its mechanism and vital endow-ments as evincing design and illustrating the Power, Wisdom and Goodness of God.* The book, published in 1832, was widely read and ran through many editions. The author sets out to show

that there is an adaptation, an established and universal relation between the instincts, organization and instruments of animals, on the one hand, and the elements in which they are to live, the position which they are to hold, and their means of obtaining food on the other:—and this holds good with respect to the animals which have existed, as well as those which now exist.

His wide knowledge of comparative anatomy and geology enables him to fulfil his purpose by innumerable examples, by no means confined to the hand, all so well described as to make very pleasant reading. There is much about muscle sense which he was the first to describe as on a parity with other senses—after his writings it was called the sixth sense—and it is pointed out that mythical creatures such as griffins, centaurs and satyrs are anatomical and physiological impossibilities.

It is difficult, nowadays, to understand the enormous popu-larity of Paley's *a posteriori* utilitarian moral philosophy. Even in the lives of many now living Paley was a subject for entrance examinations, perhaps because of his unequalled clarity of style. However, this philosophy was indeed popular; Paley's works went through more editions than can be counted. One of them often reprinted was *Paley's Natural Theology with illustra-tive notes by Henry, Lord Brougham and Sir Charles Bell, 2 vols., 1836.* It is interesting to see that only a century ago two such authors should spare time to edit this book, now as dead as mutton. Bell easily produced many examples from anatomy to illustrate Paley's doctrines. We are told that when a man tumbles sideways, the convexity of his head comes to the ground precisely on that point (the centre of the parietal bone) where the skull is thickest and most dense. Bell says:

These provisions would surely have met with earlier attention, had men con-templated in a true view the object of the animal framework; which is not to give absolute safety against inordinate violence, but to balance the chances of life,—leaving us still under the conviction that pain and injury follow violence; so that our experience of the injury, and our fear of pain, whilst they are the principal protection to life, lay the foundation of important moral qualities in our nature.

In 1819 he published *An Essay on the Forces which Circulate the Blood*. This rare tract was inscribed to Abernethy. The author emphasizes that not only the heart but also the arteries help the circulation, that tortuosity in arteries is not a provision for retarding the flow of blood and that contraction of muscles aids the passage of blood along the veins.

Fortunately, in 1835 Charles Bell was invited to, and accepted the Professorship of Surgery at, the University of Edinburgh. This enabled him to retire from the turmoil of London; in 1836, when he was sixty-one, his London house, now 30 Brook Street, was given up for 6 Ainslie Place, Edinburgh. Over a hundred London members of his profession joined in giving him a parting present. He lectured, examined, saw patients in Edinburgh, and was able to take life quietly, except that dinners were a tax—"three dinners swallowed, and six refused, is the rate of invitation last week." But the country excursions, and above all the delights of angling, alone and with Christopher North and other friends, made him very happy—"I have had some delightfully idle days." During the spring and summer of 1840 he made a tour through Italy, recording his experiences in a journal full of sketches. Hospitals and medical museums were visited, but the great joy was the beauty of scenery and of Italian works of art, the hours spent on these would, he said, enable him to enrich his book on Expression beyond belief. Soon after his return his health began to fail, and, early in the morning of April 29, 1842, he died suddenly of angina pectoris, in the house of a friend, Mrs. Holland, at Hallow Park, near Worcester. He is buried in Hallow Churchyard and the wording of the memorial to him in the church is by his old friend Jeffrey.

The *Letters of Sir Charles Bell*, published in 1870, formed the basis of a long article in the *Edinburgh Review* for April 1872, which gives an admirable account of the man, his surroundings, his relations, his friends, his industry, and his work. His portrait depicts a handsome, intellectual, dreamy, kindly face. He was unobtrusive, beloved by all who came in contact with him. His drawings and his letters show the artist to the finger tips; the *Edinburgh Review* truly says, "He sketches off passing events with a light, firm and incisive hand; and we could fill pages with his vignettes, full of spirit and life." He worshipped beauty in sculpture, painting, music and nature, witness his many accounts of the surroundings in which he fished. His gift of imagination, together with a scientific mind longing to make a great discovery, led to his work on the nervous system, so in him we find the unusual combination of artist and scientist.

Letters to George in 1807, which have already been quoted, give the first hint that Charles was thinking of the Nervous System and lecturing on it. He first put his thoughts into print in a scarce and valuable tract—only a hundred copies were printed—entitled *Idea of a New Anatomy of the Brain ; submitted for the Observations of his Friends ; by Charles Bell, F.R.S.E.* It is undated, but internal evidence from Bell's letters and a letter from the printers to Alexander Shaw prove that it was published in August 1811. Mr. Ward, writing to the *Lancet,* July 31, 1858, said he had a copy dated 1809, and John Shaw, in his paper on "Partial Paralysis" (*Med. Chi. Trans.,* April 1822), also gave the date of publication as 1809. Both were working with Charles in this year; no doubt they had seen the essay in an early stage of preparation in 1809, hence their mistake. At the meeting of the British Association in Oxford in 1868 the wish was expressed to have it reprinted. Alexander Shaw did this in the *Journal of Anatomy and Physiology* (Vol. 3, 1869), adding many interesting notes, extracts from Charles's letters to George and an admirable survey of Bell's work on the nervous system. It is allowed, on all hands, that Bell's discoveries were prior to those of others who followed him, but for which priority has been claimed.

Bell states that the prevailing doctrine then current was that the whole brain is a common sensorium, that nerves are all the same, that the nerve of the eye, for example, differs from the nerves of touch only in the degree of sensibility. But, says he:

In opposition to these opinions, I have to offer reasons for believing, that the cerebrum and cerebellum are different in function as in form: that the parts of the cerebrum have different functions ; and that the nerves we trace in the body are not single nerves possessing various powers, but bundles of different nerves, whose filaments are united for the convenience of distribution, but which are distinct in office, as they are in origin from the brain.

Aptly does he remind us that if, as believed, the sensation of light was conveyed to the brain from the retina only because the retina was more sensitive than the skin, the pain of a needle touching the retina should be so awful that "Life could not bear so great a pain," but, in fact, the needle gives "the sensation of a spark of fire." The new doctrines here enunciated were so completely at variance with the teaching of the day that it will be well to quote another statement which Bell made in 1823. "Whatever be the nature of the impulse communicated to a nerve, pressure, vibration, heat, electricity, the perception excited in the mind will have reference to the organ exercised, not to the impression made upon it." We can trace, he says, from the cerebrum by the crura cerebri downwards through the medulla oblongata to the anterior fasciculi of the spinal cord and the crura of the cerebellum downwards into the posterior fasciculi.

I found that injury done to the anterior portion of the spinal marrow, convulsed the animal. . . . On laying bare the roots of the spinal nerves, I found I could cut across the posterior fasciculus of nerves . . . without convulsing the muscles of the back; but that on touching the anterior fasciculus with the point of the knife, the muscles of the back were immediately convulsed.

The anterior and posterior roots, he says, go to form a single nerve, but clearly it is really double, one part being connected through the anterior spinal route with the cerebrum, the other through the posterior spinal root with the cerebellum, the different effects of stimulating the anterior and posterior roots suggest that the cerebrum and cerebellum have different functions. In the case of the cranial nerves, as they are not double like spinal nerves, the distant parts have two nerves, e.g. the face has the portio dura of the seventh and parts of the fifth. The surface of the cerebrum is connected with nerves of motion, but with these nerves of motion passing outwards there are nerves going inwards from the surfaces of the body, nerves of touch and nerves of peculiar sensibility. At this stage of his investigations the author did not know that nerves going inwards go by the posterior root, concerning the function of which he here gives no opinion. His discovery was that spinal nerves are mixed, containing fibres with different functions, that the anterior spinal roots are concerned with motion, the posterior are not. His "Idea" was that by tracing up to the brain nerves of which we knew the function, we could determine the functional significance of areas of the brain.

In his subsequent researches he was helped by his brother-in-law John Shaw, who was his pupil and his dear friend. He died in 1827, and John's brother Alexander, who became surgeon to the Middlesex Hospital, thereupon left Cambridge to become Charles Bell's assistant.

Ten years after the issue of the " Idea " he communicated to the Royal Society a paper read on July 12, 1821. Others brought before the same Society followed; all were gathered into *The Nervous System,* by Sir Charles Bell, the value of which is enhanced by an appendix containing numerous clinical cases supporting the author's views. The book went through several editions, the third appeared in 1844. The paper of 1821 is concerned with the fifth and seventh nerves. He asks whether each of these two nerves furnishes a double supply of the same property or endowment, as many authorities suppose, or perform different offices. An ass is used for experiment. If the seventh nerve is cut " before the ear all the muscles of the face, except those of the jaws, will be paralysed." " Thus it appears that the portio dura of the seventh nerve is the principal muscular nerve of the face; that it supplies the muscles of the cheek, the lips, the nostrils and the eyelids." Cutting it has no effect on sensation, stimulating the cut end does not cause pain but it does convulse the muscles of the face. When the sympathetic was left entire while the portio dura was cut, no sympathy pervaded the features. The sympathetic nerve is therefore not the cause of that sympathy which produces expression as has been supposed. Cutting the infra-orbital division of the fifth nerve where it emerges on to the face leads to loss of sensibility in the parts supplied by it, there is no effect on muscles of the face, stimulation of the cut end causes great pain. There is no doubt " that the fifth nerve is the sole cause or source of the common sensibility of the head and face." Bell has proved that these two great nerves have distinct functions, for one is purely motor, the other is the sensory nerve of the face. He notices that the ass could not pick up its food when the infra-orbital nerve is destroyed. He gives a large number of clinical cases to illustrate the function of each of these nerves. Paralysis of the facial nerve is universally known as Bell's palsy. " Sir Astley Cooper was the first to confirm the deductions by sending me a lady in whom, whilst cutting out a gland before the ear, he had divided the portio dura." This paper greatly enhanced his reputation; many were warm in praise of it.

Bell was aware in 1821 that the fifth nerve was, as he termed it, " the nerve of sensation and mastication," but he had not experimented on its motor root, nor traced the course of its motor fibres. He recognized the resemblance of the fifth to the spinal nerves in its having double roots with a ganglion on one, and he thought that, as would be the case with a mixed nerve proceeding from the junction of the anterior and posterior spinal roots, its branches—or some of them—contained both motor and sensory fibres and hence he considered that the reason why the ass could not take up its oats after division of the infra-orbital nerve was that the lips had lost not only sensation but some motion. Critics at once pointed out that loss of sensation alone would explain the facts. Thereupon Bell, together with his zealous and indefatigable brother-in-law, John Shaw, set out to reinvestigate the matter. John had been to Paris in 1821 to explain Bell's views and show his experiments to Majendie and others.

Bell gave their conclusions to the Royal Society in 1829, stating that reason for this communication was that in the paper of 1821 he " had attributed to one (the infra-orbital) of its (the fifth nerve) branches a function which belongs to another branch of the same nerve." He recapitulates what he had up to the time shown, namely " that nerves hitherto supposed to possess the same powers, consisted of filaments having different roots and performing different functions"; spinal nerves are made up " of two nerves derived from distinct columns, one for sensation and one for motion"; " the sensibility of the head and face depended upon the fifth pair of nerves . . . muscular branches of the fifth were for mastication . . . the portio dura . . . controlled the motions of the features." Clinical cases are described which illustrate these facts. He then gives an account of the motor root of the fifth nerve, " the root of the fifth being exposed in an ass and irritated, the jaws closed with a snap, the fifth pair being divided in an ass, the jaw fell relaxed and powerless." He then traces the motor branches of the fifth to the temporal, masseter, pterygoid, buccinator, mylohyoid and anterior belly of the digastric, muscles. Therefore the fifth nerve, by its motor root supplies the muscles which open the jaw, those which close it, and those which so move the food as to bring it under the operation of the teeth. (Bell considered that it also supplied some of the small muscles of the lips which we now know are supplied by the facial nerve.)

In short the motor portion of the fifth nerve sends no twigs with the opthalmic division, nor with the superior maxillary (infra-orbital), but only with the lower maxillary nerve, the motor function of which is masticitory. The fifth nerve is like a spinal nerve, having a sensory root with a ganglion, a motor root without one and both sensory and motor distribution.

Bell thus completely corrects his error of thinking that there were any motor fibres in the infra-orbital nerve. He several times in his writings shows that he, by now, knew, from experiment, that the posterior spinal roots were sensory. A German physiologist, Valentin, has given the name of Lex Belliana to the principle of the distinct functions of the two roots of a nerve to commemorate the name of its discoverer.

A paper which shows the originality of Bell's mind is that *On the Nervous Circle* read before the Royal Society on February 16, 1826. He is much struck by the fact that muscles have sensory nerves distributed to them; this is obvious in the face, where numerous branches from the purely sensory part of the fifth go to them. "I shall first inquire whether it be necessary to the governance of the muscular frame that there shall be a consciousness of the state or degree of action of the muscles?" His answer is Yes: "We possess the power of weighing with the hand :—what is this but estimating the muscular force? We are sensible of the most minute changes of muscular exertion, by which we know the position of the body and limbs, when there is no other means of knowledge open to us." Therefore we have "a sense of the condition of the muscles" or, as it is now called, muscle sense. By what path does this reach the central nervous system? it cannot be by the anterior roots as they are efferent, muscle sense is an afferent impulse and therefore must travel inwards by the posterior or sensory root. "Between the brain and the muscles there is a circle of nerves; one nerve conveys the influence from the brain to the muscle, another gives the sense of the condition of the muscle to the brain." The discovery by Bell of muscle sense is fundamental. His observation that when one set of muscles contract the opponents relax should also be noted.

His other writings on the nervous system, all communicated to the Royal Society, are as follows. A very full and original account of the mode of action of the external muscles of the eye, which has been neglected by many writers; he described how when the eyelids close, as in sleep, the eyeball rolls up, this is known as Bell's phenomenon. Two papers on the functions of the brain:

Sensibility and motion belong to the cerebrum—that two columns descend from each hemisphere—that one of these, the anterior, gives origin to the anterior roots of the spinal nerves, and is dedicated to voluntary motion and that the other gives origin to the posterior roots of the spinal nerves, and to the sensitive root of the fifth nerve, and is the column for sensation.

He is aware that the posterior columns are also connected with the cerebellum. He laboured under great disadvantage, for he could only trace the tracts by naked-eye dissections performed with the fine knives used for operations on the eye. A long paper *On the Nerves of Respiration* is an attempt to draw up a plan of the nerves of the body according to their evolution and function. It is well abstracted by Alexander Shaw in the *Journal of Anatomy and Physiology* for 1869. Bell recognized three divisions, an original system, which was concerned with loco-motion, prehension and mastication, over it the spinal nerves and in man the fifth exercise control, a respiratory system con-cerned with the organs of breathing which become in man the instruments of voice, speech and expression, hence Bell spoke of the portio dura as the respiratory nerve; and lastly a sympathetic system.

Bell's wonderful discoveries form a large part of the founda-tions of physiology and medicine, and it gave him great happiness that their brilliance was recognized in his lifetime. Many con-sider them only second in importance to those of Harvey. In a letter dated January 31, 1822, he writes:

Last week I went to Sir Humphry Davy's and there I found my paper had done me as much good as if I had bought a new blue coat and figured silk waistcoat. Lynn was with me, and showed his good nature by the pleasure that the civil things that were said to me gave him. In short, one gentleman —not the least important in that fraternity—Kater, called it the first discovery of the age.

He was invited to send his papers to the Institute of France and promised a prize medal if he did. When he was in Paris

M. Roux dismissed his class, to which he had taken Bell, saying, " Gentlemen, enough for to-day, you have seen Charles Bell ! " Neuburger refers to Bell's discovery as having awaked the physiology of the spinal cord from " a thousand years' slumber." But, remembering Bell was an artist, the most delicate compliment paid to him was that of Viggo Christiansen, of Copenhagen, who wrote : " He created modern clinical neurology in the same way as his contemporary Corot created modern French landscape painting."

RICHARD BRIGHT

Richard Bright, better known than any British physician since Harvey, was the third son of a family of ten, five sons and five daughters. The three elder sons were born in Queen Square, Bristol; the two younger at Ham Green, Somerset. Their father was Richard Bright, a member of the banking firm of Ames, Bright & Cove. The future great physician was born on September 28, 1789. He attended a private school near Bristol, then one at Exeter, and, in 1808, he went to Edinburgh University. During his first year he followed lectures on moral philosophy, political economy, natural philosophy and mathematics; in his second year he studied anatomy.

Young Bright and Henry Holland (afterwards Sir Henry), who had been his friend both at the school near Bristol and also at Edinburgh, learning, in 1810, that Sir George Mackenzie was planning an expedition to Iceland, asked to go with him. He " did not hesitate to meet their wishes, knowing them to be young men of very superior talents and accomplishments, in a high degree pleasing in their manners." Mackenzie published his *Travels in Iceland* and tells us that Bright was responsible for the collection, preservation and description of the plants and animals ; he also drew many of the illustrations. Owing to a storm, the ship which was to have brought them away never reached Iceland and the travellers were faced with the shortening days, oncoming winter, scanty food and clothing ; but happily a brig turned up and carried them to the Orkneys after a stormy passage and a narrow escape of shipwreck at the entrance of Hoy Sound.

On October 18, 1810, Bright entered as a student at Guy's Hospital, living for two years at the house of one of the resident officers. Among his teachers was that remarkable personality, Dr. William Babington, who so inspired the affection of his contemporaries that, on his death, a marble statue of him was erected in St. Paul's Cathedral, where it may be seen to-day.

He was one of the founders of the Geological Society, of which Bright also was an original member and read a paper before it in 1811 on the strata near Bristol. Babington and Bright became loving friends, the pupil later married the teacher's daughter, and few obituary orations have shown more feeling than that which Bright delivered on Babington's death. He and his second wife had several children, one became Master of University College, Oxford, another practised medicine at Cannes. Bright was dresser to Mr. Callaway. In January 1812 he read a paper on "Bleeding" before the Guy's Physical Society; it must have been stimulating, for the discussion of it occupied the four subsequent meetings.

Later in the same year he returned to Edinburgh and studied medicine and geology. He was a member of, and subsequently President of, the Royal Medical Society of Edinburgh and before it, in 1813, read a paper on gangrene. On September 13, 1813, he took his degree of M.D. with a thesis about Erysipelas, on which subject he had read a paper, while at Guy's, before the Royal Medico-Chirurgical Society. This was never printed, but the thesis was, and from it we learn that Bright stressed the contagiousness of the disease and its resemblance to puerperal fever. For a short time he was a member of the Edinburgh Speculative Society.

After graduation he spent two terms at Peterhouse at Cambridge, where his brother was a Fellow, but finding little of any use to him there, he came to London and became a pupil of Bateman at the London Dispensary; however, he was soon off again, for in the summer of 1814, he started on a tour through Holland, Belgium, Berlin, Vienna, Austria and Hungary, and on his way back in 1815, he arrived at Waterloo a fortnight after the battle. He observed and studied everything he came across, medical or otherwise, and in 1818 published *Travels from Vienna through Lower Hungary, with some remarks on the state of Vienna during the Congress in 1814*. The book is a well-printed quarto of over 700 pages, entertaining as an account of travel and full of detailed information which ought to be of value to students. It exemplifies Bright's wonderful power of observation and description, his wide reading, his accuracy, as is shown by the tables, maps and appendices, and his artistic ability, for it is illustrated by beautiful engravings from sketches by himself.

Medical allusions are few, but the leading doctors of Vienna are described, especially De Carro, a pupil of Jenner's, who had his own child vaccinated and was the means of introducing vaccination extensively. Most of the patients in the Viennese hospitals paid. There was a lying-in-hospital into which women were admitted secretly, and they left without any revelation of their identity.

When he returned to England, he read, before the Geological Society, a note on volcanic formations in Hungary. On December 23, 1816, he was admitted a Licentiate of the Royal College of Physicians, shortly after he became Assistant Physician to the London Fever Hospital, where he caught a severe fever from which he nearly died. In 1818 he travelled for nearly a year through Germany, Italy and France. In 1820 he was elected assistant physician to Guy's Hospital and set up in practice at 14 Bloomsbury Square, in 1821 he obtained his F.R.S., in 1824 he became full physician to Guy's.

He lectured at the Guy's Hospital Medical School on Botany and Materia Medica from 1822 to 1825, when he joined Cholmeley in lecturing on medicine. Later on Bright and Addison gave these lectures for many years. He was President of the Guy's Physical Society and in 1837 of the Royal Medico-Chirurgical Society. In 1832 he was, "with applause," elected a Fellow of the College of Physicians before whom he delivered the Gulstonian Lectures in 1833 and the Lumleian in 1837; he was a censor in both 1836 and 1839. The Académie des Sciences gave him the Monthyon prize, and in 1853 the degree of D.C.L. was conferred upon him at Oxford. He resigned his post of physician to Guy's in 1843.

By 1831 he had removed to 11 Savile Row, where he died on December 16, 1858, from heart disease, of which he had been aware for some time. He was buried at Kensal Green. There is a tablet on the south wall of St. James's, Piccadilly, with this inscription:

Sacred to the memory of Richard Bright, M.D., D.C.L., Physician Extraordinary to the Queen, Fellow of the Royal Society and other learned Bodies. He departed this life on 16 December, 1858 in the sixty ninth year of his age. He contributed to medical science many discoveries and works of great value and died while in the full practice of his profession, after a life of warm affection, unsullied purity and great usefulness.

His greatness was recognized in his lifetime, for the *Lancet* of December 25, 1858, said:

The sudden and unexpected demise of Dr. Bright has created a deep impression of grief and regret such as only a sense of irretrievable loss could occasion. In him all felt that the medical profession of England had lost one of the most original, observant and philosophic minds. A man of peculiar independence of thought, of high *morale* and untiring energy he contributed more perhaps than any other to form the medical opinion of his day. . . . By the singular devotion to pathological investigation which characterized his career, he was at once enabled to accomplish investigations which have immortalized his name.

Bright was not narrow, for we have seen that he was a traveller, a geologist, an artist, a writer and a linguist. He was an indefatigable worker and for many years spent six hours daily at Guy's Hospital. He considered no trouble too great to obtain a post-mortem examination, to do which he would willingly go into the country, and it was slow travelling then. He was a cheerful, attractive, honourable man, admired by his profession. The affectionate relations between him and the students is seen in the fact that they asked him to reprint an address he gave them in 1832. We shall see how his colleagues at Guy's liked to help him. He inspired the younger men to aid him in his researches, but was always most careful to acknowledge the assistance given. He was ungrudging in his admiration for the work of others and intensely proud of Guy's Hospital and its museum. At a dinner he had to return thanks for the toast of "The Physicians of Guy's Hospital." He said, "Gentlemen, I will return thanks: to hold the situation of Physician to Guy's Hospital is to be placed on the pinnacle of the profession. I am thankful—I am proud of a situation which has produced a Saunders, a Babington and a Cholmeley."

But Richard Bright was an infinitely greater man than this assemblage of good qualities indicates. He was an extraordinary man. It is impossible to place geniuses in order, but he is certainly among the first five or six in the medical profession. To him and to a few others an altogether marvellous power of observation has been given, but Bright's genius took him further than mere observation, however brilliant, for he could correlate his observations. It has been truly said that for one person who can see, fifty can think. Bright's power of seeing was amazing, little escaped him, but he never saw what was not there, and not a single one of his observations has been shown to be incorrect. His accuracy and truthfulness are wonderful; no preconceived idea ever tints his descriptions. Lastly his natural bent and training gave him the ability to write well. It is a pleasure to read him; the disease stands out with all its features clear, and the account he gives is still true to-day. Many times have I thought how much better it would be if some modern authors, instead of writing their picture of a disease, had transcribed Bright's words.

Let us now go to Bright himself to learn in his own words of his discoveries, beginning with the most famous, that of the disease which bears his name. In 1827 there appeared the first of the renowned two volumes entitled *Reports of Medical Cases selected with a View of Illustrating the Symptoms and Cure of Diseases by a Reference to Morbid Anatomy,* by Richard Bright. It is dedicated to Benjamin Harrison, the treasurer of Guy's Hospital, and William Babington, of whom I have already spoken. Harrison was always so willing to help Bright in his researches that it is also worth while to say something of him. He became treasurer in 1797 when he was 26 and held office till 1848—over fifty years. He was an absolute but admirable autocrat. He reformed the administration and the nursing of the hospital, he founded the medical school and the museum, he bought land adjacent to the hospital, and thus was able to greatly enlarge it when his friend Mr. Hunt left a large fortune for this purpose. He advanced considerable sums of money to the hospital, his treasurership was a constant source of expense to him, for it was unpaid, but, nevertheless, his natural generosity made him give freely to poor patients. He appointed everybody, members of the staff, lecturers and nurses; the governors always supported him, for his rule was good. The Charity Commissioners could not find any abuses. He loved the place, and devoted his whole life to trying to make it the best institution of its kind, and admirably illustrated that administration by a really good autocrat is an excellent mode of government.

In the preface to his book Bright says:

It is my wish in thus recording a number of cases, to render the labours of a large Hospital more permanently useful by bringing together such facts as seem to throw light upon each other. . . . To connect accurate and faithful observation after death with symptoms displayed during life, must be in some degree to forward the objects of our noble art. . . . The work which I now commence will not, in theory at least, be thoroughly completed, until every disease which influences the natural structure, or originates in its derangements, has been connected with the corresponding organic lesion. . . . It is a pleasing and yet no easy task, to acknowledge the kindness of those many friends who in various ways have assisted me in this undertaking. I may truly say that I have met with the most cheerful compliance in all my wishes from everyone connected with our establishment.

It is worth while to call attention to two points in this preface. Bright seeks facts, he desires to find out for every disease what is its corresponding organic lesion, so that a doctor, when he diagnoses such and such a disease, will be able to predict what will be found at a post-mortem examination if the malady is one with a morbid anatomy. The second point is that we learn of the willingness of Bright's colleagues to help him.

The subjects treated of in Volume I are diseases of the kidney in association with dropsy and albuminuria, diseases of the liver with dropsy and ascites, diseases of the thorax followed by dropsy, diseases of the lungs and diseases of the intestines in fever. Volume II was published three years later and consists of two parts, each larger than Volume I. The two volumes contain sixty-five hand-coloured plates, which are as beautifully executed as possible; the colours to-day are still perfect. The second volume is entirely occupied with diseases of the nervous system. In the preface to it Bright says :

My opportunities have increased . . . by the great augmentation of the sumptuous Hospital to which I am attached, and in which I am proud to say that my colleagues, whether medical or surgical, have, by their unremitting kindness, shown how little jealousy interferes between the two professions.

The most celebrated part of his *Reports* is the first 126 pages of Volume I dealing with the disease to which his name has become attached. This section is entitled " Cases Illustrative of Some of the Appearances observable in the Examination of Diseases terminating in Dropsical Effusion." He begins by reminding the reader that one great cause of dropsical effusion appears to be obstruction to the venous circulation. But, says Bright:

There are other appearances to which I think too little attention has hitherto been paid. They are those evidences of organic disease which occasionally present themselves in the structure of the *kidney*, and which, whether they are to be considered the cause of the dropsical effusion, or as the consequence of some other disease, cannot be unimportant. Where these conditions of the kidney to which I allude have occurred, I have often found the dropsy connected with the secretion of albuminous urine, more or less coagulable on heat. . . . I have never yet examined the body of a patient dying with dropsy attended with coagulable urine, in whom some obvious derangement was not discovered in the kidneys.

He then describes the appearance of the albumen seen when the urine is heated in a spoon, he says blood is often found in the urine and proceeds :

In all cases in which I have observed the albuminous urine, it has appeared to me that the kidney has itself acted a more important part, and has been deranged both functionally and organically more than has generally been imagined. In the latter class of cases I have always found the kidneys decidedly disorganized. In the former, when very recent I have found the kidneys gorged with blood. . . . It is now nearly twelve years since I first observed the altered structure of the kidney in a patient who had died dropsical and I still have a slight drawing that I then made. It was not, however, till within the last two years that I had an opportunity of connecting these appearances with any particular symptoms, and since that time I have added several observations.

Then follow the clinical notes of twenty-three cases to illustrate what he has said. All were patients during the years 1825, 1826 and 1827 and almost all were inmates of Guy's Hospital. Considerably over a half were fatal, a post-mortem examination was made on all that died. The account of this examination is very full, the kidneys are described and illustrated by beautiful plates. It is impossible here to give more than the first of this series which have influenced medicine so profoundly. John King, an intemperate sailor, aged 34, was admitted into Clinical Ward, Guy's Hospital on October 12, 1825, under Dr. Bright, suffering from general œdema, scanty urine and pain in the loins. He had hæmaturia, but this passed away and the urine, when clear, coagulated in heat, and the pulse was hard. The post-mortem examination revealed acute pericarditis, œdema of the lungs, pleural effusion, a large heart and ascites. " The kidneys were completely granulated throughout : externally the surface rough and uneven ; internally all traces of natural organization nearly gone, except in the tubal parts." There is a coloured plate which admirably shows a typically granular kidney. Bright says, " This is a well-marked example of a granulated condition of the kidneys connected with the secretion of coagulable urine." He inclines to the opinion that " the disease of the kidney was the first established." He considers that neither disease of the heart, lungs nor pleura was the primary condition, nor was there any disease of the liver to explain the ascites. He points out that pain in the loins is a frequent symptom of renal disease, and that " the tendency to inflammatory action in this man was a striking feature of his case, and appears to me connected immediately with the condition of the kidneys." Therefore John King becomes a classic case, presenting all the essential symptoms of chronic renal disease, and is the first recorded case in which they were successfully correlated with condition found after death.

Bright's next allusion to renal disease was in the second of his Gulstonian Lectures delivered in 1833. We learn that a century ago the now popular team-work was in existence, for he remarks, " I have lately had great assistance from the intelligent and zealous co-operation of three of my young friends and pupils, Mr. Barlow, Mr. Tweedie and Mr. Rees." He says lately because Barlow did not enter at Guy's till 1830, nor Rees till 1829. Barlow came from Trinity College, Cambridge; he was a man of great mental power and intelligence, but did not make an outstanding name for himself, as he was modest to a fault, and could not be persuaded to give an opinion. Those who knew him were fond of him, admired him, learned from him and respected his ability. He began by helping Bright in his urinary analyses and thus became much interested in Bright's disease. Rees from his entry at Guy's became attached to chemistry. Bright asked his help which he freely gave, the two becoming lifelong friends. He was generally known as Owen Rees, and many chemical papers were published by him; he proved the presence of urea in the blood and wrote in 1850 a book on *Diseases of the Kidneys.* Owen Rees was made assistant physician to Guy's in 1843, Barlow having been appointed in 1840. From reading Bright's papers it is clear that Tweedie devoted much time to helping him, but he did not come on the staff of the hospital. Bright in his papers often mentions others who aided him, he is punctilious to record the assistance given by all his helpers.

To return to the Gulstonian Lectures. Bright tells us that his three " young friends " examined the urines of 296 patients. It is pointed out that phosphates and urates must be distinguished from albumen. " In the natural and healthy condition of the urine, little or no albumen is to be detected. The specific gravity of the urine is very variable. In many cases of albuminous urine there is an excess of urea in the blood." Bright describes the varieties of nephritis found in the post-mortem room, and says that both anasarca and albuminuria may be absent in renal disease. He alludes to the enlargement of the heart, the serous effusions, the headache, the coma and cerebral hæmorrhage and he reaches this conclusion : " My conviction is complete as to existence of some decided connection between the three facts—anasarca, coagulable urine and diseased function going on to a diseased structure of the kidney."

Bright's final and most extensive communication on the subject of renal disease appeared in the first volume of the *Guy's Hospital Reports,* published in 1836. It consists of two papers. The first is entitled " Cases and Observations Illustrative of Renal Disease accompanied with the Secretion of Albuminous Urine." The second follows it immediately and is called, " Tabular View of the Morbid Appearances occurring in One Hundred Cases in Connection with Albuminous Urine." These papers occupy more than sixty pages, so they cannot be here reprinted in full, but I will give an abstract of them, using Bright's own words :

The importance and extensive prevalence of that form of disease, which, after it has continued for some time, is attended by the peculiar changes in the structure of the kidney, now pretty generally known by the names of " mottling," " white degeneration," " contraction," or " granulation," impresses itself every year more and more deeply on my mind; and whether I turn to the wards of the hospital, or reflect on the experience of private practice, I find, on every side, such examples of its fatal progress and unrelenting ravages, as induce me to consider it amongst the most frequent, as well as the most certain causes of death in some classes of the community, while it is of common occurrence in all; and I believe I speak within bounds, when I state, that not less than five hundred die of it annually in London alone. It is, indeed, an humiliating confession, that, although much attention has been directed to this disease for nearly ten years, and during that time there has probably been no period in which at least twenty cases might not have been pointed out in each of the large hospitals of the metropolis—and there is reason to believe that double that number may, at this moment, and at all times, be found in the wards of Guy's Hospital—yet little or nothing has been done towards devising a method of permanent relief, when the disease has been confirmed; and no fixed plan has been laid down, as affording a tolerable certainty of cure in the more recent cases. I believe that our want of success, in what are considered the more recent attacks, is frequently owing to the fact, that the disease is far more advanced than we suspect, when it first becomes the object of our attention; and I am most anxious, in the present communication, to impress upon the members of our profession the insidious nature of this malady, that they may be led to watch its first approaches, with all the solicitude which they would feel on discovering the first suspicious symptoms of phthisis or of epilepsy. There is great reason to suppose that the seeds of this disease are often sown at an early period; and that intervals of apparent health produce a false security in the patient, his friends, and his medical attendants, even where apprehension has been early excited.

The first indications of the tendency to this disease is often hæmaturia, of a more or less decided character; this may originate from various causes, and yet may give evidence of the same tendency: scarlatina has apparently laid the foundation for the future mischief. . . . Intemperance seems its most usual source; and exposure to cold the most common cause of its development and aggravation. . . .

The history of this disease, and its symptoms, is nearly as follows:

A child, or an adult, is affected with scarlatina, or some other acute disease; or has indulged in the intemperate use of ardent spirits for a series of months or years: he is exposed to some casual cause or habitual source of suppressed perspiration: he finds the secretion of his urine greatly increased, or he discovers that it is tinged with blood; or, without having made any such observations, he awakes in the morning with his face swollen, or his ankles puffy, or his hands œdematous. If he happen, in this condition, to fall under the care of a practitioner who suspects the nature of his disease, it is found, that already his urine contains a notable quantity of albumen: his pulse is full and hard, his skin dry, he has often headache, and sometimes a sense of weight or pain across the loins. Under treatment more or less active, or sometimes without any treatment, the more obvious and distressing of these symptoms disappear; the swelling, whether casual or constant, is no longer observed; the urine ceases to evince any admixture of red particles; and, according to the degree of importance which has been attached to these symptoms, they are gradually lost sight of, or are absolutely forgotten. Nevertheless, from time to time the countenance becomes bloated; the skin is dry; headaches occur with unusual frequency; or the calls to micturition disturb the night's repose. After a time, the healthy colour of the countenance fades; a sense of weakness or pain in the loins increases; headaches, often accompanied by vomiting, add greatly to the general want of comfort; and a sense of lassitude, of weariness, and of depression, gradually steals over the bodily and mental frame. Again, the assistance of medicine is sought. If the nature of the disease is suspected, the urine is carefully tested; and found, in almost every trial, to contain albumen, while the quantity of urea is gradually diminishing. If, in the attempt to give relief to the oppression of the system, blood is drawn, it is often buffed, or the serum is milky and opaque; and nice analysis will frequently detect a great deficiency of albumen, and sometimes manifest indications of the presence of urea. If the disease is not suspected, the liver, the stomach, or the brain divide the care of the practitioner, sometimes drawing him away entirely from the more important seat of disease. The swelling increases and decreases; the mind grows cheerful, or is sad; the secretions of the kidney or the skin are augmented or diminished, sometimes in alternate ratio, sometimes without apparent relation. Again, the patient is restored to tolerable health; again he enters on his active duties: or he is, perhaps, less fortunate;—the swelling increases, the urine becomes scanty, the powers of life seem to yield, the lungs become œdematous, and, in a state of asphyxia or coma, he sinks into the grave; or a sudden effusion of serum into the glottis closes the passages of the air, and brings on a more sudden dissolution. Should he, however, have resumed the avocations of life, he is usually subject to constant recurrence of his symptoms; or again, almost dismissing the recollection of his ailment, he is suddenly seized with an acute attack of pericarditis, or with a still more acute attack of peritonitis, which, without any renewed warning, deprives him, in eight and forty hours, of his life. Should he escape this danger likewise, other perils await him; his headaches have been observed to become more frequent; his stomach more deranged; his vision indistinct; his hearing depraved; he is suddenly seized with a convulsive fit, and becomes blind. He struggles through the attack; but again and again it returns; and before a day or a week has elapsed, worn out by convulsions, or overwhelmed by coma, the painful history of his disease is closed.

Of the appearance presented after death, enough will be said in another part of the present communication: but one question may be asked in this place— Do we always find such lesion of the kidney as to bear us out in the belief, that the peculiar condition of the urine, to which I have already referred, shows that the disease, call it what we may, is connected necessarily and essentially with the derangement of that organ? After ten years' attentive—though, perhaps, I must not say completely impartial observation—I am ready to answer this question in the affirmative; and yet I confess that I have occasionally met with anomalies which have been somewhat difficult to explain. . . .

Nothing can be more striking than the similarity which is observable in all these cases. I am not aware of any disease in which the character is more completely preserved, or in which the symptoms more clearly mark a specific form of malady. In the first eight cases, the termination, as well as the progress of the disease, bore the most perfect resemblance; and the peculiar train of cerebral symptoms, by which their advanced stages have been attended, have little analogy, when taken as a whole, with the symptoms of any other cerebral affection. The two last cases differ from the rest only in their mode of termination; and I have related them as the two most recent illustrations of a very frequent result of the disease.

Of the insidious nature of this malady, and its fatal tendency, these cases afford a pretty convincing proof: and the fact that so many of these have come within my own observation in a limited time, would be tolerable evidence of the extreme frequency of the disease. Yet the cases I have now detailed, but more especially the many more which the length of the present communication obliges me to defer, are chiefly such as I have, without any intention of publication, chanced to enter in my note-book, and form but a small portion of those which I have seen: but, in order to obtain a more accurate idea of the actual prevalence of the disease, it is necessary to have recourse to another species of evidence: and accordingly, in the winter of 1828-9, I instituted a series of experiments, by taking the patients promiscuously, as they lay in the wards, and trying the effects of heat upon the urine of each, and at the same time employing occasionally other reagents. The whole number I took amounted to a hundred and thirty; out of which no less than eighteen proved to have urine decidedly coagulable by heat: and in twelve more, traces of albumen were found: giving, therefore, an average of at least one in six, if not one in four of the whole number. In order to show how the experiment was made, and the nature of the table I constructed, I will introduce six consecutive cases out of a male, and six out of a female ward; and it is worth remarking, that in every instance, where the result allowed us to ascertain the state of the kidneys, it corresponded with the diagnosis yielded by the table. Those who had albuminous urine were found to have more or less of this disease in the kidneys; whilst those whose urine did not coagulate by heat had kidneys without disease.

The author then discusses the treatment. He doubts

whether we have it in our power, as yet, even at the earliest periods, to destroy the liability to relapse, or overcome the morbid tendency; but at all events, the management of the early stage of the disease is easy, when compared with the treatment in its more confirmed and protracted forms . . . I cannot, from my own experience, entertain a hope that diaphoretics are capable of curing any large proportion of confirmed cases. . . . Till this symptom (albuminuria) be removed the disease certainly exists: and even when it is removed, it is often absent but a short time, and it is, for many years, liable to return. It can never be sufficiently impressed on the minds of practitioners, that the anasarca . . . is but a symptom.

But he says anasarca may be absent throughout or it may disappear and yet the disease be fatal. As diaphoretics he used antimonial powders, compound ipecacuanha powder and liquor ammoniæ acetatis, with the warmth of the bed, a warm bath, fomentations and large linseed poultices. He is particularly insistent on the necessity of keeping the skin warm; hence he advises an inner dress of flannel and residence in a suitable climate. Bleeding may be useful in the earlier stages, but with regard to the later periods

when we call to mind the constant loss of albuminous matter which the system is sustaining by the kidneys, and the peculiar pallid hue which the patient assumes, we shall pause before we venture to afford temporary alleviation, at a still further expense of the more nutritious and stimulating portions of the blood.

Cupping the nape of the neck may relieve the headache, and a few leeches to the loins may assuage the pain there. He calls attention to the value of acupuncture for œdema, but " all attempts to draw off the serum by mechanical means should be most cautiously conducted; for the powers of repair are weak and there is a great tendency to erythematous inflammation." He is opposed to the use of mercury. Elaterium used with care may be beneficial.

With regard to diuretics, I have generally wished to abstain from all except digitalis. . . . I look upon this class of remedies, however, in the light of a necessary evil in some cases; and do not feel authorized in recommending their employment. . . . A great deal still further depends upon diet. Where milk is grateful, if it sits easily on the stomach, and is freely digested, I believe it to be one of the best aliments which can be taken. . . .

The great rule is to avoid everything which obviously deranges the stomach, and to take tonic and nutritive food. " The less of wine and spirituous liquors is taken, the better."

Every precaution must be taken to avoid chill to the surface or check perspiration. If exercise be taken, it must be gentle. This surely is a masterly exposition of the treatment of what was then a new disease, and now nearly a century later we cannot do much better.

Bright's second paper in the *Guy's Hospital Reports* begins with a tabular view of the morbid appearances occurring in one hundred cases. The details are extraordinarily complete.

In almost all I have been present at the examination after death. . . . The first circumstance which strikes the mind, is the extent and frequency to which the derangement of one organ is connected with the derangement of several others. Yet we are not at liberty to assume, that the disease of the kidney has been the primary cause on which the disease of the rest depended. It may be, that some other organ has first suffered, and that the kidneys, together with the rest, have become involved. I confess I am inclined to believe that the kidney is the chief promoter of the other derangements. . . . I do not therefore by any means assert, that all the lesions . . . flow as a consequence from the kidney alone; but that they are such derangements as generally co-exist with this peculiar disease of that organ.

Then follows an account of the post-mortem appearances, other than renal, in Bright's disease. They are inflammation of the pleura, pericardium and peritoneum, hypertrophy of the heart, œdema of the lungs and bronchitis, enteritis and cerebral hæmorrhage. Some of these lesions are the cause of death, but the commonest is that producing the cerebral symptoms we call uræmia.

Bright's enthusiasm for the study of renal disease continued, and in 1842, with the willing permission of Mr. Harrison and his hearty co-operation, the whole of the forty-one beds in the

clinical wards—then in the building now exclusively surgical—
were, from May to October 1842 set aside for the admission of
renal cases under the care of Bright. This, as he says, is "the
first experiment which, as far as I know, has yet been made in
this country to turn the ample resources of a hospital to the
investigation of a particular disease, by bringing the patients
labouring under it into one ward properly arranged for observation." A small laboratory "was fitted up and decorated entirely
to our purpose." He was helped by Barlow and Rees, and
these two published in the *Guy's Hospital Reports*, for 1843,
the results of their labours which corroborated Bright's original
statements. In the *Medical Gazette* for January 28, 1843, is a
letter from Bright saying that since 1839 he and Mr. George
Robinson had been making microscopic investigations of 1,000
specimens from kidneys of about 100 patients suffering from
nephritis, and that they hope to publish a work on the Anatomy
and Pathology of the Kidney; unfortunately they never did this.

Assuredly this is one of the most wonderful series of papers
in medical literature. In 1826 nothing was known about
chronic nephritis, by 1836 Bright had established the existence
of a common disease, which presents symptoms of derangement
of most of the organs of the body and had unerringly correlated
these symptoms with changes in the kidney. He describes all
the very numerous and diverse symptoms—even the alterations
in the blood—and tells us how to recognize the disease; he
advises as to its treatment and describes its post-mortem appearances, all with such completeness and accuracy that, although
in the century which has elapsed very many hundreds of papers
have been written about the disease, no error has been detected
in Bright's description, and nothing of importance has been
added, except facts, such as retinitis, that have been revealed
by instruments he did not possess, but the hard pulse is recorded
by him, so is occasional blindness. When we reflect upon the
multitude and diversity of the symptoms, many of which are
often absent, we are filled with astonishment that anyone should
have had the genius to see that they are all indications of one
disease; but not only did Bright do this, he saw that the fundamental lesion was in the kidney, he gave the correct treatment
and wrote a masterly description.

Barlow, Rees, Gull, Wilks, Mahomed, Goodhart, Starling

and Osman at Bright's own school have continued to work at the subject of the kidney and its disorders. Much investigation by workers all over the world has been devoted to trying to obtain a better understanding of Bright's disease and much discussion has taken place as to whether the diseased kidney is the cause, not only of the symptoms, but also of the other organic disorders seen after death, or whether all these and the disease of the kidney are due to some cause of wide effect. The matter is undecided, I only mention it because it is sometimes asserted Bright considered the kidney to be the primary cause of all else that is found wrong with the patient. This may have been so, but it is by no means certain, although it is true that he seemed to consider the disease of the kidney to be the cause of the albumen and anasarca. Thus he says, " My conviction is complete as to the existence of some decided connection between the three facts—anasarca, coagulable urine and diseased function going on to diseased structure of the kidney." On the other hand he appears to have had in his mind the possibility that the alteration in the kidney might be only one of several results from an unknown cause, for he says, " Yet we are not at liberty to assume that the disease of the kidney has been the primary cause on which the disease of the rest depended."

Had he done no work on the subject of renal disease Bright would have been among the really famous physicians because of his other original observations.

He published a series of papers in the *Guy's Hospital Reports* on " Abdominal Tumours." These received the honour of being reprinted as a separate book. The second chapter contains a description of fifteen cases of abdominal hydatid disease. Here again we see his originality, for Barlow says:

It is but due to the memory of Bright to state, though without any desire of imputing plagiarism to more recent continental pathologists, that the description of acephalocyst hydatids is altogether original, and certainly an anticipation of similar observations which have since been published in Germany.

Chapter III contains twenty-nine cases of ovarian tumour and is worth reading, for, now that ovarian tumours are removed, many practitioners do not appreciate the huge size they may attain. What proportion of this mass of clinical observations on a hundred and seventeen cases is original it is impossible to say, for we cannot be sure of the exact state of knowledge at the time, but the whole series should be read as we read classical clinical lectures, namely, to enjoy and to learn from the description of a master who is an observer and can appreciate the value and relation of the facts he records.

Bright's most original paper among his many on abdominal diseases was "Cases and Observations connected with Disease of the Pancreas and Duodenum" (*Medico-Chi. Trans.*, XVIII, 1832–33). These cases he says,

are chiefly intended to call the attention of the Members to a particular symptom in disease which I believe to have been but little noticed . . . The symptom to which I refer is a peculiar condition of the alvine evacuation, a portion more or less considerable assuming the character of an oily substance resembling fat, which either passes separately from the bowels or soon divides itself from the general mass, and lies upon the surface, sometimes forming a thick crust particularly about the edges of the vessel, if the fæces are of a semi-fluid consistence, sometimes floating like globules of tallow which have been melted and become cold, and sometimes assuming the form of a thin fatty pellicle over the whole or over the fluid parts, in which the more solid figured fæces are deposited. This oily matter has generally a slight yellow tinge and a most disgustingly fetid odour.

The first case was that of a man aged forty-five, who had considerable glycosuria; this Bright abolished by diminishing the carbohydrates in the food. He shows that he knew that pancreatic disease causes glycosuria. The patient was jaundiced; a tumour was felt in the upper right part of the abdomen, and on several occasions during the last few weeks of his life he passed "a quantity of yellowish fatty matter much resembling butter that had been melted and had again become solid. This matter followed the fæces and, as it was evacuated in a melting state, it was perceived on the surface of the dejection." The sectio cadaveris revealed malignant disease of the head of the pancreas, firmly adherent to the duodenum on the inner surface of which it formed an ulceration. Bright had during the patient's life shown that the fatty stools could not proceed from fat taken by the mouth, for, when this was stopped, the stools remained fatty. The second patient, a woman, aged fifty, passed similar motions; she was jaundiced. Bright was much interested and predicted that the condition would resemble that of the first case. As her husband would not let her remain in the hospital, Bright persuaded him to let him know when she died, so that he might make a post-mortem examination.

The husband did; Bright at once went to Gravesend and found malignant disease of the pancreas ulcerating into the duodenum. The third patient, a woman aged twenty-one, passed similar motions and was jaundiced; in her case also a tumour of the pancreas and duodenal ulceration were found. The rest of the paper consists of a masterly discussion of these cases and a consideration of the possible causes for these stools. Bright reaches the original and correct conclusion that their occurrence is symptomatic of pancreatic disease.

In a paper entitled " Observations on Jaundice" (*Guy's Hosp. Rep.* vol. I, 1836) he mentions that fatty stools are present when the pancreatic duct is implicated in disease. There is an admirable description of jaundice and its causes. Cirrhosis of the liver due to alcohol is given as one cause of jaundice, and Bright knew that the liver in this disease may be at first large and then contract.

In this paper we have the first description of acute yellow atrophy of the liver; although Bright did not name the disease, he described it and its post-mortem appearances, for he speaks of a febrile form of jaundice with cerebral symptoms and an excessive tendency to hæmorrhage. Two cases are described. Case 5 is headed *Jaundice of a most intense Character, without Mechanical Obstructions ; and apparently depending on Inflammatory Action in the Liver.* " The liver only weighed two pounds, five ounces. It was soft and flaccid to the touch. . . . Its external appearance was mottled dark red liver colour with stone yellow colour." Case 6 is headed *Intense Jaundice without Mechanical Obstruction and apparently depending upon Inflammatory Action in the Substance of the Liver.* A girl aged eighteen suffered from jaundice and torpor; later she was delirious, had a rapid pulse and soon died. The liver was unusually small, " of a brightish yellow colour with portions marked with purple or deep brown." It is quite possible that Case 4 was also an example of this disease, for her liver was small, she was jaundiced and died from hæmorrhage. The last two cases in this paper are examples of pyæmic abscesses in the liver secondary to portal phlebitis, but it is clear that Bright did not recognize the relationship between the two conditions; he was inclined to regard multiple abscesses in the liver as a later stage of acute yellow atrophy and the condition of the portal vein as secondary to that of the liver. In the same volume he records an extraordinary case of diaphragmatic hernia, which has escaped the notice of nearly all who are interested in the subject.

Bright was the first to describe Chronic Proliferative Peritonitis. He begins by saying that he has discovered a new sign, namely the crepitation that may be felt by the hand on the abdomen and is caused by the adhesions. He then gives in the *Medico-Chirurgical Transactions*, Vol. XIX, 1833–5, p. 176, the following perfect account of the condition:

One of the most frequent morbid changes in the peritoneum is when the whole is covered with an evenly distributed false membrane, which renders it, in its general appearance, opake, and is apt to contract the loose folds of the membrane and those by which the various viscera are suspended or attached, and likewise to form a kind of compressing ligature about all the viscera themselves; the result of which is, that the omentum gradually becomes shortened and corrugated, ultimately forming but a narrow band along the arch of the stomach and the colon—the mesentery becomes shortened, and the intestines, by this means drawn towards the spine—the calibre of the intestines themselves becomes diminished and they are most obviously shortened in their course—the liver is drawn close to the diaphragm and the spleen to the stomach—while the kidneys are fixed more firmly into the cavities formed by the muscles of the loins,—and all these viscera are compressed in a degree which often produces alteration in their shape. . . . This false membrane is polished, like the peritoneum, and at first sight gives the idea of a thickening and opacity of the membrane itself; but upon examination it is found capable of being removed and stripped off in large flakes, leaving the surface of the peritoneum polished and entire. This I should consider the product of a very low stage of chronic inflammation.

The author then points out that the condition can be diagnosed if there is fluid in the abdomen, for then, owing to the intestines being retracted, there will be a dull note in front. He remarks upon the honeycomb appearance of the membrane over the liver and spleen.

To Bright must be given the credit of being the first to describe Addison's disease, but in no sense did he discover the disease, for he did not connect the symptoms with disease of the suprarenals. The merit of this is entirely due to Addison. Bright's case was that of a woman admitted into Guy's in July 1829. She was greatly emaciated and apparently sinking. "Her complexion was very dark." She had vomiting, became drowsy and died. At the sectio cadaveris slight evidence of chronic phthisis was found, but the only marked disease was in the renal capsules, both of which were enlarged, lobulated, and the seat of morbid deposits apparently of a scrofulous character; they were at least four times their natural thickness, feeling solid and hard; on the left side one part had gone into suppuration, containing two drams of yellow pus.

This specimen is still in the Guy's Museum and is probably the earliest specimen illustrating Addison's disease.

In London in 1839 was published Volume I of *Elements of the Practise of Medicine,* by Richard Bright, M.D., and Thomas Addison, M.D. It contains the first accurate account of appendicitis, but this will be referred to in the life of Addison.

In Volume II of his *Reports of Medical Cases* Bright gives an admirable account of chorea, mentioning hemichorea and the paralysis associated with chorea, and also the mental symptoms which may occur. He finds no explanation for the disease in the post-mortem room. As long ago as 1802 Babington and Curry had taught that rheumatism was a cause of chorea. Bright did much to enforce that rheumatism, cardiac disease and chorea are associated, he records pericarditis with chorea and was the first to describe the mitral murmur that accompanies chorea. Probably too he was the first to describe the bronchopneumonia and pulmonary collapse seen in whooping cough.

A large portion of Bright's observations were made upon nervous diseases. They will be found chiefly in the second volume of his *Reports to Medical Cases* and in papers in the *Guy's Hospital Reports.* As it is now, so then, for speaking of diseases called functional, he says, " This view has often been an unintentional cloak for ignorance and has materially retarded investigation." He was constantly preaching that by carefully observing symptoms we could predict in what position in the brain or spinal cord the lesion would be found, that is to say he was a pioneer in the doctrine of cerebral localization. He was insistent that certain epileptic seizures, or as we should now call them, attacks of Jacksonian epilepsy, are due to organic disease of the brain, and he showed how to tell such attacks from ordinary epilepsy. In his *Reports of Medical Cases*, Vol. II, p. 514, he says:

As far as I have been able to infer from my own observation, I should say that the organic causes of epilepsy, connected immediately with the brain, are more frequently such as affect its surface, than such as are deep seated in its substance. Thus we find that morbid growth, taking place in the skull, showing itself by a thickened heavy state of bone, or by a roughened surface either internally or externally, or a remarkable prominence in the natural projections at the base is often associated with epilepsy. Slow changes, producing a thickened condition of the membranes, will not unfrequently be found attendant upon epileptic attacks. Tumours pressing on the surface, or amalgamated with the cineritious substance will also be found in cases of epilepsy.

Case 265 is an example in point. A man, aged 37, liable to severe headaches, had fits, ushered in by an aura, which took the form of a tremor and cramp-like sensation in the calf of the right leg which was partially paralysed; in the fits the patient lost consciousness. The aura was so sure a herald of a fit that, when it appeared, a tourniquet " was applied at the lower part of the thigh, with the complete effect, apparently, of putting a stop to the fit." The patient experienced so much relief from the tourniquet that he kept it " constantly loose on the limb, screwing it tight when he was aroused by the painful sensations usually preceeding a fit." Again in Volume I of the *Guy's Hospital Reports* he records the case of a man who had right-sided fits, saying

"I now gave it as my opinion that these fits were owing to some local disorganization affecting the membrane and cineritious portion of the brain on the left side. . . . My reason, then, for supposing that the epileptic attacks, in this case, depended rather on a local affection . . . was the degree of consciousness that was observed to be retained during the fits."

Other similar cases are mentioned. Here we have the brilliant observation that retention of consciousness in a fit suggests a local lesion, but we must hasten to add that Bright was well aware that occasionally consciousness may be lost when fits are due to a local lesion.

The paper in Volume II of the *Guy's Hospital Reports* continues the same subject. The first two cases in it had many symptoms and were difficult to analyse, but both had a tumour in the cerebellum and both had impairment of taste, which Bright had " no doubt arose from pressure made by the tumour on the fifth pair of nerves," for this was found at the post-mortem examination. Then follow examples of disease of the spinal column, which illustrate how particular symptoms can be precisely explained by pressure on the cord or on the nerves derived from it. After these come two admirably recorded cases of aphasia: the woman

had total inability of connecting her words, when she could utter them, with the ideas she wished to express, or the things to which she meant to refer. . . .

When asked, for instance, the name of her hand, to which I pointed, she said "a pin," but immediately signified her knowledge that this was not the right word, though she could not tell what the right name was.

At the autopsy a cerebral hæmorrhage was found: "its occupying chiefly the posterior part of the corpus striatum is further in accordance with an impression I have received from observation, and inculcated, with regard to the lesions which influence the articulation." The man had a similar form of aphasia: "the great and striking peculiarity was the difficulty of bringing the right words into play when he spoke." The full description exemplifies this and might be copied into a modern text-book. The last case is that of a man, who during life had deranged sense of touch on the right side together with disorder of vision. The only cerebral abnormality found was an old hæmorrhage in the "posterior part of the right thalamus nervi optici (corpus geniculatum inferius)," and Bright concludes the paper by saying "that the symptoms which arise in cerebral and spinal disease are actually the results . . . of the lesions which the different parts of the nervous system have suffered." These references show that he was one of the earliest enunciators of the doctrine of cerebral localization. This is not known by many who write on the subject. He describes two cases of tumour of the brain in which the legs were stiff and the spinal cord was "remarkably firm throughout, almost like cartilage. . . . It appears probable that this condition of the cord was chiefly instrumental in producing . . . the peculiar spasmodic extension of the limbs." This observation that secondary degeneration of the cord is associated with spastic paraplegia is entirely original. He records very carefully with excellent plates over forty cases of cerebral hæmorrhage, and he notes that the patient may have hemiopia.

This is a brief account of the chief observations made by the marvellous insight of a man who wrote to his father that " he was very fond of seeing," who told his students " acute cases must be seen at least once a day by those who wish to learn. In many cases twice a day will not be too often," and who had, in addition, the rarest gift given to a scientist, namely that of interpreting correctly the experiments of nature. His writings show him to have been a wise practitioner of the art of medicine; he was cultivated, modest, high minded, much beloved, generous and possessed a dignified simplicity. When urged to protect himself against the statements of a quack of the same name, he declined, saying that the matter was beneath his notice.

At no time during the last hundred years has his fame lessened. The centenary of the publication of Bright's *Medical Reports* came round in 1927, it was commemorated by a reception at the Royal College of Physicians and by a celebration at Guy's Hospital on July 8. In the morning an address was given by Professor Ludwig Aschoff on the Pathology of Bright's disease and one by Professor Lemierre on its clinical aspects. After a lunch, at which the Prime Minister, the Earl of Balfour, a governor of Guy's Hospital, and many distinguished guests were present, a meeting, under the chairmanship of Lord Balfour, was held. The Chairman referred in particular to Bright's introduction of team-work and to Bright himself as " an observer of unequalled perseverance and accuracy, who knew how to turn his observations to account. Those are, in some respects, different arts. It is only when they are combined that humanity gains such services as those rendered to it by Bright." Bright Memorial gold medals were presented to Professor Thayer, Professor Aschoff, Professor Lemierre (on behalf of Professor Widal, who was unable to attend), Sir John Rose-Bradford, and Dr. Hurst (on behalf of Professor Starling, who had died since the medal was awarded). At this meeting Professor W. S. Thayer, Emeritus Professor of Medicine at the Johns Hopkins University, delivered the Bright Memorial Oration. This admirable tribute to Bright should be read by all who wish to learn more about him. The *Guy's Hospital Reports* devoted numbers 3 and 4 of Volume 77 to papers about Bright's disease as a memorial to him. Among these may be found Professor Thayer's oration, the addresses by Professor Aschoff and Professor Lemierre and a full account of the celebrations at Guy's Hospital.

A fitting conclusion to this account of Bright is a quotation from Thayer: " Observe, record, tabulate, communicate."

MARSHALL HALL

John Fitzwilliam was attached to the court of William the Conqueror. Marshall Hall claimed descent from him, the name, at some period, being gradually changed from Fitzwilliam to Hall on account of the place of residence of a member of the family, which had for a long time lived on the adjacent border of the shires of Nottingham and Lincoln. His father, Robert Hall a cotton manufacturer, was a remarkable man, a friend of Wesley's and a member of the New Connection Methodists. It was suggested in the House of Commons that this sect was disaffected with the government; the member for Nottingham, afterwards Lord Carrington, said: "As long as that gentleman [Mr. Hall] is connected with the disaffected body, all will be safe and right, there will be nothing wrong." The leader of the Luddite rioters wrote to him to say not a hair of his head should be touched, so much was he beloved and respected. He had much scientific learning, and was the first to employ chlorine for bleaching; he was so laughed at for trying this that his works were called Bedlam. He died in 1827 at the age of 72. His wife was an admirable woman. Their second son, Samuel, followed in the business, to which he contributed many excellent inventions.

Marshall, the sixth of their eight children, was born at Basford, near Nottingham, on February 18, 1790. His father, wrapped up in his business, neglected the education of his precocious, brave son who, when a child, inquired if hell was under the sea, for if so why not bore holes in the bottom of the sea to put out the fire, and who, like Keats, thrashed a schoolfellow much bigger than himself. He taught himself Latin, got up at five in the morning to read, studied chemistry and after some desultory schooling was in October 1809 sent to learn medicine in Edinburgh.

Here his industry, which was unremitting, continued; he obtained permission to dissect early in the morning before the ordinary hour of opening the dissecting-room, he contributed articles on chemistry to *Nicholson's Journal,* he entered into the discussions at that venerable students' institution "The Royal Medical Society," of which he was elected Senior President and to his delight made an Honorary Fellow shortly before his death; he made few friends, his sojourn in Edinburgh suggests that all work and no play makes Jack a dull boy; anyhow, his fellow-students appear to have been proud of his knowledge and attainments; he took his degree in June 1812, whereupon he returned to Nottingham. Hardly had he arrived when he was recalled to fill the post of Senior Clerk, otherwise Resident House Physician, to the Edinburgh Royal Infirmary. The appointment was for two years, the salary £20 a year, with board. He continued his labour, it "was always going on and knew no suspension." Of his own free will he gave a private course of lectures to any who wished to hear him; fifty came.

After leaving Edinburgh, visits were paid to the hospitals in Paris, Berlin, Göttingen and other places on the Continent. He evidently admired walking, for he records in a letter that he saw the Chancellor of the Exchequer walking to London, six miles off, and he, all alone, walked the 600 miles from Paris to Göttingen, carrying a cocked pistol for fear of wolves. On his return, he practised at Bridgwater for six months, but as there was no scope he put up his plate as a physician in Nottingham in February 1817, being then scarcely 27 years old.

The news of the reputation he made in Edinburgh had reached Nottingham, his family was well known, he was skilful and thorough in his work, kind and considerate to his patients; soon he was doing a very large practice which extended into the Dukeries and even as far as Derby and Leicester and included the best families in the neighbourhood. He was an ambitious man, and in 1825 was elected Physician to the General Hospital, Nottingham. At first he rode, being a good horse-man, but soon he was driven about in a gig, thus gaining leisure to read during the drive. He never dined out as it was a waste of time; in the evening he read, wrote and made experiments, indeed he slaved at work, being filled with the desire to be somebody of note.

His close neighbour, the Vicar, says he was stout, of middling stature, simple, neat, cheerful and always seemed to be thinking of something. This Vicar, Dr. Wilkins, wrote a treatise called *Body and Soul*. Hall was asked to read the proof, but, keeping it a long while, received a note from the author asking him to return his body and soul. Hall's manservant, who read the note, rushed into the kitchen saying to the cook that he could not stay in his place any longer as his master had the Vicar's body and soul.

Writing came easily to Marshall Hall; during the first year of his practice in Nottingham *On Diagnosis* was published. It is a book of considerable size. Many doctors only treated symptoms empirically without any thought of what was really the matter with the patient; indeed, it is highly probable that most of them did not know what the word diagnosis meant, for the first book on the subject, *A Treatise on Diagnosis and Prognosis*, by J. J. Price, had not appeared till 1791. Hall's book laid down the principle that the first thing is to find out the disorder from which a patient suffers. This is to be done by observing symptoms, of which a great many are given. He deserves great credit for teaching that the art of medicine is to reason correctly from observation. Matthew Baillie at once saw the importance of the book. It chanced that Hall, being in London, one day called on him. Baillie said to him, " I hope your father is well; I, for one, am much indebted to him for his extraordinary work *On Diagnosis*." Hall modestly said he was the author. Baillie exclaimed, " Impossible ! it would have done credit to the greyest-headed philosopher in our profession." After this Baillie, then at the height of his fame, did much for Hall's advancement. Baillie, a nephew of the Hunters, was celebrated as the author of the first treatise on Morbid Anatomy; it had been published in 1795. Hall in his book had seized its importance, saying, " Nothing has contributed so much . . . to raise medicine from its condition of a conjectural art, to the rank of a science as the investigations into Morbid Anatomy." A second edition of Hall's book appeared in 1834; it was thoroughly brought up to date; in it we are told we must use the stethoscope. A second edition of the first part only, dedicated to Matthew Baillie, had been issued in 1822.

A year after the first edition of the book *On Diagnosis* he published one entitled *On the Mimoses ; or a Descriptive, Diag-*

nostic and Practical Essay on the Affections usually denominated Bilious, Nervous, etc. In a second edition, also dedicated to Matthew Baillie, the title was changed to *Essays on Disorders of the Digestive Organs and General Health and on their Complications.* By calling the cases described mimoses he wished to express that they imitated disease of the liver or nervous system, but really they were examples of disorder either of the general health or of the digestive system and could be cured by improving the first and regulating the second. It is not of the same value as the work on diagnosis, but when we remember the ignorant vague way in which such words as bilious and nervous were then used the book did much good. He saw many who illustrated his contention because of the large numbers in Nottingham employed in sedentary work in the factories. Yet two more publications were about this time dedicated to Baillie, one a small volume called *On the Symptoms and History of Diseases,* the other an essay concerned with the prevalent reckless bleeding after parturition. This and his other publications on venesection influenced medicine for good so greatly that they will be described separately. Lastly, during his Nottingham days he contributed some papers to the *Transactions* of the Medico-Chirurgical Society; the most noteworthy is an account of four children who drank hot water from the spout of a kettle, the result being inflammation of the glottis, epiglottis and larynx, spasmodic contraction of the muscles of the pharynx preventing any damage to the œsophagus.

Desire to make a name for himself drew Marshall Hall to London. Knowing that his friends in Nottingham would oppose his going, he left without saying a word to anyone. A week after arrival in London he wrote to his brother-in-law in Nottingham, telling him to sell his effects and pay his few debts. He took a house—15 Keppel Street—where friends of his, a Mr. and Mrs. Burnside, lived with him, relieving him of the trouble of housekeeping. He moved from there, on his marriage in 1829, to 14 Manchester Square, and twenty years later to 38 Grosvenor Street, where he remained till his retirement from practice early in 1853. Many of his patients from Nottingham consulted him when they came to town, so that quickly he was busy. He set up a carriage and earned £800 the first year in London. Baillie was dead, but Sir Henry

Halford helped him. The seventh year yielded over £2,000, then his income fell a little, for his numerous scientific publications led to the belief that he was concerning himself less with clinical medicine; then it rose again reaching its maximum of £4,000 a year after twenty-three years in London. He practised because he had to earn his living and because he liked clinical work, feeling that he could often do good by correcting the prevailing errors. In a little book of commentaries published soon after arrival in London he says every pain is not inflammatory, every attack of palpitation is not due to organic disease, every icteroide hue does not come from disease of the liver, every case of muscular debility does not originate in disease of the spine; because of failure to recognize these facts friends are unduly alarmed and patients are bled, blistered, leeched and afflicted with setons painfully and fruitlessly, health is impaired by depletion, digitalis and mercurials, and sufferers from muscular weakness are kept for months or years in the recumbent position. Such preaching was a healthy beneficent breeze blowing away the fog of the thinkingless, ignorant, rule-of-thumb mentality that passed for medicine with many practitioners about a century ago. Hall was not a money-grubber, he saw many gratuitous patients, but made a rule to charge his full fee or none in order not to interfere with the fee of the family practitioners, to whom he was always courteous; if he arrived at the patient's house before the family doctor, Hall sat in his carriage till he came. His examination of the patient was careful and thorough, his directions were precise. Those who consulted him liked him for the trouble he took over them, for his honesty, his kindness, his charm and his cheerfulness. Seeing him was a different matter from an interview with a pompous, long-winded doctor who ascribed most ailments to inflammation and bled you on every possible and impossible occasion.

The family led a quiet life—invitations to dinner and to parties were declined—its circle was therefore small. Patients at home in the morning, visits to them in the afternoon, writing or experiments in the evening, practice sacrificed for a tour on the Continent once a year. Hall spoke French well and liked going to Paris, Dr. Louis there was a man for whom he had a great admiration. This secluded existence was made the more so by the fact that, except for the post of consulting physician to an asylum near Uxbridge, he had no hospital appointment. It is therefore noteworthy that he lectured at the Aldersgate Medical School, Webb Street Medical School and Sydenham College, the last two on the same evening; the exertion led to clergyman's sore throat and his consequent resignation in 1839. It is remarkable that he was invited to lecture on the Practice of Medicine at St. Thomas's Hospital which had its own staff and its own Medical School. He began in 1842, lecturing there for four years, when he resigned. In 1839 he was a candidate for the post of physician to University College Hospital, but was not elected, although he presented admirable testimonials from Louis and Flourens of Paris and Müller of Berlin.

Shortly after coming to London Marshall Hall became a Licentiate of the Royal College of Physicians, the Fellowship did not follow until 1841, but he delivered both the Gulstonian and Croonian Lectures before the College. They were reprinted with the title of *Synopsis of the Nervous System*. All his lectures were extempore, great stress was laid on accurate diagnosis; many letters from old pupils show him to have been a fine impressive lecturer who took an immense amount of trouble. He would spend an hour after lecture answering questions; a few listeners were invited to breakfast the next day in order that they might afterwards see illustrative cases among his patients; a student was prevented from coming to lecture by illness— Marshall Hall called on him to give him an account of the lecture he had missed.

Perfect health till middle life enabled him to do much writing and experimental work, the last between dinner and bedtime, the writing for an hour before breakfast and in his carriage, hence it was sometimes almost illegible, then it was transcribed by his wife, who relieved him of all domestic matters. His interest in the effects of loss of blood led to the publication in 1831 of *A Critical and Experimental Essay on the Circulation of the Blood*. This essay was founded on papers previously read before the Royal Society which had been refused publication in its *Transactions*. The coach in which the manuscript was sent to the printers was burgled during its passage through the crowds assembled for the coronation of William the Fourth, and the manuscript was stolen. The author had to rewrite his essay, in which we are told that if batrachian reptiles are placed in water of 108° F. the action of the heart continues, so, movement of the animal being abolished, it is easy, under the microscope, to observe for four hours the circulation in the mesentery or lung of a salamander. Then it will be seen that the capillaries " do not become smaller by subdivision, nor larger by conjunction, but they are characterized by continual and successive union and division or anastomis while they retain a nearly uniform diameter." The author claimed that this was the first accurate account of the capillary vessels and the circulation in them, and the first of any sort of the capillary vessels and the circulation in them in the lungs. The retarded flow in the capillaries is noticed, as are the effects on it of the heart, nervous system, heat, alcohol, opium and irritants. Beautiful plates illustrate the essay. Elsewhere he says arteries and veins are merely machinery for conveying blood, the capillaries bring the blood in contact with the tissues and here nutrition and absorption are effected, in the lung it is in the capillaries that the blood is exposed to the influence of the air. He proposed to call capillaries methæmata, or methæmatous blood channels, to indicate their function. Müller described this entirely original paper as of extraordinary interest. Many came to see the beauty of the circulation under the microscope. Bransby Cooper attended on several evenings. Marshall Hall said to him, " The arteries divide, divide, divide; the capillaries divide, unite, divide, unite; the veins unite, unite, unite." Bransby Cooper was delighted and said, " I shall tell that to my pupils in my next lecture." Without doubt these investigations revealed the capillaries and their function to many who were before ignorant of them.

Although aggrieved that this work was not given a place in the *Philosophical Transactions* Marshall Hall read two further papers before the Royal Society next year. One was entitled *Theory of the Inverse Ratio which subsists between the Respiration and Irritability in the Animal Kingdom*. It was laid down as a law, applicable to the whole animal kingdom, that the quantity of respiration is inversely as the degree of the irritability of the muscle fibre. An ingenious instrument, a pneumatometer, was invented to measure the amount of oxygen used by the animal. This paper received great praise from Flourens and others, its author thought highly of it and twenty-one years later he returned to the same subject, when before the Smithsonian Society at Washington, he delivered a lecture on Zoonomia, or the Law of Life. This was reprinted in the *Lancet*; in it the author lays down the law as follows : All living beings possess peculiar *dynamic* properties which respond to appropriate *stimuli* in inverse proportion, the higher the dynamic the lower the stimuli and *vice versa*. Such is the *Law of Animal Life*. There are two forms of dynamics, in the nervous system and muscles respectively. The other paper was on *Hybernation*, in it are many interesting observations which show great industry, especially as they were made when he was in busy practice. How far his observations are new is difficult to say, but he tells us that the breathing during hybernation is reduced to almost nothing, that the animal's temperature rises and falls with that of the atmosphere, that muscular mobility is unimpaired; by an ingenious device the circulation in the wing of a hybernating bat was observed, the heart's beat falling to 28 per minute. A hedgehog, which had been hybernating, was killed, whilst still hybernating, by section of the upper cervical cord, its heart continued to beat almost twelve hours, but after the same experiment on a lively hedgehog it only beat 2 hours. Marshall Hall regards this as an illustration of his law of life. Both these papers were printed in the *Philosophical Transactions*; shortly after their appearance he was elected to the Fellowship of the Royal Society.

At a meeting of the Committee of Science of the Zoological Society held on November 27, 1832, Marshall Hall first made known his theory of reflex action, and, on June 30, 1833, he read before the Royal Society his famous paper, *The Reflex Function of the Medulla Oblongata and Medulla Spinalis,* which was printed in the *Philosophical Transactions* for that year. He was thrilled by his discovery and continued to work at the subject for many years. Fortunately his friend, Mr. Henry Smith, was likewise thrilled; every evening, when an experiment was due, Smith's knock could be heard on the door, punctually at seven, announcing his coming, to act as assistant, for the evening investigations. In 1837 Marshall Hall offered a second paper on reflex action to the Royal Society, it was rejected by the Council. Marshall Hall begged some of the Council to see his experiments for themselves, a request which was unanswered. In 1847 another paper of his was refused. This induced him to write to the Earl of Rosse, the President, a letter which must have been considered to be of importance, for it was printed and reached a second edition. In it Marshall Hall sets forth his reasons for thinking that he has been unfairly treated; certainly, if what he says is correct, he was rudely and scoffingly rebuffed. However, the letter apparently had effect, for, in 1850, he was put upon the Council of the Society, but he contributed no further papers to it. In this country there was a clique in the medical profession which attacked him, some said there was nothing new in his work, others said it was new but wrong. Much the same sort of criticism as that from which Harvey, Newton and other great men had suffered. It is difficult to see why he was thus pilloried, anyhow the controversy wasted his time and tired him. Happily against these detractors can be set great praise from many whose opinion was well worth having. The *Lancet* always upheld Marshall Hall, fighting his battles against his enemies; Le Gros Clark, lecturer at St. Thomas's, at once publicly announced that a great discovery had been made; several years later he said he remembered how the discoverer was an object of obloquy and was denounced as the propagator of absurd and idle theories. Sharpey and Watson at University College both recognized the discovery, so did Faraday, Sir Henry Holland, Budd, Hughes Bennett and many others. Abroad, the paper on reflex action was at once translated for publication in the *Archiv für Anatomie und Physiologie*, and Müller alluded to the discovery as new, in his well-known Handbook; Van Deen said, "You alone are the discoverer of the reflex function"; the discovery was welcomed warmly in Paris by Flourens, who highly praised the second paper, which the Royal Society had refused for its *Transactions*; this paper was also published in the *Archiv*. Hall's discoveries were immediately appreciated in America; his papers were translated into the German, Dutch and Italian languages; when English doctors travelled abroad they found their colleagues there always regarded Marshall Hall as one of the greatest of their profession, and when these colleagues came to England, Marshall Hall was the man they wanted to see. He was made an honorary member of several continental and American medical societies; what pleased him most was that he was elected a foreign Associate of the Academy of Medicine of Paris and a corresponding member of the Institute of France: the single vacancy here produced five candidates, Marshall Hall received 39 votes out of a possible 41. For a while his practice lessened, but soon he was looked upon as an authority on diseases of the nervous system, then practice became larger than before, patients with nervous complaints even came from the Continent and America to consult him.

A bibliography of Marshall Hall's writings would contain about a hundred and fifty entries. The investigations on the spinal cord led to lectures and publications on diseases of the nervous system, some of these appeared in French periodicals; epilepsy in particular attracted him, the suggestion being made that it depended upon altered circulation in the brain caused by contraction of the muscles of the neck compressing the vessels there. The wide extent of his interests is shown by papers on the oxidation of iron, the production of intense cold, the movements of the barometer, the higher powers of numbers and the signs of algebra, and the Greek nouns and verbs. In the middle of the nineteenth century, the inhabitants of Great Britain were with justice seriously alarmed by cholera. There were, in 1849, 14,000 deaths from it in London alone. Marshall Hall's active mind was stirred, and in 1850 a pamphlet by him appeared with the title *Principles of the Sewerage of London and Other Large Cities with Suggested Works on the Thames.* It is a wonderful production from a busy doctor, deeply engaged in physiological research, for it contains closely reasoned detailed suggestions, the result of much thought. It reached a third edition and many of the suggestions were adopted. He belonged to that useful group of people, who when they see anything wrong feel an over-whelming desire to reform it. In 1840 we find him lecturing on medical reform; later he wrote to *The Times* to point out the cruelty of using open second-class carriages in bitter cold weather; in three weeks the offending company had closed them. A soldier died, in 1846, at Hounslow Barracks twenty-six days after receiving 150 lashes. The public was horrified, *The Times* could not print one-fiftieth of the letters it received upon the subject, nevertheless it printed two from Marshall Hall protesting against the wickedness of such a sentence. Two instances of poisoning owing to mistakes on the part of the druggist led him to write urging a reform in the strength of pharmacopœial preparations.

It will be remembered that in 1839 he had to desist from lecturing on account of what was called clergyman's sore throat; he also complained of difficulty in swallowing, he improved for a time and was able to work very hard for several years, gradually the difficulty of swallowing became more troublesome, and his general health began to fail; consequently early in 1853, at the age of 63, he retired from practice, disposing of the lease of his house, 38 Grosvenor Street, to Dr. Russell Reynolds.

On February 12, 1853, he and his wife started for New York to meet their son, then in the United States. During the voyage he wrote a paper on "Sea-sickness" for the *Comptes Rendus*. Rather more than a year was spent touring through the United States, Canada and Cuba. Wherever he went he found his books were widely read and that his reputation was considerable. The medical profession welcomed him enthusiastically, generally asking him for a lecture or two, which he gave before packed audiences; in fact, he discovered that he was in the North American Continent a famous man. In spite of the fatigue of so much travelling his health improved.

Shortly after his return he published *The Twofold Slavery of the United States*, in which it is suggested that the best solution of the slave question is first to educate the negro, secondly to facilitate in every way his saving for the purpose of ultimately buying his freedom; when this is attained he will probably continue in the employment of his master as a free man paid for his labour. The severity of cholera on the Continent detained Marshall Hall and his wife in this country. An invitation to give a short course of lectures on the Spinal System at Manchester was accepted; his voice only just held out until the third of the three lectures. The winter of 1854-5 was spent travelling through France and Italy; occasionally a patient was seen on the journey; in Rome, where he gave a lecture on the Spinal System, he was seized with a wish to learn Hebrew—so he studied it assiduously with a tutor. He stayed in Paris some months on the way back, seeing much of his many French friends; when he arrived in England in the autumn he was better than he had been for a long while.

Unhappily in a few weeks, difficulty of swallowing returned

and expectoration tinged with blood occurred. His energy was unchecked; chancing to read the Annual Report of the Royal Humane Society, in which directions for dealing with drowned persons were given, he remarked " There is nothing in this treatment to restore respiration "; he immediately set to work to evolve his well-known treatment of the drowned which will be described presently. One of the most fascinating of celebrated murder trials is that of William Palmer for murdering John Parsons Cook with strychnine in November 1855. Everyone in the country was excited, it was the first time strychnine had been used for murder. Marshall Hall had already studied the effect of strychnine on the frog, publishing his observations in the *Comptes Rendus*. It now struck him that the susceptibility of this animal's spinal cord to this poison is so great that the effect of the drug might be used as a test for its presence. He found that a young frog might be affected by as little as a fivethousandth of a grain of strychnine. This is the earliest suggestion of a physiological test, it is now advised in text-books on toxicology. Marshall Hall was among the many doctors briefed for the defence but not called, for he would have had to say that the symptoms were those of strychnine poisoning.

The last year of Marshall Hall's life was spent mostly in bed; the increasing difficulty in swallowing meant slow starvation. He bore this tedious distressing time with great fortitude, occupying himself with letters to the *Lancet* on various subjects; he prepared an address to be read at the Harveian Society, continued his study of Hebrew and conducted a considerable correspondence. He was greatly cheered by being made an Honorary Member of the Royal Medical Society of Edinburgh a few months before his death on August 11, 1857. The postmortem examination showed a stricture of the œsophagus at the level of the eighth ring of the trachea. The œsophagus was dilated and ulcerated for three inches above the stricture, there were perforations in several places leading to pouches and sinuses among the muscles of the neck. The substance of the lungs was healthy. No opinion was expressed as to the nature of the stricture. His widow, who has written a life of him, and his only child, a barrister, also named Marshall, survived him.

Marshall Hall was of middle height, he had a fine forehead above kindly eyes. His habits were simple; money-making did not attract him; politics did not interest him; but he was always ready to reform abuses and would freely spend time and energy in helping others. He was ambitious to make a name for himself in science; in this he was helped by his genius for seeing, at once, the fundamentals, e.g. that diagnosis was essential to clinical medicine, that patients were often more damaged by bleeding than by the disease for which they were bled, that capillaries were vital, for in them changes took place between the blood and the tissues, that the spinal cord was the centre of reflex action and that drowned people were suffocated. His power of work was prodigious; he used in the evening to write in the family drawing-room with talking and piano-playing going on around him. He thought clearly, expressed himself clearly, he disliked controversy and was not naturally quarrelsome, but he felt keenly a sneer or a rebuke, and, when attacked, defended himself with indomitable perseverance and courage. J. F. Clarke describes a debate at which Marshall Hall's opinions on the spinal reflex were adversely criticized, saying " In a speech of unsurpassable clearness and true eloquence he quickly grappled with the arguments against him. In epigrammatic sentences he demonstrated the truth of his theory. He met with great applause at the end of his address."

His death called forth speeches and addresses in praise of him from London, Paris, Berlin and New York. Some years after it £500 was collected to found a memorial to him. At a meeting of the subscribers held in 1870 with Sir William Gull in the chair, it was decided to hand the money over to the Council of the Royal Medico-Chirurgical Society to commemorate Marshall Hall, as it thought fit. This the Council did by founding the Marshall Hall Prize to be awarded at intervals of five years for the best original anatomical, physiological or pathological work on the nervous system published in the English language within the preceding five years. It was awarded in order to Hughlings Jackson, Ferrier, Gaskell, Gowers, Sherrington and Head—such a galaxy of talent was a distinguished compliment to the memory of Marshall Hall. When the Society became merged in the Royal Society of Medicine, the money was put into the building fund and a room in the library of the new present building was named the Marshall Hall room and a Marshall Hall bookplate was provided for neurological books. The door of this room has his name on it and inside is a tablet commemorating him. Thus he is, no doubt to the surprise of the ghosts of his detractors, permanently honoured. Marshall Hall is, to-day, remembered for, in order of their publication, his writings on bleeding, on reflex action and on artificial respiration.

Bleeding has been in use for 3,000 years. During the later part of the eighteenth century and well on into the nineteenth, doctors indulged in an orgy of it. People were bled at the spring and fall, just as a precautionary measure, whether they needed it or not; they could be seen, lying on the floor of the surgery of hospitals, recovering from these venesections. A doctor was prosecuted for malpractice because he did not bleed a patient suffering from pneumonia. A medical student at a hospital bled seventeen patients in one afternoon. Leeches cost the Nottingham Hospital £50 a year. Marshall Hall gives many cases of this sanguinary treatment, a few may be quoted. A physician had laryngitis, he was bled freely on two successive mornings at his own request, on the afternoon of the second day he was bled a third time to thirty-four ounces, he then suddenly fell on the floor violently convulsed and recovered with difficulty. A man, aged 57, fractured three ribs, he was bled to eighteen ounces, at noon to twenty, next day bled twice to eighteen ounces, the third day to twenty after which he died; ninety-four ounces of blood in all were taken; at the post-mortem examination the organs were found to be light-coloured from loss of blood—the man was bled to death. A young woman was frequently wet-cupped after confinement, often to twenty ounces at a time, she suffered from all the symptoms of loss of blood, it was proposed for these to bleed from the arm, she refused and recovered. A lady was bled at short intervals for several months, she was nearly dead before this treatment was stopped, she at once improved and recovered. A man, aged 40, fractured two ribs, he was bled twice to sixteen ounces, in the night he bled himself freely, next day seventeen leeches were applied, on the third day he was bled to twenty-four ounces, on the fourth to seven ounces, up to now he had lost 120 ounces and was suffering from the consequent symptoms from which he died. A man had an abdominal pain, in three days he lost nearly seventy ounces of blood by lancet, cupping and leeches, he nearly died from this. A woman suffering from fever after confinement was profusely bled and leeched, she died. Another woman under the same treatment died also. A man of 70 was bled, his pulse sank, nevertheless he was bled again the next morning and died. A woman bled freely after delivery, in spite of this she was freely venesected and died.

Such was medical custom, when, soon after beginning to practise at Nottingham, Marshall Hall was called to some patients suffering from abdominal pain after confinement, they had been bled for this because the opinion of the time was that pain indicated inflammation which always necessitated bleeding. He recognized that what these women needed was an aperient and, further, this great point, that many of the symptoms, after the bleeding, were due to loss of blood. This was an immense advance, for the symptoms due to loss of blood had hitherto been regarded as those of the supposed inflammation and therefore the unfortunate patient was still further bled, even unto death. Especially were the reaction symptoms of great loss of blood misinterpreted and ascribed to inflammation. Marshall Hall established his view by experiments upon animals and by a careful study of clinical cases. His book, *Researches Principally Relative to the Morbid and Curative Effect of Loss of Blood*, gives numbers of cases in which each of the well-known symptoms of loss of blood such as syncope, convulsions, delirium, coma, amaurosis were due to bleeding by the lancet, leeches or wet-cupping, and he details how, if the patient was not too far gone, he recovered when the medicinal loss of blood was stopped. It is terrible to think of the mismanagement of children who, being already exhausted from, say, diarrhœa, were further exhausted by the doctor; Marshall Hall says:

Of the whole number of fatal cases of disease in infancy a great proportion occur from this inappropriate or undue application of exhausting remedies. This observation may have a salutary effect in checking the ardour of many young practitioners, who are apt to think that if they have only bled, and purged, and given calomel enough, they have done their duty; when in fact . . . they have excited a new disease, which they have not understood, and which has led to a fatal result.

This is perfectly true, a little child aged two years had six leeches applied to the head, the bites were allowed to bleed freely.

Marshall Hall remonstrated strongly against the plan of applying leeches in infancy and allowing the bites to continue to bleed, and against that of applying leeches late at night, for the bleeding may continue during the night. Patients were often bled when lying down. Marshall Hall protested, stating that the patient should be bled when erect, then the moment he feels faint, enough has been taken, and he should be laid down, which is very sound advice. He wrote many papers on this subject; soon his views became known; doctors saw that "the slaughtering practice of blood-letting" was very wrong. Others took up the campaign against it; medicinal bleeding became less and less until by the time of Marshall Hall's death it was hardly ever performed. To him must be given the honour of having saved a multitude of lives by arresting a mode of treatment thousands of years old. He did not urge its complete abolition, indeed he gives cases for which he thinks it suitable, the almost total extinction of it was not his fault, his disciples were more full of fervour than he was. Gradually the practice returned and the valuable remedy of venesection is now rightly applied to appropriate instances. Some of the patients Marshall Hall would have bled we should certainly not bleed to-day, but that does not detract from the fact that he was the first to attempt to put bleeding in its right place, which, being widely misunderstood and misapplied, caused the death of many patients. The chief points in his correct teaching were that symptoms thought to be due to the disease were caused by the bleeding used for the treatment of it, and that in thousands of cases for which it was used it did no good and great harm.

Marshall Hall had been examining the pulmonary circulation of the triton about the beginning of 1832. During his last illness he dictated as follows:

The decapitated triton lay on the table. I divided it between the anterior and posterior extremities, and I separated the tail. I now touched the external integument with the point of a needle; it moved with energy, assuming various curvilinean forms! What was the nature of this phenomenon? I had not touched a muscle; I had not touched a muscular nerve; I had not touched the spinal marrow. That the influence of this touch was excited through the spinal marrow was demonstrated by the fact that the phenomenon ceased when the spinal marrow was destroyed. It was obvious that the same influence was reflected along the muscular nerve to the muscles, for the phenomenon again ceased when these nerves were divided. And thus we had the most perfect evidence of a reflex or diastaltic or diacentric action.

Thus in 1832 he began to study reflex action, continuing to do so for nearly a quarter of a century. He computed that he had devoted 25,000 leisure hours to it. The following is a brief account of his findings, most of which were announced in the paper on *The Reflex Function of the Medulla Oblongata and the Medulla Spinalis,* read before the Royal Society, June 20, 1833. Many kinds of animals were used—frogs, turtles, guinea-pigs, hedgehogs and snakes. By destruction or section of the appropriate parts of the central nervous system, he was able to demonstrate local examples of purely reflex action. He truly says that many phenomena seen in the limbs and which depend upon reflex function had long been known to physiologists, but he is able to give other examples: for instance, much of the act of swallowing is reflex, so are some movements of the iris, of the eyelid and eyeball; it was a new discovery that these movements can be obtained from a separated reptilian head but cease on destruction of the brain. He makes the following important statement:

But the reflex function exists as a continuous muscular action, as a power presiding over organs not actually in a state of motion, preserving in some, as the glottis, an open, in others, as the sphincters, a closed form, and in the limbs a due degree of equilibrium or balanced muscular action,—a function, not, I think hitherto recognized by physiologists.

This is a just claim, and to him is due the discovery of the reflex nature of balanced muscular action and the reflex nature of the " principle which presides over the orifices and sphincters of the internal canals." In this connection it is interesting to note that he observed that some patients cannot walk in the dark or with their eyes closed. The next point he makes is that previous writers had mixed volition, sensation and instinct with reflex action, whereas he contends that not one of these plays any part in it, reflex action only requires a stimulus, an afferent nerve, an efferent nerve going to muscle and a corresponding portion of the medulla oblongata and medulla spinalis, independent of the brain. This he calls the spinal system, and he first employs the word arc to it. He regards it as distinct from the cerebral system. Subsequent research has shown that he relied too much on absolute separation of these two. His writings did much good, for he furnished the basis of the conception of a reflex arc which could act independently of the

brain, he emphasized that the cerebro-spinal axis was, functionally, a segmental series of reflex arcs. He refers to Whytt,
Legallois, Mayo, and others, saying that they were aware of
many reflex phenomena, but he contends that until he described
these they had " never been accurately distinguished from sensation and volition." To ascertain whether this was a just claim
it is necessary to read all the older authors, but even when this
is done it is by no means easy to be sure of their meaning.
There is no doubt he believed his conception of a reflex arc
to be original. He was furiously attacked, particularly in the
London Medical Gazette, being accused of dishonest plagiarism;
the *Lancet* valiantly defended him. The controversy became
personal, people took sides, but inasmuch as it was conducted,
by some of the disputants, in a way discreditable to science
and good manners it would be a pity to disinter it. Why such
a disagreeable, unnecessary quarrel was ever started, is hard to
say. That Marshall Hall was honest there can be no doubt,
and I have previously given evidence that many distinguished
people, capable of forming an opinion, believed in his originality. Certainly we owe our conception of a reflex arc and
balanced muscular action to him.

Turning now to Marshall Hall's other investigations on the
nervous system we find that he was a pioneer in the study of
the effects of drugs on it; in his own words

> If a frog be made to swallow a watery solution of strychnine or opium . . . the
> animal soon becomes affected with symptoms perfectly similar to those of tetanus.
> The surface becomes highly susceptible to the impression of stimuli, and the
> muscles of the limbs become affected with continued spasmodic action. The
> affection is obviously one of augmented reflex action of the medulla (spinalis).
> It accordingly ceases instantly on destroying the nervous masses.

He divided a frog, made tetanic by opium or strychnine, into
three portions, the head, the anterior, and the posterior extremities
and tail. "Each part remained tetanic, impressible by the
slightest touch, and spasmodically contracted on any application of stimulus. The tetanus in each is instantaneously terminated by destroying the corresponding portion of the spinal
marrow." Later on he says: "If a few drops of dilute hydro-
cyanic acid be placed upon the tongue of a frog, a state of
things the reverse of that just described as the effect of opium
or strychnine is induced." These experiments, he points out,

show reflex function to admit of exaltation and of diminution. He also observed that removal of the cerebral hemispheres augments reflex action, a fact that has stimulated much research, also that " If in a frog the spinal marrow be divided just behind the occiput, there are for a very short time no diastaltic actions in the extremities. The diastaltic actions speedily return. This phenomenon he calls ' shock.' " It was known before, but the giving of the name shock to it was new. He pointed out that the tone of muscles was lessened when the hemispheres are destroyed, and he maintained that tonus and reflex actions are but modifications of one and the same function of the spinal cord; he noted that a stronger stimulus was necessary to evoke reflex action if applied to the trunk of the nerve than if applied to the periphery. Nor are we without evidence, he says, that the same principles obtain in the human subject. The infant born without cerebrum or cerebellum, and breathing from the influence of the medulla oblongata, is an example of reflex function, with the addition of respiration. Such a case is quoted, and we are reminded that parturition can take place normally in a woman whose thoracic spinal cord is completely severed, which shows that it is a reflex function. The principles of the movements in the anatomical economy are thus enumerated: 1, cerebrum, the source of voluntary motions; 2, medulla oblongata, the source of the respiratory motions; 3, medulla spinalis, the source of reflex function; 4, the neuro-muscular fibre, the seat of irritability; 5, the sympathetic, the source of nutrition and secretions. These functions disappear in this order in death, an order which is inverted when the same functions gradually came into existence in the foetal and natal states and in the progressive series of the animal kingdom.

In a *New Memoir on the Nervous System* Marshall Hall answers his critics and expands his opinions. The book contains tables and beautiful plates showing the reflexes from that acting through the optic nerve and the tubercula quadrigemina to the iris, down to those of the extremity of the spinal cord. Our knowledge of nervous diseases has advanced so far since his time that his pathological explanations have not now much interest. Being convinced of the importance of reflex action he tried to make disorder of it explain almost anything. For example, convulsions in children were ascribed to the reflex action originating in the oncoming teeth, hence scarification of the gums was advised. Asthma, tetanus, some forms of epilepsy, hysteria and puerperal convulsions are supposed to be reflex phenomena, but it is only fair to add that other forms of epilepsy and hydrophia were recognized to be of central origin.

The treatment of the apparently drowned advised by the Royal Humane Society was to carry the body to the nearest house and then to apply warmth, if possible by a warm bath at about 100° F. Marshall Hall chanced in 1855 to read these directions, and at once saw they were all wrong, because the cause of death was suffocation, not loss of heat. In spite of severe illness he investigated the subject, and next year published his results in the *Lancet* and in a pamphlet which he sent to the Royal Humane Society. He wrote a paper on Asphyxia for the *Comptes Rendus,* his plan of treatment was copied into the *Journal des Débats.* In this country it was adopted at once by the profession. In the pamphlet which is entitled *Prone and Postural Respiration in Drowning,* the author begins by telling his readers that normal respiration is reflex, carbonic acid exhaled from the blood in the air cells of the lungs, acting as a stimulus on nerves in the lungs, reflexly excites the muscles of respiration, but, in apnœa, the carbonic acid accumulating in the blood for want of normal respiration poisons the spinal centres of respiration. Therefore, the first thing to do for the drowned is to excite respiration. He then says the inhalation of oxygen may be long nearly suspended without proving fatal; the suspension of the exhalation of carbonic acid, even if incomplete, destroys life in a short time; next he gives experiments designed to show that the effects of apnœa are not the result of want of oxygen but of the retention of carbonic acid; next come figures indicating that both high and low temperatures are injurious to life. The rules of the Humane Society are examined. No. 1 said, "Convey the body carefully, with the head and shoulders raised, to the nearest house"; Marshall Hall comments justly that this is a bad position because the tongue will fall backwards, so closing the glottis and thus making the entry of air difficult, fluids in the mouth will stay there, or even go into the lungs, but, says he, turn the body into the prone, i.e. face downwards, position, then the tongue will come forward and the water run out. Further, in the prone position, the weight of the trunk will compress the abdomen and thorax, this pressure will induce expiration, additional pressure by the hands on the posterior portion of the thorax and on the abdomen will render expiration more complete. " This pressure is then to be removed. Its removal will be followed by slight inspiration. The weight of the body is then to be removed from the thorax and abdomen, by gently turning it on the side and a little beyond, placing one hand under the shoulder and the other under the hip of the side moved." These measures are to be repeated gently, deliberately but efficiently and perseveringly sixteen times in the minute only. " And thus without instruments of any kind and with the hands alone, if not too late we accomplish that respiration which is the sole, but sure effective means of the elimination of the blood poison." Treatment must be begun immediately after the body is taken out of the water: why waste precious time by carrying it to the nearest house? If the weather is not too cold do not wrap up the drowned man, for cool air, impinging on the skin, reflexly helps to start respiration. Snuff, hartshorn, tickling the nostrils with a feather and dashing hot and then cold water on the face help a little in the same way. Those not engaged in performing artificial respiration should energetically stroke the limbs upwards, to promote the flow in the veins and thus aid the elimination of carbonic acid gas. Stillborn infants are to be treated in the same way. The warm bath is perfectly useless, not to say injurious. This plan for restoring the apparently drowned was first known as the Ready Method, later as the Marshall Hall method. Its author was much annoyed because the Royal Humane Society advised that it should be tried after the warm bath had failed, although thereby much valuable time is lost. Later the Society followed his directions. The Marshall Hall method held the field for many years until Silvester and Sharpey-Schafer devised other ways of restarting respiration. To Marshall Hall is due the entire credit of pointing out this is what must be done. It is pleasant to think that the last original thing he did before his death was to originate a method whereby thousands of lives have been saved.

THOMAS ADDISON

The home of the Addisons was at Lanercost, about eight miles east of Carlisle. In 1612 Sir Thomas Addison resisted payment of dues to Lord William Howard, and in 1618 Matthew Addison was convicted of horse-stealing. In Commonwealth times Addisons were living at Banks House and St. Mary Holme, both houses close to the Priory or Abbey of Lanercost. One of this family was Thomas Addison, who was born in 1636 and had Mary for his spouse. Their oak chest, with, carved on it, their initials, the date 1676 and the inscription "When God doth thee in store, remember thou the poor," still exists. In the direct male line a great-grandson named Joseph was a farmer; he married Sarah Shaw, the daughter of a grocer of Long Benton, near Newcastle-on-Tyne. They lived for a time at the grocer's house at Long Benton, where the future physician, Thomas Addison, was born in April of 1795—some say 1793, but that is almost certainly incorrect. He had one brother, John. How long the family lived at Long Benton is not known, but Joseph was living at the Banks before his marriage, and this certainly became the family home, for Addison always regarded himself as a Cumberland man; his father in 1823 and his mother in 1841 both died at the Banks. The house in which Addison was born, now a supply store, shows few changes, the chief is that the small panes of the shop front have been replaced by a single large pane.

The Banks is an oblong stone house, there is a central door with a porch, a window on each side, and a ground and first floor; it stands a stone's throw to the south of the Roman Wall, high up on the right bank of the River Irthing, which, half a mile away, separates Naworth Castle from Lanercost Priory. The view from the house is marvellous; in the distance, Solway Firth, Skiddaw, Saddleback and Helvellyn; in the foreground, the river, the trees surrounding Naworth Castle and, standing on the level green grass by the river, the beautiful ruins of the great Priory of Lanercost, fortunately now in the hands of the National Trust. No wonder Addison always spent his holidays at the Banks, and wished to be buried in the churchyard of the Priory, part of which is Lanercost Parish Church. There is his tomb, under some old yew-trees, for a time neglected, but now looked after by Guy's Hospital. It is surrounded by the tombs of many Addisons. The parish registers contain more than sixty entries under the name of Addison between the years 1731 and 1837.

Addison was first sent to a school, kept by a John Rutter, in a roadside cottage at Kellingworth, near Long Benton, the same school in which Robert, the son of George Stephenson, was educated. From there he went to the Grammar School of Newcastle-on-Tyne: here he learned Latin so well that he was able later to take down lectures in that language and to speak and write it fluently. The head master, Mr. E. R. Thomas, recently told me that no records of Addison's career can be found save a Greek book with his name in it.

His father wished him to follow law, but allowed his son to have his own way and study medicine, offering to make him a pupil of Dr. John Thomson of Edinburgh for three years, at an annual premium of £100 a year, but young Addison preferred to go straight to the University of that city, where he entered as a medical student October 1812. He was never President of the Medical Society, as stated by Lonsdale, nor did he distinguish himself specially when a student. On August 1, 1815, Thomas Addison graduated Doctor of Medicine, the subject of his thesis being *De Syphilide et Hydrargyro*.

It is generally supposed that he next visited some of the continental schools of medicine, but this is doubtful. His father's means had been increased by the opening of collieries in his neighbourhood, so young Addison was able to try his fortune in London, where he had but one friend, a fellow-student who had lived in Edinburgh. He began by holding the office of House Surgeon to the Lock Hospital. When this appointment ended he first lived in Skinner Street, Snow Hill, in a haunted house; moving to Hatton Garden he became a pupil, and later on physician, at the General Dispensary, studying diseases of the skin under the celebrated Dr. Bateman. He was attached to this Dispensary for eight years, and on his retirement the Governors were so well pleased with him that they gave him a silver claret jug. When at Hatton Garden he made by practice £50 in his first year, and in his second about a hundred. He obtained the licentiateship of the Royal College of Physicians on December 22, 1819, and was elected a Fellow on July 4, 1838. He never became a Censor nor held any office at the College.

It is said that he began to study at Guy's Hospital about 1820. The correct date is 1817, for the books of the Guy's Medical School have this entry: "Dec. 13, 1817, from Edinburgh, T. Addison, M.D., paid £22 1s. to be a perpetual Physician's Pupil." There is another payment of £57 18s. from him to the School. What this was for we do not know. He soon attracted the notice of that beneficent despot, Mr. Harrison, the Treasurer, who did as much as any man for the good of Guy's, not the least of his benefactions being that, through his influence, Addison was appointed assistant physician on January 14, 1824, there being a vacancy consequent upon the promotion of Dr. Bright to be full physician because of the retirement, owing to ill health, of Dr. James Laird. Wilks says:

There were other candidates for the appointment, and amongst them, we believe, Dr. Seymour, well known for his good West End practice. He worked up great interest on his own behalf among Governors, and actually got a recommendation from the future King William IV. Showing the estimation in which Addison was held, Dr. Seymour sent his son some years afterwards to Guy's in order to study under his former rival.

The Minutes of the Court of Governors held on January 14 show that there were five candidates; all were interviewed, three after this retired from the contest and a ballot was taken, Addison received 38 votes and Seymour 6.

In 1827 Addison became lecturer on Materia Medica. In 1837 he was elected full physician, filling the vacancy caused by the death of Dr. Cholmeley. He was at the same time appointed joint lecturer on Medicine with Bright. In 1840, on Bright's retirement from the lectureship, Addison became sole lecturer and held this position until 1854 or 1855. During the years 1849 and 1850 he was President of the Royal Medico-Chirurgical Society.

In September 1847 he was married at Lanercost Church to Elizabeth Catherine, widow of W. W. Hauxwell, Esq., who had two children by her first marriage but none by that with Addison. She died in May 1872. In the Parish Register of marriages, neither Addison nor his wife give their age; both state that they are " of full age."

Generally his health was good, but towards the end of his life he suffered from gall-stones and jaundice. Early in 1860 he resigned his post of Physician to Guy's Hospital. So greatly did the students value his teaching that a deputation of them waited upon him to urge him to withdraw his resignation, but he, poor man, knowing that he had a threatening disease of the brain, was compelled to persist. He had recently removed from Spring Gardens, where he had lived near Bransby Cooper's house for more than twenty years, to Berkeley Square, from whence he went to Brighton for the benefit of his health. He died there on June 29, 1860, and was buried at Lanercost on July 5.

The long epitaph on the tablet placed in Lanercost Church by his wife is printed in Lonsdale's *The Worthies of Cumberland,* where also will be found the words on the tablet in the gallery of the Chapel of Guy's Hospital, and those below his bust— for which a subscription among the profession was raised—in the hospital, where one of the medical wards was named after him and exists with the same name to-day. In the hall of the Counting House at Guy's there is a portrait of him; the front of the hospital forms the background and his hand is resting on a book, *The Practsie of Medicine.* This picture was given by Mr. Jonathan Hutchinson to Mr. Clement Lucas for Guy's. Mr. Hutchinson, in a letter dated July 19, 1875, said that his brother bought it at an auction in Newcastle and that it was " by Bewick of Newcastle, whose life has, I believe, been recently written." This is incorrect, it is most likely by a portrait painter, William Bewick, who worked much in London. Mr. Arthur Durham, who knew Addison, said it was a very good likeness. A stained-glass window to his memory was placed in the east end of Long Benton Church and remained there till about thirty years ago, when it was removed to the south wall of the Church, where it is now the organ chamber window. There is no inscription on it and the figures have badly faded. His will, dated September 26, 1855, showed personalty under £60,000. The executors were his brother, John Addison of Banks House, and Alfred Brooke Barnes, surgeon, King's Road, Chelsea. To his wife he left his freehold estate and residence at Brighton, with its furniture, an annuity of £350 and his shares in the Indemnity Mutual Marine Assurance Company, and to her son and daughter an annuity of £100. His presentation plate was left to his brother to be kept as an heirloom.

Addison's elder brother John left the Banks estate to John Joseph Addison, son of his cousin William Addison. From John Joseph it descended to Dr. Haygarth Maling Addison, whose brother sold it to Mr. G. E. Henderson, who was living in Banks House when I went to Lanercost in 1926; then I could not find any Addison living in the neighbourhood.

What kind of a man was he? The two best able to answer are Wilks, his pupil, and Lonsdale, his doctor friend in Cumberland. The first tells us:

The personal power which he possessed was the secret of his position, much superior to what Bright could ever claim, and equal, if not greater, than that of Sir Astley Cooper. For many years he was the leading light of Guy's, so that every Guy's man during the thirty or forty years of his teaching was a disciple of Addison, holding his name in the greatest reverence, and regarding his authority as the best guide in the practice of the profession. . . . He was dogmatic in his teaching, and thus the pupils accepted as pure gospel every word which flowed from his lips. The force of his words was enhanced by his mode of delivery and by the presence of the man himself. Addison was of good height and well made, stood erect, with coat buttoned up very high, over which hung his guard and eyeglass. He wore a black stock with scarcely visible shirt-collar, and this further elevated his head. He had a well-proportioned good head, with dark hair and side whiskers, large bushy eyebrows and smallish dark eyes, nose thick, as were also his lips, which enclosed his firmly knit mouth. His features were not refined, but belonged to a powerful mind and showed no trace of any kind of sentiment. His penetrating glance seemed to look through you, and his whole demeanour was that of a leader of men, enhanced by his somewhat martial attitude.

The students worshipped him, feared rather than loved him. He was melancholy and liable to fits of depression, and at times appeared haughty, unapproachable and even rude. Addison knew of this failing, by him said to be a cloak for his nervousness, which was such that he was all his life nervous when he began a lecture or address. But he could throw this off. When he was President of the Royal Medico-Chirurgical Society, he invited the reporters of the medical press to meet some of the leaders of the medical profession. J. F. Clarke says:

The evening was one of the most delightful I ever spent. Addison I had never met in private before; I had only known him as the great physician of Guy's Hospital, and the somewhat haughty and pompous President of two medical Societies, the Westminster and the Royal Medico-Chirurgical. I was astonished at his bonhomie, his hospitality, and his powers of conversation. . . . Foote joined me in eulogizing Addison.

Wilks maintains that in reality he was an amiable man. " In his professional life no character on record has presented in a higher degree the sterling hard qualities of true professional honesty. We have never heard a single instance in which a word of disparagement of a professional brother escaped him." Lonsdale tells us how he loathed advertisement, indignantly refusing to write what he called " puffery," that he was musical, in politics a Tory, and considers that he would have risen to the top of any profession he had entered. He often did kindness by stealth, and the degree to which he was idolized by the students is shown by the fact that, when his health broke down, they sent him a letter of condolence; the touching answer from him, given in Lonsdale's book, reveals his deep affection for them.

Astley Cooper had retired from the hospital in 1825, so Addison reigned as the supreme teacher. He even made the dry bones of Materia Medica attractive, for his fees derived from lectures on this subject were between £700 and £800 a year. Wilks says:

As a teacher, it is difficult to conceive a better. His lectures were of a very superior order, extempore, couched in good language, which amounted sometimes to real eloquence. The clinical lectures were most excellent . . . arguing both from positive and negative reasons, he placed the diagnosis on a sure foundation.

Lonsdale writes:

Guy's Hospital had long had a deservedly high reputation, to which Sir Astley Cooper, Dr. Bright and others lent additional lustre; but some are of opinion that Addison, single-handed, raised a higher column than any of his predecessors of the present century. He was admitted to be one of the most impressive teachers of his day and assuredly popular among the students, many of whom were attracted to Guy's on his account alone.

In 1828 Addison introduced the practice of making the clerks systematically write reports of the cases, and thus it is to him we owe the whole practice of clinical reports made by students. Always interested in them, he had a way of getting the best out of them, and instilling professional ardour into them. "Addison carried the pupils of Guy's as if by subtle traction." Great in himself, he strove to make others great, and he was always mindful of the fame of the school. Golding Bird dedicated his book on *Urinary Deposits* to him, saying:

It is now thirteen years since I found myself within the walls of Guy's Hospital, a stranger and unknown. In a short time my admiration and respect were excited for your profound knowledge and experience as a physician and for your zeal as a teacher. But I soon experienced another feeling, that of gratitude for numerous acts of most disinterested friendship, for which I must ever remain your debtor.

After taking his degree, his chief interest was in diseases of the skin; this accorded with his work at the Lock Hospital, and at the Dispensary under Dr. Bateman. He always remained one of the best authorities in this department of medicine; it was he who superintended the making of the marvellous wax models of diseases of the skin that are the pride of the Guy's Museum, and at Guy's he used to give a course of demonstrations on cutaneous diseases during the summer session. But he was hostile to specialism; his mind was too great and his interest was too wide for him ever to be content with studying diseases of only a part of the body. He trained himself to take an infinitude of pains and to cultivate the art of exact observation; he was always at work either in the wards or the dead-house, and so attained an enormous experience, on which he relied far more than on book knowledge; he had the supreme gift, not only of acquiring all the possible evidence about a case, but of using it with great judgment, unerringly separating that which was relevant from that which was not. All this, together with his exceptional sagacity, gave him the reputation of being the most skilful man of his day in unravelling a difficult case, and the reputation was deserved. He seemed to search deep into the innermost parts of the human body, much as a man would try to discover the derangement of a complicated machine, and he appeared literally to drag the malady to light. No time was too long for the investigation of a case; he must solve the problem. Once in the middle of the night and to the astonishment of the Sister he appeared in the Clinical ward because, when he got into bed at home, he remembered that he had not satisfied himself that a patient, whom he had seen in the afternoon, had not got a hernia. Naturally such a man compelled himself to be an accomplished auscultator; being this, he was aware of the difficulties of the subject. Nevertheless, the audience were surprised when, in a paper read before the Physical Society on February 28, 1846, *On the Difficulties and Fallacies attending Physical Diagnosis of Diseases of the Chest,* he enumerated forty-two difficulties and fallacies, but his doing so was characteristic of his carefulness and thoroughness.

Some blamed him because, having made a diagnosis, he did not always prescribe for the patient, but this, as Lonsdale says, arose from the best of motives, for often Addison, being honest, had to admit that he did not know any drug which would be of benefit.

He was not successful in building up a large practice, and he was almost unknown to the general public. So much the better for the science of medicine, for he was left free to teach and to make his discoveries. Still, one fact connected with private practice is worth recording. He was called to see a member of the Rothschild family in Paris. Trousseau, Nelaton, and all the élite of the profession in that city attended a public dinner in his honour. His health was proposed, and Addison replied in excellent French. Truly a prophet is not without honour save in his own country.

No man has ever been held in greater esteem at Guy's than Addison. Yet, because he was of a retiring, somewhat forbidding nature, the medical public in England, outside those with whom he was in immediate contact, paid little attention to him or to his discoveries in his lifetime. Neither the *Lancet* nor *British Medical Journal* published an obituary notice of him when he died; the College of Physicians did not elect him as a Fellow till nineteen years after he had become a Licentiate; he never lectured or held any office at the College; his name never appeared among the list of candidates for the fellowship of the Royal Society; no University gave him an honorary degree; he held no Court appointment; he was not a member of the newly formed Pathological Society, and the Royal Medico-

Chirurgical Society refused to publish some of his papers, even after he had been President of it.

Now his fame is world-wide, for not only was he a great personality, a brilliant teacher and an exceptionally skilful diagnostician, but he made fundamental discoveries in several departments of medicine. The writer of the obituary notice of Addison in the *Medical Times and Gazette,* the only medical paper that thought it worth while to notice the great man's death, put his work on pneumonia and phthisis first in importance, and Wilks did also. Addison's teaching on these and other subjects is now so completely the familiar knowledge of every student that it is difficult to imagine ourselves without it.

I will now give, in Addison's own words, an account of his original discoveries in the order of their publication. They relate to fatty liver, appendicitis, pneumonia, carnification of the lung, phthisis, xanthoma, Addison's anæmia and Addison's disease.

The appearances of a fatty liver were well *known before Addison's time, but medical authors were ignorant of any clinical symptoms which would enable them to predict its presence. Characteristically, Addison applied himself to the problem and published a paper in which he said that a fatty liver might be predicted during life if

to the eye the skin presents a bloodless, almost semitransparent and waxy appearance; when this is associated with mere pallor, it is not unlike fine polished ivory; but when combined with a more sallow tinge, as is now and then the case, it more resembles a common wax model. To the touch, the general integument, for the most part, feels smooth, loose and often flabby; whilst in some well-marked cases all its natural asperities would appear to be obliterated, and it becomes so exquisitely smooth and soft as to convey a sensation resembling that experienced on handling a piece of the softest satin.

All subsequent physicians have confirmed the accuracy of this entirely original observation, which could only have been made for the first time by one endowed with an altogether exceptional gift for seeing. Addison tells us that the above condition of the skin is first to be noticed on the face and the backs of the hands. He gives cases in which he correctly foretold a fatty liver from the aspect of the skin, and he remarks that a fatty liver may have other causes than phthisis, one of which is alcoholism. The paper is illustrated with a beautiful chromolithograph of a fatty liver.

Appendicitis.—In 1839 there was published the *Elements of Practical Medicine,* by Richard Bright, M.D., and Thomas Addison, M.D., Physicians to Guy's Hospital and Lecturers on the Practice of Medicine. Only Volume I ever appeared; hence, as the book is incomplete, it is rare. In the Preface the authors state that they have felt the want of an elementary and practical book, to which they could refer their pupils, and that in this work they have endeavoured, "to state, with as much conciseness as is consistent with perspicuity, the history, symptoms and treatment of each disease, as established in their own minds, by what they have read as well as by what they have seen." The result is admirable; the *Elements* are just what a text-book should be, not a conglomeration of what this or that person has said, but a plain statement in excellent English of the experience of two great teachers.

From what I have read and from what I have heard said by my teachers, the general opinion was that most of this first volume was written by Addison, so that almost certainly he is responsible for what I am going to quote, and at any rate he is jointly responsible for the earliest accurate account of appendicitis. No reference to this occurs in the first six modern text-books I took up by chance, and Deaver in his very full history of the disease does not mention it, but Kelly does in these words: "descriptions so clear and well presented that they could not be surpassed to-day."

On page 498 of the *Elements,* under the heading "Inflammation of the Cæcum and Appendix Vermiformis," we find the following:

The history of this affection is often as follows: The patient has complained, more or less, for some time past, of pain and uneasiness in this part, increased on exertion, or after neglect of the bowels, or excess in eating or drinking; he has, however, retained such a share of health that he has not been interrupted in his daily avocations, till, after some unusual exposure to cold, or some long walk, or other over-exertion, he has been suddenly seized with more severe pain, attended with rigors, chills, and sometimes with sickness and violent vomiting. The pain and tenderness become excessive, and extend to the neighbouring parts of the abdomen. A hardness and tumefaction are soon very evident to the hand in the part first affected: this continuing, general symptoms of peritonitis often take place, and terminate fatally; but under careful treatment the inflammation remains circumscribed, and becomes even less extensive, assuming the form of a local, deep-seated abscess. The threatening symptoms of peritonitis subside; the tumefaction just above the crest of the ilium on the right side is more and more obvious to the touch, and gradually shows a tendency to point; the constitution still suffering severely. In process of time it either opens of its own accord, or is assisted by the lancet, and a discharge of ill-conditioned pus follows, which from its peculiar fetid smell, and from its appearance, is soon discovered to be mingled with feculent matter. The discharge continues for many weeks and the patient often sinks at length from exhaustion. In other cases, when the powers of the system are previously unbroken, the abscess closes and permanent recovery is obtained.

Morbid appearances.—From numerous dissections it is proved that the fæcal abscess thus formed in the right iliac region arises, in a large majority of cases, from disease set up in the appendix cæci. It is found that this organ is very subject to inflammation, to ulceration, and even to gangrene . . . this little worm-like body is often detected in the midst of the abscess, with a perforation at its extremity; or by ulceration higher up in its parietes; a considerable portion of it, nearly or entirely separated, is found in a disorganized condition among the pus and fæces which fill the abscess . . . it sometimes points at a considerable distance from the original source of the disease.

About forty years ago the profession thought that some of its members had discovered appendicitis; they discussed whether it was a new disease, but Addison had given a perfect description of it before most of the supposed discoverers were born.

Diseases of the Lungs.—Addison devoted more attention to diseases of the lungs than to any other branch of medicine. The collection of his published works contains five papers bearing on this subject. He had the greatest reverence and admiration for Laennec; he acknowledged " himself indebted for almost all he knows of thoracic diseases to that truly great man, at once the most distinguished and most successful cultivator of medical science that ever adorned the profession." Nevertheless, in two important matters, namely, pneumonia and phthisis, his teaching differed from that of Laennec.

Before Addison's time it was universally believed that pneumonia consisted of an exudate into the interstitial structure of the lungs. It was defined by Laennec as " inflammation of the lung tissue." Opinions as to the structure of the lungs were variable and inaccurate. Addison made matters plain; he wrote:

Accompanied by a corresponding branch of the pulmonary artery, I trace a filiform bronchial tube to a lobule or bunch of (air) cells, in which it abruptly terminates; the blood distributed over these cells being received by the pulmonary veins, which pass exteriorly to the air cells, in a loose and very distinct interlobular cellular tissue. I entirely fail to discover any structure to which the term interstitial or parenchyma can be fairly applied.

This quotation is from a paper read before the Guy's Physical Society in 1843, and is a condensed statement, the details of which he had previously published and had often mentioned when teaching orally. On the same occasion (1843) he reiterated his earlier announced views on pneumonia thus:

There are probably some present who remember the time and occasion when, in this Society, and in opposition to all existing authorities, I ventured to call into question the long-cherished notion that pneumonia had its seat in a sup-posed parenchyma of the lungs and that the products of pneumonic inflammation were poured into that parenchyma.

The occasion to which he refers was in 1837, when before the same Society he said: " I entertain no doubt whatever of its (pneumonic inflammation) being primarily and essentially seated in the (air) cells themselves," and his discovery can be best briefly expressed by a few words taken from the work by Bright and himself.

Pneumonia may be defined to be an inflammation of the air cells of the lungs, speedily producing an effusion into them of a serous-looking fluid commonly mixed with blood; causing, if unchecked, such a degree of thickening of their parietes as apparently to fill them up entirely for a time; or leading to the deposi-tion of an albuminous matter, which is either solid or of a puriform character; and seldom, if ever, terminating in the formation of a genuine abscess.

There follows an admirable detailed description of the stages of engorgement, red hepatization and grey hepatization. Addison, as a result of careful dissection of healthy lungs, had given an accurate and correct account of the minute anatomy of the lungs, and, by diligent examination after death of the lungs of those afflicted with pneumonia, he was able to show that the universal opinion as to its morbid anatomy was entirely wrong, and he was able to describe the morbid anatomy with an accuracy which no one has since challenged. He insisted that the same morbid anatomy is true of lobular pneumonia. He alluded to the condition of lung described by Laennec as carnification and regarded by him as the result of pneumonic inflammation modified by pleural effusion. Addison demon-strates that this is not so, that the whole condition of carnification is due to compression by fluid, and that inflammation plays no part.

In his clinical description of pneumonia he lays much emphasis on his experience that cough and expectoration may be entirely absent. He also says, " But of all the symptoms of pneumonia, the most constant and conclusive, in a diagnostic point of view, is a pungent heat of surface." It is difficult to say who is the first to observe a symptom, but certainly this one was not generally known before Addison's time.

Turning now to phthisis, Laennec, it is true, admitted that pneumonic consolidation may occasionally be found in persons dead of phthisis, but he did not lay stress on this, nor did he think it common. The cavities and most of the features usually seen in the lungs of phthisical patients were in his opinion due to the softening of, or the presence of, tuberculous matter. Addison disagreed, and taught that most of the changes seen in a phthisical lung are due to pneumonic inflammation. Thus the last words in his article " On the Pathology of Phthisis " are : " inflammation constitutes the great instrument of destruction in every form of phthisis." In the same communication he says, " I very much question whether there ever was a single instance of tubercular disease of the lung proving fatal, in which more or less of this pneumonic change might not have been distinctly recognized, if the prevailing notions respecting tubercular infiltration had not obscured the perception of the beholder." He tells us that the inflammatory products may contract, leading to a diminution in the size of the lung and flattening of the ribs ; this contraction, he says, is a favourable sign in every form of phthisis, for it indicates an attempt at repair, or they may lead to mere induration, which in some cases is also a stage towards repair, or they may break down to form a cavity.

Those who read Addison's *Pathology of Phthisis* nowadays may be inclined to urge that he underestimates the importance of the tubercles, for he maintains that in some forms of phthisis no tubercles can be found, but this criticism is hardly fair, because nearly all his work was done by observation of the naked-eye morbid anatomy of the lung; microscopy was then in its infancy and tubercle bacilli had not been discovered. What he did was to enunciate that in phthisis there are two processes at work, the tubercles and ordinary inflammation. This was an immense step forward, and although his work dates back more than eighty years his conclusions are the same as are taught to-day. But this entirely original and revolutionary doctrine spread very slowly, for when in 1870 Baumler translated Niemeyer's *Clinical Lectures on Pulmonary Consumption,* second edition, 1867, into English, for the Sydenham Society, he said:

The views insisted on by Professor Niemeyer have almost to their whole extent been confirmed by the results of recent investigations. But the renewed study of the whole question has led also to more just appreciation of the works of former observers. In this country the labours of Thomas Addison, which had almost been forgotten, and which had remained almost entirely unknown on the Continent, have been brought to light again, and show that already, at a period when Laennec's teaching had just commenced to dominate over the pathology of lung diseases, an independent observer arrived at and firmly held the opinion which in more recent times was established by Reinhardt, Virchow, and his disciples, and which forms the key-note of these lectures—namely, that, to use Addison's own words, " inflammation constitutes the great instrument of destruction in every form of phthisis."

In Niemeyer's lectures themselves there is no reference to Addison or to his teaching. A reviewer of the translation notes this and says, " Dr. Baumler has done justice to our countryman, Dr. Thomas Addison," and previously the *British and Foreign Medico-Chirurgical Review,* in reviewing Niemeyer's work in 1870, said, " Dr. Addison perhaps did more than anyone else in England to advance the doctrine of ' pneumonic phthisis.' "

Vitiligoidea (Xanthoma).—A paper entitled *On a Certain Affection of the Skin Vitiligoidea—Plana, Tuberosa* was published by Addison and Gull. It is almost certainly chiefly by Addison, and Wilks and Daldy state that Addison was the first to describe Vitiligoidea. This disease became known later as Xanthalasma and is now called Xanthoma. This entirely original paper contains an admirable description of a new clinical entity, the association of which with jaundice is noticed.

Addison's Disease and Addison's Anæmia.—Only once has a physician achieved the distinction of discovering two diseases, and of having them both named after him, and that physician was Addison.

The story is as follows: On March 15, 1849, at a meeting of the South London Medical Society, John Hilton, Addison's colleague, being in the chair, he read a paper on what he described as a "remarkable form of anæmia," whose approach is indicated by languor and restlessness; next follow pallor and loss of strength and enfeeblement of pulse; all these symptoms progress, shortness of breath succeeds, and "the whole surface bears some relation to a bad wax figure." The patient dies from sheer weakness, not from wasting. In only three cases was there an inspection after death, and in all of them a diseased condition of the supra-renal capsules was found. The author had a strong impression that the disease of the supra-renals was the cause of the malady, "at all events he felt the time had come for directing the attention of the profession to these facts." It will be noticed that there is no mention of pigmentation nor of vomiting in this preliminary communication, which, however, is of great historical importance, for in it is the first evidence that the supra-renals are essential to life, and the whole of endocrinology dates from March 15, 1849. It is interesting to notice that, Addison's colleague, Wilk· son King the pathologist, had, in the *Guy's Hospital Report* for 1836, when writing on the uses of the thyroid secretion, f·reshown the doctrine of internal secretion by saying,

"Yet we may one day be able to show that a particular material principle is slowly formed . . . and that this principle is also supplementary, when poured into the descending cava, to important subsequent functions in the course of the circulation."

Addison continued to work at the subject; he got Wilks, then a young man about the hospital, to collect cases, and in 1855 he published the famous thin book, illustrated with chromo-lithographs, entitled, *On the Constitutional and Local Effects of Disease of the Supra-renal Capsules*. In the preface he remarks that occasionally the pathologist may be able to give a more decisive reply as to the function of an organ than the physiologist, and that pathology and physiology mutually advance and illustrate each other. Addison puts forward his book as a "first and feeble step" in the inquiry as to the function of the supra-renal capsules.

After a few preliminary sentences, the author, "as a preface to my subject," announces the discovery of another new disease, which is now universally known as "idiopathic anæmia,"

" pernicious anæmia," or " Addison's anæmia." He says that
for a long period he had observed a remarkable general anæmia,
which had no discoverable cause, which he was accustomed to
call " idiopathic."

It makes its approach in so slow and insidious a manner that the patient can
hardly fix a date to his earliest feeling of that languor which is shortly to become
so extreme. The countenance gets pale, the whites of the eyes become pearly,
the general frame flabby rather than wasted; the pulse perhaps large, but remarkably soft and compressible . . . there is an increasing indisposition to exertion,
with an uncomfortable feeling of faintness or breathlessness on attempting it;
the heart is readily made to palpitate; the whole surface of the body presents a
blanched, smooth and waxy appearance; the lips, gums and tongue seem bloodless; the appetite fails; extreme languor and faintness supervene, breathlessness
and palpitations being produced by the most trifling exertion or emotion; some
slight œdema is probably perceived about the ankles; the debility becomes
extreme. The patient can no longer rise from his bed, the mind occasionally
wanders, he falls into a prostrate and half-torpid state, and at length expires.
Nevertheless, to the very last, and after a sickness of perhaps several months'
duration, the bulkiness of the general frame and the obesity often present a most
striking contrast to the failure and exhaustion observable in every other respect.
   With perhaps a single exception the disease . . . sooner or later terminated
fatally. . . . After death I have failed to discover any organic lesion that could
properly or reasonably be assigned as an adequate cause of such serious con-
sequences.

Whilst seeking to throw light on this disease, Addison, to
use his own words, " stumbled upon" another malady, now
universally known as " Addison's disease," but which he called
either " Bronzed skin" or " Melasma Suprarenale." Expand-
ing the account he had given in 1849, he begins thus:—" The
leading and characteristic features of the morbid state to which
I would direct attention are, anæmia, general languor and
debility, remarkable feebleness of the heart's action, irritability
of the stomach, a peculiar change of colour of the skin, occurring
in connection with a diseased condition of the supra-renal
capsules." Then follows a perfect description of the languor,
feebleness of pulse, occasional vomiting, weakness, pigmentation of the skin and lips, all foreshadowing a fatal termination
without at any time any physical signs. The cases are given
in detail; the first four are undoubted examples of the disorder
and are those on which Addison founds his discovery; the
fifth he quotes from Bright, who had observed the cutaneous
discoloration and other symptoms, and had noticed the diseased

condition of the supra-renals shown after death, but he was unaware of the connection between this and the symptoms. There are six others given; Addison evidently regarded these as doubtful, and I think most readers would agree that they are not examples of the disease in question.

This thin quarto book of less than forty pages of large print, and mostly occupied with reports of individual cases, thus contains the first description of two diseases now known all over the world. Addison's account of each is so perfect that nothing has been found wrong in his clinical picture, and nothing has been added except facts that have been obtained by instruments which he did not possess, and a few occasional symptoms not present in the cases he described.

There was no review of this book in the *British Medical Journal*. That in the *Lancet* was half-hearted and rather foolish, the reviewer not understanding that two diseases were described. That in the *Medical Times and Gazette* warmly praised it, saying, "We believe that Dr. Addison has made a discovery which is one of the most important practical medicine has produced for many years, and one in every way worthy of the untiring zeal and energy in professional pursuits which have characterized his life."

It took a long while to convince people of the reality of Addison's anæmia. This was partly because he called it " idiopathic," and partly because later writers called it " pernicious anæmia." Two worse adjectives could not have been found, for any anæmia of which the cause was not evident was called idiopathic, and any severe case was naturally called pernicious. As recently as 1887 its existence was denied, but now it is universally recognized as a distinct malady, and further confusion will be avoided if it is called " Addison's anæmia." Addison's successors at Guy's have contributed considerably to our knowledge of Addison's Anæmia and Addison's Disease. Since his time about twenty papers dealing with these diseases have appeared in the *Guy's Hospital Reports*.

Although Greenhow, in his Croonian Lectures on Addison's Disease delivered before the Royal College of Physicians twenty years after the publication of Addison's discovery, thought that the knowledge of it had spread slowly, there is no doubt the profession acknowledge the truth that a new disease had been found much more quickly in the case of Addison's Disease than in that of Addison's Anæmia. It is true that many denied its existence, but Trousseau quickly appreciated the discovery and named the malady Addison's Disease, by which designation it has since always been known. Addison's Disease has passed into general literature. Readers of Wendell Holmes' *Poet at the Breakfast Table* will remember that the poet consults Dr. Franklin for a discoloration on the forehead.

"The colour reminds me," said Dr. Franklin, "of what I have seen in a case of Addison's Disease, Morbus Addisonii."

I said I thought the author of the *Spectator* was afflicted with a dropsy to which persons of sedentary and bibacious habits are liable !

"The author of the *Spectator* !" cried out Dr. Franklin; "I mean the celebrated Dr. Addison, the inventor, I would say, discoverer, of the wonderful new disease called after him !"

His other publications were few and of far less importance. Reference to them will be found in the life of him in the *Guy's Hospital Reports* for July 1926.

Addison was a lonely man, he did not marry till he was over fifty and he had no children. His mind delighted in the beauty of Lanercost and in the science and art of medicine.

It was a pleasing thought of the Border Counties Branch of the British Medical Association to arrange for a meeting, in commemoration of him, at Lanercost. This was held on June 19, 1926. There was a large gathering, doctors came from afar: London, Edinburgh, Newcastle, Whitehaven. After a short service in the Abbey, papers on Addison were read in the adjoining ancient Dacre Hall and afterwards there was a pleasant tea-party in the garden. The meeting caused great interest in the neighbourhood and was fully reported in the *Carlisle Journal*. We have seen how—outside his own hospital—Addison was grossly neglected in his time, therefore if his spirit looked down on the scene, it must have been with pleasure, for here, in his own beloved Lanercost, was a gathering of doctors proclaiming his greatness.

WILLIAM STOKES

Gabriel Stokes, a celebrated engineer, came from Shropshire to Dublin in 1680, practising his profession there for the greater part of his life. He had two sons, both Scholars and Fellows of Trinity College. The elder, John, became Professor of Greek there; John's son was the father of Sir George Gabriel Stokes, Professor of Mathematics at Cambridge and President of the Royal Society. The younger son of the engineer was likewise named Gabriel and was also a Professor of Mathematics, but at Trinity College, Dublin; his eldest son, Whitley, born 1763, was a Scholar and Fellow of the same College, and ultimately Regius Professor of Medicine. In early life he became a member of the Society of United Irishmen, but retired when he found that its efforts to effect reforms were not confined to peaceful and constitutional means. Nevertheless, he was cited to appear before Lord Clare, the Vice-Chancellor, and suspended from his Fellowship for a year. He must have been a remarkable man, for, although he left the Society of United Irishmen, one of its most prominent members, Theobald Wolfe Tone, said he loved Stokes most sincerely and regarded him as one of the best men he had ever known. Whitley was a principal founder of the Botanical Gardens and the famous Zoological Gardens in Phœnix Park; he translated the New Testament into Irish, was an accomplished physician and medical writer who insisted on the contagiousness of typhus and the necessity for its isolation, a philanthropist and lastly a distinguished member of the brilliant and witty society which existed in Dublin in the early part of the nineteenth century.

William Stokes, the great physician, the second son of Whitley, was born in Dublin, July 1804. His childhood was spent at the family country house, Ballinteer, among the Dublin hills. He cared nothing about games and sport, but loved to be out of doors learning Scottish ballads and reading the Waverley novels, which he delighted in for the rest of his life. His father, who had much influence on him, considered home education far superior to school and college, so William had a tutor from whom he learned Latin, Greek and Mathematics. He studied clinical medicine and scientific subjects bearing on it at the Meath Hospital, Dublin, then for two years at Glasgow, and finally at Edinburgh, which he reached at the age of 21. Here he fell under the influence of Professor Alison, for whom he had ever after the greatest affection and regard. Sir Henry Acland thus describes how the two first met:

He [Stokes] was walking one wet night down the old Cowgate; he observed a crowd at the entrance of a dark passage; he stopped to see what it could mean; he entered a low room filled with sick poor, Professor Alison being seated among them; he watched the scene; a young man evidently suffering from advanced fever stepped forward. Alison said, " Go to your bed and when I have done here I will come to you." Young Stokes then stepped forward and said, " Sir, I will take the poor man to his home." " Who are you ? " asked Alison. " One of your pupils; my name is Stokes." " I never saw you before," said Alison. " Perhaps not, but I have seen you, for I go to your lectures. Let me take the poor man home and I will come and tell you how he goes on." " Very well," said Alison, " you may go." From that time they were companions and friends.

I have given elsewhere an account of Laennec's discoveries and a biography of him, but I may remind the reader that his famous book was published in Paris in 1819. In it he tells us that in 1816, wishing to listen to a girl's heart, he recalled a well-known acoustic phenomenon: namely, if you place your ear against one end of a wooden beam the scratch of a pin at the other extremity is most distinctly audible. He took a sheaf of paper, rolled it into a very tight roll, one end of which he placed over the præcordial region, and put his ear to the other. He was both surprised and gratified at being able to hear the beating of the heart with much greater clearness and distinctness than he had ever done before by the direct application of his ear. Laennec in his book describes how from this paper stethoscope he evolved one of wood; in addition, from his astonishing power of observation he gives perfect, precise and original descriptions of the clinical symptom and post-mortem appearances of diseases of the chest. Most of these descriptions refer to conditions then unknown or imperfectly understood. The book is and will always remain a classic; from it dates all our knowledge of diseases of the chest. Laennec had wretched health, but, in spite of this, his clinical dissertations at the Necker Hospital were so brilliant that they attracted many foreigners, among whom was Hodgkin, who attended them in 1822, and in the same year read a paper before the Guy's Physical Society entitled *The Application of the Stethoscope.* This was probably the earliest introduction of the instrument to a medical society in this country. Stokes must have read Laennec's book, because in 1825, when only 21 years old, he published in Edinburgh a small treatise on the use of the stethoscope for which he received £70. Three years later saw the publication by him of two lectures, delivered at the Meath Hospital, on the use of the stethoscope. Forbes, in 1821, published a translation of part of Laennec's book in which he made scornful references to the stethoscope, but to Stokes is due the credit of being the first person to publish in the English language a treatise on the instrument, a remarkable achievement for one so young. Laennec's book directed Stokes to the study of diseases of the chest, the department of medicine in which he became famous, as will be presently shown.

In the autumn of 1825 he took his degree at Edinburgh and returned to Dublin, where he was elected Physician to the Dublin General Dispensary. Next year his father resigned his physiciancy to the Meath Hospital; his son was appointed in his place, having for a colleague the illustrious Robert James Graves. They became great friends. Sir William Stokes, the son of the physician, says:

> For years they worked together in the Meath Hospital, assisting one another in their clinical researches, and in the initiation and carrying out of a system of clinical instruction till then unknown in this country, which eventually acquired a world-wide fame for the Dublin School of Medicine. Never did any disagreement arise between them.

Robert James Graves was descended from Colonel Graves, an officer in Cromwell's army in Ireland. Robert's father, Richard Graves, Senior Fellow of Trinity College, Regius Professor of Divinity in the University of Dublin and Dean of Ardagh, had three sons, all of great distinction; Robert James, the youngest, born in 1796, after studying arts and medicine in Trinity College, Dublin, took his M.B. there in 1818, he next studied in London and from there went to the Continent for three years to learn at the medical schools of Berlin, Göttingen,

Vienna, Copenhagen and those of France and Italy. At all these places he studied hard and made many friendships which lasted his lifetime. He acquired languages with such facility that when walking in Austria without his passport on him, he was arrested and thrown into prison for ten days, as a spy, for it was said no Englishman could speak German so well as he.

Graves was travelling in a diligence in the Alps when a man who looked like the mate of a ship got in, sat beside him, and soon took from his pocket a note-book across which his hand from time to time passed with the rapidity of lightning. Graves wondered if the man was insane, he looked, saw that the stranger had been noting the forms of clouds as they passed and that he was no common artist. The two travelled and sketched together for months before they found each other's name, Graves's companion was J. M. W. Turner. He tells that Turner would outline a scene, sit doing nothing for two or three days, then suddenly "perhaps on the third day, he would exclaim, 'There it is' and seizing his colours, work rapidly till he had noted down the peculiar effect he wished to fix in his memory."

On one occasion Graves was lying in his bunk when a violent storm sprang up, a man rushed in to tell him that the crew were taking to the only boat, leaving the passengers to their fate; he tore on deck, seized an axe, stove in the boat, virtually took command of the ship, mended the pumps with leather from his own boots, stopped the leak and brought her into port. He returned to Dublin in 1821.

Stokes made a selection from Graves's writings after his death. He edited them and published them under the title of *Studies in Physiology and Medicine*, prefixing a biographical notice of Graves, in which he gives a short account of the Dublin Medical School. For a century before 1821 there had been a Medi.. i Faculty in the University of Dublin, with a Regius Professor of Medicine. Nevertheless, Stokes says, " Dublin was little more than a school of elementary anatomy, of book medicine and book surgery." " Clinical investigation and clinical teaching could scarcely be said to exist, and so the great path of the advancement of the healing art was almost untrodden." Graves, in 1821, was elected physician to the Meath Hospital, and at once began to found a new School of Medicine in Park

Street. In his first lecture he told his audience that few students are impressed with the great difficulty of becoming good practitioners, many misbehave in the wards, seeming to consider a hospital a place of amusement; they are to blame, so also are their teachers who do not teach, but only turn out practitioners who have never practised. The result is that numbers of patients die annually in consequence of bad medical treatment, "their immolation is never long delayed when a successful candidate for a dispensary commences the discharge of his duty." Doctors, he says, do not seem to have thought it their duty to try to restore the sick to health. Graves quotes, as what he calls "this foul blot on medical practice," the fact that out of 10,272 sick children sent to the Dublin Foundling Hospital, 45 recovered.

He insists that the only way to alter this appalling state of things is to teach better. Mere walking the hospital must go. The Edinburgh system, in which the teacher interrogates the patient in a loud voice, the clerk repeats the patient's answer in a similar voice, the crowd of students round the bed, most of whom cannot see the patient, hears all this and makes notes, is of no use. Students must examine patients for themselves under the guidance of their teachers, they must make suggestions as to diagnosis, morbid anatomy and treatment to their teacher who will discuss the cases with them.

This is real clinical teaching; to Graves belongs the honour of having introduced it into the British Isles; Stokes joined in the reformation five years later; these two are the founders of British Clinical teaching; they made the Dublin School of Medicine famous all over the world.

Graves's *Clinical Lectures* were published in 1843, and quickly spread knowledge of him over Europe. A second edition appeared in 1848. He received the Honorary Membership of the Medical Societies in Berlin, Vienna, Hamburg, Tübingen, Bruges, Montreal and the Fellowship of the Royal Society of London. The *Lectures* were translated into French. Trousseau wrote the preface; he entreated his pupils to consider the book as their breviary; he declared that of all the practical works published in his time, there was none more useful, more intellectual. He had incessantly read and reread it, he knew it almost by heart, but still could not refrain from perusing a book which never left his study.

The reader of to-day must remember the state of the practice of medicine when Graves began to teach. It was founded on all kinds of " doctrines," each without the shadow of proof. All fever was supposed to depend upon inflammation—what this was was nowhere stated—which must be subdued. Hence starvation, purges, and bleeding. Graves's teaching was like fresh air in a foul room. He would not even consider doctrines; he depended solely on his observations. He called attention to what happens to a healthy man who has little food for three weeks, his loss of strength and flesh, yet a man sick of fever was starved for three weeks. Many fever patients, he is sure, have died because of this. Feed them to aid them to combat the loss of strength and flesh due to the fever; remember that their bad digestion is evidence of the feebleness of the gastric function; food will strengthen it. A gentleman, having much purulent discharge and high fever, owing to a psoas abscess was greatly emaciated and sinking rapidly under the usual treatment; he took his case into his own hands, ate six meals a day consisting of beef steak, mutton, fowl and other solids, washed down with wine and porter. His pulse improved, his strength increased, the sweats disappeared and he recovered completely. Graves going round his ward expatiating on the healthy appearance of some who had recovered from severe typhus made a remark which has become celebrated " This is all the effect of our good feeding and lest when I am gone, you may be at a loss for an epitaph for me, let me give you one in three words: He fed fevers."

If a fevered patient had a furred tongue, it was assumed that the inflammation had attacked the bowel so he was purged violently, this, says Graves, is absurd. He states that during a typhus epidemic in Dublin the mortality was greater among the rich than the poor because they received more drugs. His remarks upon excessive bleeding, the importance of sleep, the proper ventilation of the sick-room and the ill health that follows upon the continuous use of large doses of mercury were, at the time they were made, all novel. Nothing has done more to improve treatment of disease than Graves's *Clinical Lectures*. Many hundreds of thousands of the sick owe their lives to them.

There is not a dull page in these lectures, the frequent reference to individual cases carries the reader on, even to-day; they are unlike a modern text-book, for they can be read with enjoyment in an easy chair before the fire. At the end of the forty-ninth lecture there is a description of a young lady of 20, who suffered from exophthalmic goitre. It is a single case, recorded without comment. Trousseau on the strength of it suggested that exophthalmic goitre should be called Graves' Disease.

He was a prolific writer of essays. One on how to use opium appeared as a small book, more than fifty years before the advent of abdominal surgery, and when this drug was the only powerful remedy for all varieties of acute peritonitis. Opium has been called one of God's great gifts to mankind, and so it is. Graves did immense good by teaching how to use it. Many doctors use it badly even at the present day, and many patients are denied the relief it can give in a multitude of conditions. Cholera ravaged the British Isles in Graves's time, he devoted more attention to this than to any malady. It was strongly asserted to be epidemic and not contagious. Graves wrote to show that this was wrong; it certainly was contagious and quarantine was useless. He did much good by teaching the value of acetate of lead in this disease. Some of his essays deal with subjects outside medicine; the most notable of these are two on the war in Afghanistan which he had studied closely.

He was President of the College of Physicians in Dublin during 1843 and 1844. His health began to fail in the autumn of 1852 and he died on March 20, 1853. Graves was an eloquent, forcible lecturer who held the attention of his audience. He was tall, dark, with expressive features, a good talker, with the power of converting others to his way of thinking; his kindness, his total want of arrogance and his love of truth made this really great man popular.

Inspired by what he saw of the methods of Graves and stimulated by what he read of Laennec, Stokes now began his life's work at Dublin. In clinical teaching he followed Graves, immense pains were taken with lectures; on the night before the first he sat up, working at it, till past three in the morning, from sheer fatigue then to bed, rising again at six to continue. It was an immense success, everybody congratulated him upon it; other lectures were equally good and at the age of 22 he became noted as a great teacher. In a letter he describes a day's work thus:

I rise early, write till breakfast, then go to the dispensary, where I sit in judgement on disease for an hour; then to the hospital, where I go round the wards attended by a crowd of pupils; from the hospital I return home, write again till two, and then go round and visit my patients through different parts of the town attended by a pupil. My patients have all one great defect, viz., that, instead of giving money, they too often, unfortunate beings, have to solicit it from their medical attendant; and who, with the heart of a man, would refuse to relieve their sufferings when he has a shilling in his pocket? A poor woman, whom I attended for long, and who ultimately recovered, said, "Oh, doctor you have given me a good stomach, but I have nothing to put into it."

His heart was deeply touched by suffering; Acland, his friend, says he is to be thought of, above all else, as the physician of the poor. In the summer of 1826 there was great distress owing to the failure of the potato crop; in the autumn and winter typhus raged in Dublin. The poor lay dying in the streets with typhus on them. Stokes writes:

I walked out the other night, and on passing by a lane my attention was arrested by a crowd of persons gathered in a circle round a group which occupied the steps of a hall door. This was a family, consisting of a father, mother and three wretched children, who had just been expelled from their lodgings as having fever. The father was in high delirium, and as I approached him started off and ran down the street; the mother was lying at the foot of the door perfectly insensible, with an infant screaming on the breast, where it had sought milk in vain, and the other two filled the air with their lamentations. It was a shocking sight indeed. No one would go near them to bring them even a drop of cold water. In a short time, however, I succeeded in having them all carried to the hospital; they have since recovered.

The epidemic was severe; there were 1,414 beds for fever patients in Dublin; were these five times the number "they would be filled in a day." Stokes worked away at teaching, lecturing and attending the sick from half-past seven in the morning till midnight all through the winter. In the spring of 1828, a dissection wound made him dangerously ill, he went to his father's country house to convalesce; on his return in April he married Mary Black of Glasgow—they had been engaged three years. He brought his wife home to his father's house, 16 Harcourt Street, Dublin, where they remained for upwards of three years.

Unfortunate Ireland was, in 1832, for the first time in its history, afflicted with cholera; the epidemic was serious and disastrous. It so chanced that Stokes saw the first case, as is thus described by his son, Sir William Stokes, the surgeon. His father, together with Mr. Rumley,

had been sent to inquire into the cause of a sudden and mysterious death which had occurred at Kingstown, then little more than a seaside village. Neither of these physicians had ever seen a case of this disease either before or after death. The result of their inspection, however, was that they pronounced the deceased to have died of the worse type of asiatic cholera. Outside the house, in which the body lay, a crowd was anxiously awaiting their decision. The announcement was first received with silent dismay, then came a burst of frenzy and indignation. A furious crowd of men, women and children hurled stones, mud and brickbats at them from all sides. They escaped injury almost by a miracle; their carriage was battered and broken by the missiles thrown at them, and it was only by whip and spur that their postillions outstripped their pursuers.

Some of Stokes's lectures delivered at the Meath Hospital and the Park Street School between 1832 and 1835 appeared in the *London Medical and Surgical Journal*. They were highly praised and reprinted in America, where they became one of the standard medical treatises. At this time he contributed seven articles to the *Cyclopædia of Medicine,* and various papers to the *Dublin Journal of Medical and Chemical Science*; the most important is one on the proper use of large doses of opium. Stokes and Graves were the first to state that bleeding and purging were harmful but that plenty of opium was beneficial for acute abdominal disease; by doing so they saved thousands of lives. In 1834 he became an editor of this Journal. By the time he was 30 he was celebrated as a distinguished clinical teacher, far beyond his native city. Next year he began writing the great work of his life, namely, his book on *Diseases of the Chest*. Towards the end of the year he showed signs of breaking down under such a stress of work; accordingly he took a long holiday abroad with several friends. Returning home, he was immediately in the thick of work, lectures, clinical teaching, large practice; nevertheless, he was able early in 1837 to announce that the book on *Diseases of the Chest* would be finished in three days. It so enhanced his reputation that he was awarded the M.D. (honoris causa) of the University of Dublin and made a member of the Medical Societies of Vienna, Berlin, Leipsic, Edinburgh, Ghent, Baden, Hamburg and Philadelphia.

Practice in Ireland led to queer experiences. During the Fenian disturbances, James Stephens escaped from Kilmainham Gaol. The Government offered £2,000 for his apprehension. Stokes and Dr. Hatchell were called into the country to a patient. On their return they lost their way, as it was very dark. Hatchell knocked at a cottage door and asked the tall, ragged woman who opened it, for someone to show them the way. "Show you the way is it?" replied the virago; "there's no one here to do it, himself is in bed these two days with a stuffin in his chest, and the boy's away." Then "himself" appeared, Hatchell whispered in his ear, "Don't ask me the name of the man in the carriage, it begins with an S." "Holy mother of God," said the man. "Patsy," he cried to the boy who was asleep, "git up and show the gentleman the way." which he did for some miles so that the two doctors reached home safely. Stokes had many Irish stories; he, talking to a man he met, said he heard that So-and-so had had his coffin made. The man replied that was true and it was presumptuous of him to have done it. "Why?" asked Stokes. "Because," came the answer, "how does he know he will live long enough to want it." He asked a woman what she thought of the soup the Government distributed during the famine. "Soup, is it, your honour! sure it isn't soup at all." Said Stokes, "What is it then." "It's nothin', your honour, but a quart of water biled down to a pint, to make it sthrong!"

Space does not allow of any more stories, nor of the harrowing accounts in Stokes's letters of the destitution from famine and typhus. The mortality from this last among Irish doctors was 24 per cent. He went to London to intercede with the Government for some monetary compensation for their families; he was only partially successful. Those who wish to learn of Irish life should read the life of Stokes written by his son, Sir William.

The Pathological Society of Dublin, the first of its kind, was founded by him in 1838. He contributed many papers on diseases of the heart to the *Dublin Quarterly Journal of Medical Sciences*. These formed the basis of his work on *Diseases of the Heart and Aorta* published in 1854. It was translated into German, Italian and French. In 1861 he went to Edinburgh to receive the degree of LL.D.; he took a holiday in Scotland, next year one abroad. On his return he was appointed one of the Physicians in Ordinary to the Queen in Ireland, and the following year he was elected F.R.S. He was also a member of the General Medical Council. Two subjects which interested him much about this time were Medical Education and Sanitary Science; the outcome was much improved attention by the University of Dublin to the medical school and in 1871 the granting of a diploma in state medicine. His *Lectures on Fever* appeared in 1874. He pleaded strongly for the view that fevers change their type and that typhoid and typhus were the same one fever. Although in these matters he was wrong, yet the book is valuable because of the fine clinical information in it. He was now 70 years old, and this book was his last contribution to medicine.

He made no great discovery, but, by his character, teaching and personality occupied an outstanding position. This is shown by the distinctions conferred upon him. In addition to those already mentioned he was a D.C.L. of Oxford, an LL.D. of Cambridge, President of the meeting of the British Medical Association in Dublin, President of the Royal Irish Academy and a member of the Prussian order "Pour la Mérite": the two last are rare honours. He and Graves will always be famous because, both orally and in writing, they were great teachers, who immensely raised the standard of clinical medicine.

Trouble came upon him; he lost his wife, then his daughter Janet; he suffered from spinal concussion following a fall from a car; weakness increased, so that, in 1876, he resigned all professional work and retired to his country house at Howth, where he died on January 6, 1878. There is a fine statue of him by Foley in the hall of the College of Physicians in Dublin.

Stokes must have been a happy man, for beauty in nature and beauty in every form of art gave him great joy. He had the gift of writing beautiful prose. Sir Henry Acland transcribes a letter picturing a sunset on the west coast of Ireland. Here is a quotation from a family letter written without any thought of publication.

A perfect rainbow of the most beautiful colours suddenly spanned the Rhine, and seemed to rise to an extraordinary height in the heavens. This was succeeded by another and by a third. So that we had a triple rainbow of the most surpassing beauty, and between each arch a mass of iris colours that seemed to have lost their way, erring spirits that had no guide. By and by the black curtain rose more and more from the west, and curling upwards, with round masses like drapery, disclosed the brilliant sunset. The sunnier Tyrol had a clearness like diamond, and the trees and flowers all the richness of colouring and distinctness of outline we wonder at in Both's landscapes. The clouds after forming masses hanging in the clear æther, like pendants in a Gothic cathedral, gradually rolled away. The sun sank, gilding the Drachenfels, and night rapidly set in.

It is not surprising that such a writer had for his friends Burton, who became Director of the National Gallery, and that singular man George Petrie, notable artist, learned antiquarian and fine musician, who helped in the survey of Ireland and was awarded a Civil List pension. He was constantly touring his native country, painting, carefully describing its antiquities, and taking down its native airs. Stokes often went with him, each had a deep affection for the other. Petrie died in January 1865. Three years later *The Life of George Petrie, LL.D.*, by William Stokes, appeared. It is a large book, remarkable for the very wide knowledge of painting, archæology and music shown by Stokes and also for the care he takes to make the reader understand the high position of his friend as an authority in all three subjects. The writer, who contributes the biography of Petrie in the *Dictionary of National Biography*, agrees fully with Stokes. How he found time, in the busiest period of his life, to write such a book passes comprehension. That he did so is a magnificent tribute to the love he bore his friend. Only one incident from it can be quoted. Petrie, with manuscript music book and violin, Stokes and another friend, O'Curry, went on a musical tour in the Islands of Arran. When they came to a village they inquired " who had music." Being told who, it was arranged they should go in the evening to the cottage where music could be heard. A huge peat fire was blazing; outside was a crowd of islanders; inside, the room was packed with more, their handsome faces, rich-coloured dresses making a wonderful picture by firelight. The minstrel, man or girl, sat on a stool in the chimney corner, O'Curry and Petrie on stools opposite, everyone else stood. The song having been given, O'Curry wrote it down in Irish. Then the singer sang it again and again slowly till Petrie had taken down the tune correctly. He published a volume of 147 native Irish airs which he thus rescued from oblivion; it was he who gave Moore several which he used. His best-known anti-

quarian work is that in connection with The Hill of Tara
and that about the Round Towers. He painted many pictures.

Stokes's love of art is shown in many ways—in his letters
written when travelling, in his description of continental pictures
which he saw, in his review of Kugler's *Handbook of Painting,* in
his friendship with Helen Faucit and in his membership of the
Shakespeare Reading Society, at which he used himself to read.
Good literature he thoroughly enjoyed, especially poetry; Wordsworth and Scott were particular favourites. An invalid cobbler,
named Denny, was a friend to whom he used to lend a volume
of Scott's novels; one day he asked Denny what he thought
of the last he had read. Denny replied, " It's a great book
intirely, docther, an' Sir Walter Scott's a true historian"; Stokes
asked him why. He answered, " I mane, your honour, he's a
thrue historian, because he makes you love your kind." Stokes
always said that this was one of the finest comments he had
ever heard on Scott.

As might have been expected he was constantly urging that
a proper medical curriculum should provide for intending
doctors to be persons of wide interests and general culture. It
is easy to comprehend why he was elected President of the Irish
Academy, a position almost always reserved for one eminent in
the arts or abstract science.

During the first quarter of the nineteenth century, the mind
of Ireland was sunk in apathy and dejection, gradually these
passed away and Dublin contained brilliant intellectual society
in which Stokes fully played his part. Mahaffy tells us that
his house became the resort of all the wit and learning which
Ireland possessed. Stokes's fame brought many foreign visitors
of literary celebrity to see him. He kept open house. Carlyle
came to a dinner party, Stokes thought him a bore; Carlyle considered Mrs. Stokes to be one and he was, as he says, unlucky,
for he quoted Johnson's saying " Did I say anything that you
understood, Sir ?" she thought he addressed her and soon left
the room " my enemy for ever." He liked Petrie, but was
quite out of it by recording that he was " old bachelor you
could see," for Petrie was married and had several children.
The dinner was indeed "rather unsuccessful." His unfavour-
able criticism of everything Irish was much resented and considered to be in bad taste as he was the guest of Irishmen. All

this was a pity, because, in congenial company, Stokes was a fine talker, it was a great treat to hear the pathos with which he told a serious Irish story or the humour with which he related others. He particularly enjoyed the company of young men, his influence brought out the best in them, yet he never preached nor gave formal moral advice. He was far too subtle and original a teacher to follow such a well-beaten and futile track.

A characteristic story of Stokes is that of the tragic death of Clarence Mangan, Ireland's great poet. Unhappily he was an opium addict and an incorrigible drunkard, generally on the verge of starvation. Nothing had been heard of him for months when a half-naked, wretched-looking man sought admission to the Meath Hospital; the resident, Dr. O'Reilly, saw him, had him washed and put to bed. Shortly afterwards Stokes came; for a moment he was bewildered before he recognized his friend, Mangan; he spoke to him, Mangan answered, " You are the first who has spoken one kind word to me for many years." A terrible reply. Stokes told those around who the patient was, had him put into a private room, and himself provided extra clothes and food. He only lived a few days. Immediately after his death, which took place at night, Stokes was struck with the beauty of his features, so he hurried off early next morning for Burton, whom he brought back and who made a sketch, now in the National Gallery of Ireland. A plaster cast was also taken. Stokes paid the funeral expenses. So completely had poor Mangan—whose beautiful poems have given pleasure to many—cut himself off that only three persons attended his funeral. Those who wish to see a copy of Burton's beautiful portrait and to study the mind of an extraordinary genius should read *The Life and Letters of James Clarence Mangan,* by D. J. O'Donoghue.

Medicine participated in the general intellectual activity of Dublin at this time. The Pathological Society, the *Dublin Hospital Reports* and the *Dublin Journal of Medical Science* all flourished. The last had 400 names on its subscription list, it reviewed many books and received numerous journals in exchange. Clinical medicine was closely studied in it. Many participated, Stokes and Graves were the soul of this revival.

In the nineteenth century three books appeared, one written by Laennec, two by Stokes, which are the foundation of our knowledge and every-day diagnosis of diseases of the chest. Before Laennec physicians generally did not or would not examine the chest; they speculated. Sydenham's saying, " True practice consists in the observations of nature; these are finer than any speculations," had fallen on stony ground. Readers of Stokes must not turn away from him when they come across opinions which experience has not confirmed; he was a pioneer, most pioneers make mistakes, he made very few, which count as nothing in comparison with the truths he enunciated as a result of his own observation and which he drove home with a terseness and clarity not surpassed by any other writer. The enormous advance made in medicine from 1820 to 1870 was in diagnosis and morbid anatomy; in this advance no one played a greater part than Stokes.

As we have seen, he began at the age of 21 by the publication of a little book *An Introduction to the Use of the Stethoscope.* From the wording of the dedication to Cullen it is clear that this one of Stokes's teachers had attentively studied the use of the instrument. The object of the book is to properly connect the different signs obtained by the stethoscope with the pathological state of the viscera to which they owe their origin. There is much more in it than this, percussion, varieties of breathing, morbid anatomy and diseases of the heart are all described. Illustrative cases copied from the French are included. It must be rare for such an admirable short text-book to have been written at the age of 21. As you read it you feel that it foreshadows a great teacher. Three years later it was followed by another small book called *Two Lectures on the Application of the Stethoscope.* This instrument, he says, has " added more to the facility, certainty and utility of diagnosis than anything which has been done for centuries. By the stethoscope we substitute the ear for the eye; penetrate into the mysteries of hidden disease."

The characteristics of both Stokes's large books are his elevation of the science and art of diagnosis, his appeal to morbid anatomy, his banishment of unsupported dogma, his insistence that neither the presence nor the absence of any sign is pathognomonic, but for accurate diagnosis every negative and every positive fact must be considered, his teaching that the place to learn clinical medicine is the bedside where it rarely corresponds with the teaching in books, the large number of illustrative cases which he quotes, the admirable recapitulations he gives at the end of each chapter, his wide reading of foreign literature and, lastly, the total absence of egotism, for he says :

There can be nothing more commendable than to avoid controversy when the object is to establish mere priority of discovery . . . it matters little to the right-thinking man who, having discovered a new truth, finds it claimed by another, if it be established and made available for good.

The two books occupy more than 600 pages each, therefore only a few extracts can be given.

The *Treatise on the Diagnosis and Treatment of Diseases of the Chest* was published in 1837; it soon went out of print. A new edition, edited by Dr. Hudson, with a memoir by Sir Henry Acland, appeared in 1882. The book deals only with the respiratory apparatus.

There are many masterly descriptions; one that struck me as superb was that of emphysema. Stokes thinks dilatation of the air cells is a better name than that of pulmonary emphysema, introduced by Laennec. He observes that there is no monograph on " Foreign Bodies in the Lungs, Trachea and Bronchial tubes," therefore he writes one, in which the account of the difference in symptoms between partial and complete obstruction of the right bronchus is very good, the importance of auscultation is stressed. Anyone writing a monograph on the subject to-day ought to refer to this by Stokes.

The discussion on the diagnosis between bronchiectasis and phthisis is admirable; a pithy saying is that in phthisis we have first dullness, then a cavity, whereas in bronchiectasis there is first a cavity, then dullness. There is an account of the influence of destruction of the ciliated epithelium in the production of dilated tubes. There are no physical signs peculiar to tubercle, of the signs of incipient phthisis none is more important than feebleness of respiration. The discussion of the prognosis of phthisis is excellent. There may be contraction of the side of the chest in which fluid is present.

Many patients would recover from fevers were it not for the accompanying bronchitis. Violent primary bronchitis is common in children, rare in adults; the reverse is true of chronic bronchitis, which is a species of gleet of the mucous membrane. In chronic bronchitis the circulatory and digestive functions remain healthy, in phthisis they do not. The necessity of bringing young infants into the open air is not sufficiently known and many lives are sacrificed to an absurd, ignorant and destructive prejudice against this. The greatest practical improvement which modern medicine owes to clinical study is our disuse of the lancet in a vast number of cases.

The Diseases of the Heart and Aorta was published in Dublin in 1854. Stokes says in the preface, "It seeks to embody the results of my clinical observations, continued almost unremittingly for upwards of a quarter of a century." But it does more, for like the previous book it shows his wide reading, for example he quotes from Wilkinson King—hardly known to most physicians. About a sixth of the book is occupied by the subject of pericarditis, the account of which is one of the best I have ever read. In this disease the heart is not impeded by the pressure of effused fluid, but by the spread of inflammation into the cardiac muscle, which is the cause of death when it is due directly to pericarditis. The mere obliteration of the pericardial space by adhesions does not lead to hypertrophy and dilatation of the heart. By far the most frequent cause of pericarditis is rheumatic fever, in this disease the heart should be examined daily. No special condition of pulse belongs to any one form or stage of pericarditis. No symptom is constant; even pain, often the first and most important may be absent. Difficulty of breathing is frequent. How to distinguish whether these last two symptoms are due to pleurisy or pericarditis is skilfully debated.

One of the most melancholy reproaches to medicine is the fact that innumerable persons have been condemned to invalidism merely because a doctor heard a cardiac murmur. Would to goodness such doctors had read Stokes who, a century ago, taught that organic change in the valves may be arrested and then, if the condition of the muscle of the heart remains unaltered, the individual may enjoy perfect health and be able to undergo great fatigue. Stokes says a loud murmur is detected and a twofold error is then commonly committed; first it is supposed to indicate recent and progressive disease, secondly the patient is told that he has organic heart disease. He gives a realistic account of the replacement of the happy healthy life often led by a man who has a murmur, by one in which, owing to the discovery of a murmur by a doctor, the constant fear of sudden death is combined with drastic treatment which slowly kills the patient. The unpardonable error has been committed of treating a fixed and incurable organic change as a recent and progressive disorganization. Many examples of this error, in which Stokes was happily able to put the patients back on to the right road, are described. Over and over again he lays down that the key to the understanding and treating disease of the heart is the state of the cardiac muscle. Valvular disease of the heart has little influence on health so long as the muscle is sound. The loudness of a murmur is no guide to the seriousness of the valvular disease, which may be considerable when no murmur is audible. Sudden death in heart disease is infrequent, uncomplicated dilatation of the heart is excessively rare, fremitus over the heart almost invariably indicates organic disease, there are inorganic murmurs indistinguishable from some which indicate mitral regurgitation, loss of tone in the first sound is common in fever, this is known as Stokes's sign. Among his cases of functional disorder of the heart are some good examples of the effect of excessive tea-drinking.

Stokes was one of the first to give a full description of the signs and symptoms of abdominal aneurysm. Starvation diet was then, and for a long while after, thought to be desirable for patients with aneurysm. He remarks that many patients with this disease continue quite well till they have the misfortune to consult a doctor who orders the fashionable starvation. The diet for aneurysm should be nutritious and generous.

The chapter on fatty heart is the best known, as it contains accounts of Cheyne-Stokes breathing and Stokes-Adams disease. Dr. J. Cheyne, in the *Dublin Hospital Reports*, Vol. 2, pt. 2, p. 216, for the year 1818, recorded " *A case of Apoplexy in which the fleshy part of the heart was converted into fat.*" The patient was a man aged 60. The respiration is thus described:

For several days his breathing was irregular; it would entirely cease for a quarter of a minute, then it would become perceptible, though very low, then by degrees it became heaving and quick, and then would gradually cease again: this revolution in the state of his breathing occupied about a minute, during which there were about thirty acts of respiration.

Stokes reprints this and says he has seen this variety of respiration in many cases of fatty degeneration, but that he has never seen it except in this condition. He describes it fully, and, in the recapitulation, says that it is

A form of respiratory distress . . . consisting of a period of apparently perfect apnœa, succeeded by feeble and short inspirations, which gradually increase in strength and depth until the respiratory act is carried to the highest pitch of which it seems capable, when the respirations, pursuing a descending scale, regularly diminish until the commencement of another apnœal period.

Cheyne does not show that he connected the phenomenon with the state of the heart, Stokes rescued his observation from obscurity and ever since this variety of breathing has been known as Cheyne-Stokes respiration.

Robert Adams, in the *Dublin Hospital Reports,* Vol. 4, 1827, published a paper entitled *Cases of Diseases of the Heart accompanied by Pathological Observations.* It is a long rambling paper, in which no special attention is paid to the slowness of the pulse in the three cases in which it occurred. The best reported is that of a man, aged 68, who had had many attacks of insensibility, his pulse rate was 30, after death the heart was found to be fatty; another man, aged 60, had usually a pulse rate of 90 but it would drop to 30, he suffered from enormous cardiac hypertrophy; the last case was that of a physician who had had many fainting attacks and for the last six weeks of his life no pulse could be felt. Extreme atheroma of the coronary arteries was found. Adams suggests that the cause of the symptoms was imperfect supply of blood to the heart.

Stokes, in the *Dublin Quarterly Journal of Medical Science,* Vol. 2, p. 73, 1846, in a paper entitled *Observations on Some Cases of Permanently Slow Pulse,* reports the case of a man, aged 68, who had at least fifty fainting attacks, and a pulse that varied from 28 to 32, and another of a man who apparently had only one faint and that fatal, his pulse varied from 35 to 40. Putting together Adams's cases, his own cases and those he had heard of, Stokes then knew of seven cases of fainting attacks associated with a slow pulse. It was this paper by Stokes that disinterred Adams's cases and first drew attention to the combination of syncopal attacks with slow pulse, which is now known as Stokes-Adams disease. Properly it is not a disease, but a syndrome. Stokes did not call it a disease, as far as he then knew it was a symptom of fatty heart and it is under this heading that he describes it in his book.

SIR JAMES YOUNG SIMPSON

It has been claimed by many that, in his day, Sir James Simpson was the best-known doctor in the world.

Alexander Simpson, a farmer who lived at Torphichen, two and a half miles from Bathgate, which is eighteen miles west of Edinburgh, married Isabella Grindley, and lived to be 91. Of his several children, David, the fourth son, who was born in 1760, became a baker, working as a journeyman in London, Glasgow and Leith. In 1792 he married Mary, the daughter of John Jarvie, a farmer, who was descended from the Huguenots; some of his ancestors had been people of note in Scotland.

David opened business on his own account as a baker in Bathgate in 1810 after two unsuccessful attempts in other places. He had one daughter, Mary, and seven sons, two of whom died early. James Young, the seventh son, was born on June 7, 1811, at Bathgate. By this time the business here was as bad as the others had been, David had no money and was in debt; he had concealed his financial trouble from his wife but now he had to tell her. She took the management of the business into her own hands; immediately it improved and soon it was fairly successful. She appears to have combined the virtues of Martha with those of Mary. James and her other children had a deep affection for her. When she died in 1820, the daughter Mary, who was the eldest child, took competent and loving charge of the household and became a second mother to her brothers. They were a happy family, each doing his best for the whole, so united were they that, when one of them needed money, he just took it out of the till in the shop.

In Scotland it was the ambition of families for their sons to enter a profession. If want of money forbade that more than one should do so, it was usually the youngest who was chosen, because, as the others had started in life, it was possible to spend a little more on his education, and often, as with the Simpsons, the elders took a pride in the career of the youngest and were willing to help. Therefore it was according to custom that James should, after attendance at two village schools, go to Edinburgh University at the age of 14. As a child he was loved, popular, gentle, good tempered and industrious.

In Edinburgh he lodged at the top of a large house, No. 1 Adam Street, with John Reid, who became Professor of Anatomy at St. Andrew's, and with Dr. Macarthur, both from Bathgate. Simpson showed only average ability in the arts courses; he obtained a Bursary of £10 a year and decided to study medicine, but nearly altered his resolutions after seeing an amputation of the breast. Liston was his favourite teacher; his obstetric studies began in 1829 in Dr. Hamilton's class. His father died in 1830, he himself qualified as a member of the Royal College of Surgeons in Edinburgh the same year. He tried for the post of ship's surgeon and also for a practice on the Clyde; both applications were unsuccessful, so, on the strength of his small bursary, he returned to the University as assistant to Dr. Gairdner; his brother David having begun business in Edinburgh he lodged with him. In 1832 he received his M.D. for a thesis on "Death from Inflammation."

Fortunately the thesis was read by Dr. John Thompson, who thereupon wrote to Simpson offering him the post of assistant to himself at a salary of £50 a year, which situation was joyfully accepted. It was very helpful to a young man to be associated with Thompson, for he was a person of much consequence, wide knowledge and active in advancing the medical school. He held three Professorships, that of Surgery at the Royal College of Surgeons, that of Military Surgery to the University and that of Pathology to the University, hence Robert Knox sarcastically called him "the old Chairmaker." He was also an extramural lecturer on medicine. Simpson now resolved, largely on the advice of Thompson, to try to make his living by practising obstetric medicine in Edinburgh and began hard work in real earnest. Happily for him he had the rare faculty of being able to concentrate on reading and writing in a room full of people who were talking. Alexander, his favourite brother, and his brother John, chiefly from affection and partly from family pride, helped him financially, so that he was able to buy many books on the subject he had selected to practise and these he studied assiduously. In 1833 he joined the Royal

Medical Society of Edinburgh, which venerable students' society is now nearly 200 years old. Three years later he was President, delivering his Inaugural Dissertation on Diseases of the Placenta.

During the spring of 1835 he went on a tour of England and parts of the Continent, devoting the chief part of his time to visiting hospitals and museums.

The following year he considered a proposal from Dr. Mackintosh, an extramural lecturer on Midwifery, that he should take over his lectures, together with his museum; again Alexander and John came forward with an offer to find the £200 or £300 asked for by Dr. Mackintosh. Simpson did not do so because he would have to lecture also on Medical Jurisprudence. Nevertheless he was determined to lecture on midwifery as soon as possible. Practice in this department was coming to him; in June 1836 he writes to Alexander from 2 Teviot Row "I am scarcely off my feet from morning to night, running after this and that. I saw fourteen patients on Tuesday in every different quarter of the town. . . . And then the sitting up all night; but my mind is made up for it all and I am contented." To expand his experience, he attended Hamilton's lectures on midwifery a second time and, in addition to his practice, acted as house surgeon to the Lying-in Hospital for twelve months; doing so increased the number of his private patients considerably. He took boarders in his lodgings, wrote papers on his subject for medical journals, including one on Hermaphroditism for *Todd's Cyclopædia of Anatomy and Physiology*, altogether he worked desperately hard, either sitting up till two or three or getting up at four in the morning when not out at a midwifery case. He acted for a session as interim lecturer on Pathology for Dr. Thompson, and in 1838 began to lecture on Obstetrics in the extramural school. He could always hold an audience, and the lectures were a success; his biographer, J. Duns, says, "this was the reward of work, not the triumph of genius," which is undoubtedly true.

Dr. Hamilton resigned his Professorship of Midwifery at the University in the autumn of 1839. Simpson, writing to the Lord Provost, Magistrates and Town Council, from his lodgings, 1 Dean Terrace, on November 15, 1839, sent in his application for the post. Elections to Edinburgh Professorships were then terrible affairs. The electors, who were the thirty-three members of the Edinburgh Town Council, could know little of the candidates' suitability for the post, therefore personal considerations and especially politics operated powerfully. It was not long since James Wilson (Christopher North), who knew no moral philosophy, was elected by two to one against the famous philosopher, Sir William Hamilton. With the energy so characteristic of him, Simpson threw himself into the work of canvassing, and collecting support in every way he could, he speaks of having canvassed and written for nearly seventy consecutive hours. His youth and his being unmarried were urged against him. He had been betrothed for some time to Miss Jessie Grindlay of Liverpool; to get rid of the second objection he wrote to her father honestly telling him that he was in debt to his brothers for over £300, but that as his prospects of practice were very good he believed he could " maintain a wife respectably," would his future father-in-law give consent to an immediate marriage ? He did, and Simpson married Miss Grindlay on December 26, 1839. The contest for the Chair was keen and bitter. His serious opponent was Dr. Kennedy of Dublin, of whom it was said that he was a poor lecturer. To dispel this opinion his supporters persuaded him to give a lecture, his doing so did no harm to Simpson who on February 4, 1840, received 17 votes to 16 recorded for Kennedy. Every voter voted. The battle had been extremely strenuous, Simpson left no stone unturned, he collected every testimonial he could, printed them and spread them broadcast. His election expenses were £500. Unfortunately he had been vehemently opposed by Syme and all his future colleagues at the University; they did not wish the appointment to go to a youngster, the son of a baker, therefore he began his duties in an atmosphere of unfriendliness amounting often to hostility. Misunderstandings were frequent; he writes of having to battle with his brother Professors.

His new position and his marriage prompted him to move into a larger house, more suitable for his increasing practice; he went to 22 Albany Street. A carriage became a necessity, he insured his life for £2,000. The expense of all this was met by a loan from his father-in-law on which he paid interest. In October 1840 his first child, a daughter, was born.

The extramural lectures were discontinued and in November 1840 began those which he delivered as Professor. They were an immense success, he received £600 for the first course. Unhappily he had not come to love his colleagues, who certainly did not love him, for he writes :

It is very satisfactory to have beat in the race not only my friends in the Medical Faculty, but all the thirty bald and grey-headed professors. Dr. Alison who changed his hour to lecture at the same one with me, has a very small class. Don't he deserve it ? He has broken his own head and missed mine.

For success in practice industry, experience and painstaking thoroughness are required and in addition, the gift, given to certain persons, of inspiring confidence, the ability properly to value and apply all the evidence as to the nature of his malady which each separate patient presents, and lastly the insight to appreciate how different persons react to the same disorder. Simpson possessed all these qualities, hence his practice was enormous. It was chiefly concerned with midwifery, to a less extent with gynæcology and to some degree with general medicine. The hotel keepers in Edinburgh had derived much money from patients who came from afar to consult Hamilton ; the appointment of so young a successor filled them with dismay, but they soon found he was worth far more ; when Simpson died they lost many thousands of pounds. By the time he was thirty he was keeping two horses and attending many aristocratic ladies. Three years later he writes, " I have been exceedingly fortunate in getting the Princess as a patient because it quietly places me at the top of the practice on this side of the Tweed." This was Princess Marie of Baden, wife of the Duke of Hamilton. Letters to his relatives mention Duchesses, Marchionesses and Countesses in numbers among his patients. At the age of thirty-three his income was well over £4,000 a year and it grew rapidly after this. His debts were all paid. He bought a house, 52 Queen Street, for £2,150 and enlarged it considerably. He travelled professionally all over Great Britain ; we find him several times at the house of the Duchess of Sutherland in London, in the north of Scotland and many other distant places ; often these visits for confinements occupied some days. At home he saw patients from one o'clock till 5 p.m. and sometimes later. Attempts to restrict the number of patients failed.

Not long after Simpson had started in practice Sir Robert Christison called on him on a professional matter ; he writes :

Simpson was at this period in the full swing of his marvellous practice. When I called for him, his two reception-rooms were, as usual, full of patients, more were seated in the lobby, female faces stared from all the windows in vacant expectancy, and a lady was ringing at the door bell. But the doctor brushed through the crowd to join me, and left them all kicking their heels at their leisure for the next two hours.

Such a large practice ought to have been conducted by method, but he had none, he kept no visiting list, some patients complained that they were neglected, some doctors, who sent him patients, were made to wait a long while before they heard from him, but it is only fair to say that the discontented were a very small proportion of those who consulted him. His professional success led to his being appointed, in 1847, one of Her Majesty's physicians in Scotland. In 1848 several of the staff of St. Bartholomew's Hospital in London suggested that he should be a candidate for the vacant chair of midwifery there, but he declined. He was not a money-grubber; very many times he returned fees; he willingly helped all sorts of people, often throwing his money away because he had not enquired into the circumstances of the application. It is noteworthy that although when poor he was careful of money and kept accounts, when he had abundance he was exceedingly careless, he would take anybody's advice about investments, consequently he lost a great part of his earnings. It is pathetic to read in a letter to his son at Cambridge in 1867 that he is in great distress, for he has squandered much money in some manufacturing business, which money he ought to have saved so that his son could support the baronetcy.

When he was at the height of his fame every visitor to Edinburgh who was anybody brought an introduction to him. He kept open house at luncheon-time, for he was hospitable to all visitors and especially cordial to members of his own profession. Ten, twenty or even fifty people, statesmen, noblemen, doctors, scientists, artists, clergymen and politicians from all over the world were assembled at the table awaiting their host, whose busy professional life always made him late. The atmosphere was chill till he came, then, under his genial influence, all tongues were set talking and the meal progressed enjoyably. Lunch over, all quickly dispersed, for Simpson had crowds of patients waiting for him. During the daytime his house was more like a busy public office than a home.

He was a good operator, full of resource. The tale is told that on one occasion, the chloroform bottle was knocked over and broken during an operation. Simpson at once cut out the piece of carpet on which it was all spilled, put this over the patient's face and thus the operation was completed. It has already been mentioned that he was an excellent lecturer, he was also an admirable teacher in the wards.

Before the days of anæsthetics every doctor must have prayed for the discovery of some means of deadening the awful pain of operations, the only advantage of which was that it forbade unnecessary operations and led to the extraordinary skill of master surgeons. Liston would complete a lithotomy " in two or three minutes at most."

Early in his career Simpson studied mesmerism in the hope of relieving pain during operation by it; he was unaware that Cloquet, in 1829, successfully removed a cancer of the breast of a woman in whom hypnotic analgesia had been induced, and that Esdaile, about two years his senior as a medical student at Edinburgh, was studying mesmerism in India and had, in 1845, painlessly injected a hydrocele in a hypnotized patient and had, in the year following painlessly performed 100 operations—many severe—in the hypnotic state. However, experience has shown hypnotism to be of little use in midwifery, for it is difficult to hypnotize a woman in labour pains.

The attempt to diminish pain by drugs is a practice of great antiquity; opium, Indian hemp and mandragora were often used. The Romans crucified rebels by the thousand, and while on the cross sour wine with drugs in it was given to those crucified to lessen pain. It is thought that the vinegar (sour wine) and hyssop were offered to Christ for this purpose.

A full account of the early history of modern anæsthesia, with extensive references, is given in volume two of F. R. Packard's *The History of Medicine in the United States.* Sir Humphry Davy in 1799 inhaled nitrous oxide gas, he found that it was respirable and that " it absolutely intoxicated me." Next year, after continuing his experiments, he wrote, " as nitrous oxide, in its extensive operation, seems capable of destroying physical pain, it may probably be used with advantage in surgical operations." He is said to have had a tooth pulled out when under this gas. In 1818 Faraday demonstrated that ether produced loss of consciousness and loss of reaction to painful stimuli; in 1824 a young Englishman, Henry Hill Hickman, published a pamphlet entitled *A letter on Suspended Animation showing that it may be Safely Employed during Operations on Animals, with a view to Ascertaining its Probable Utility in Surgical Operations on the Human Subject*. He produced unconsciousness in animals by the exclusion of air, with the inhalation of carbon dioxide and later nitrous oxide. No one in England paid any attention to him, so he went to Paris in 1828, and tried to get his methods investigated by the Académie de Médecine, but failed; he returned to England and died a disappointed man in 1829. In 1844, Horace Wells, an American dentist, heard a lecture on nitrous oxide, next day he gave himself the gas and allowed Dr. Riggs to pull out one of his teeth while under it.

Ether was first used by Dr. C. W. Long in 1842 when he removed a small cystic tumour under it, no pain was felt; in 1848 he read a paper on the subject. In 1846 Morton, a dentist, extracted a tooth while the patient was under ether, in the same year he painlessly removed a tumour from the neck in the same way. Oliver Wendell Holmes hearing of this wrote to suggest the name " Anæsthetic " for the drug. It is to him, therefore, we owe this common word.

On December 21, 1846, in University College Hospital, London, Liston amputated a thigh, and removed by evulsion both sides of the great toe-nail while the patients were under ether, and on January 19, 1847, Simpson, for the first time, used it in midwifery; in the *Monthly Journal of Medical Sciences* for March 1847 he published a paper with the title *Notes on Sulphuric Ether in the Practice of Midwifery*, in which he writes: " I am not aware that anyone has hitherto ventured to test its applicability to the practice of Midwifery. . . . Within the last few months I have had opportunities of using the inhalation of ether, in many cases of great difficulty, as well as in ordinary cases." These " Notes " were reprinted and widely distributed to doctors at home and abroad, so anxious was he to make known that the pains of labour could be eased by anæsthetics. He was full of enthusiasm and early noticed " some of the inconveniences pertaining to sulphuric ether, particularly its disagreeable and persistent smell, its occasional tendency to irritation of the bronchi during its first inspirations and the large quantity of it required." Therefore, during the summer and autumn of 1847, he and his assistants, Dr. George Keith and Dr. Matthews Duncan, met at his house in Queen Street on many nights to inhale " several chemical liquids of a more fragrant or agreeable odour." Mr. Waldie suggested that chloroform should be investigated. Duncan and Flockhart supplied some. It lay in Simpson's house several days before it was tried because such " a heavy, unvolatile liquid" did not look promising. Late at night, on November 4, 1847, the trio met as usual in the dining-room, after a hard day's work, to resume their inhalation of various drugs out of tumblers. The first experiments led to nothing, then chloroform was remembered; Simpson dis-interred the bottle of it from among a heap of waste paper, each tumbler was charged with it, Simpson was the first to inhale, seeing that no harm followed the others breathed the drug.

Immediately an unwonted hilarity seized the inhalers; they became bright eyed, very happy and very loquacious, expatiating on the delicious aroma of the new fluid. The conversation was of unusual intelligence and quite charmed the listeners—some ladies of the family and a naval officer, brother-in-law of Dr. Simpson. But suddenly there was a talk of sounds being heard like those of a cotton mill.

In a moment all was quiet, then there was a crash as all three fell from their chairs. As Simpson came round he said to himself " This is far stronger and better than ether," he then noticed that he was prostrate on the floor, that Matthews Duncan was snoring heavily and that Keith was violently kicking the table above him. Mrs. Simpson and others present were in a state of con-fusion and alarm. Nevertheless, the ardour of the experimenters led to several more trials that eventful night. They " were so satisfied with the results that the festivities of the evening did not terminate till the late hour, 3 a.m." His niece Miss Petrie who was present joined in inhaling the drug, as she fell asleep she cried out, "I am an angel. Oh, I am an angel." What a dramatic story of a great discovery.

Simpson's impulsiveness to find a better anæsthetic than ether made him rashly bold, he never tried any drug on animals before experimenting on himself. Playfair, the chemist, says he came to his laboratory and wanted to inhale some liquid there and then, but Playfair insisted that it should be first tried on two rabbits who quickly died under it. Once after swallowing some decoction Simpson was insensible for two hours; on another occasion, after the discovery of chloroform, he tried on himself a substance which brought on such irritation of breathing that he had to be kept under chloroform to relieve him. He tried the effect of drinking a mixture of aerated water with chloroform, the butler gave the cook some; she fell down insensible and he rushed to fetch Simpson to revive her. It really was a great piece of good luck that no fatal tragedy followed all these experiments.

The first child to be born under the influence of chloroform was the daughter of a doctor, she was christened Anæsthesia; when she was 17 she sent her photograph to Simpson, who with pride hung it over his desk. The initiatory public demonstration of the use of chloroform was at the Edinburgh Infirmary on November 15, 1847. A boy, four or five years old, was to be operated on by Professor Miller. When Simpson held a handkerchief, on which some chloroform had been sprinkled, to his face, he became frightened and wrestled to be away. He was gently held by Simpson and obliged to inhale. After a few inspirations he ceased to cry or move and fell into a sound snoring sleep. Nearly the whole of the radius was necrosed and was extracted. Not the slightest evidence of pain was given, the child was carried back to the ward sound asleep, when he awoke he said he had felt no pain. Two other severe operations were performed under chloroform immediately after that on the child, in these Simpson poured the chloroform into a hollow sponge, in neither was any pain felt. " A great collection of professional gentlemen and students witnessed these results, and among the number was Professor Dumas of Paris, the chemist who first ascertained and established the chemical composition of chloroform."

A pamphlet by Simpson at once appeared with the title *Account of a New Anæsthetic Agent, as a Substitute for Sulphuric Ether, in Surgery and Midwifery*. It was inscribed to Dumas. Four thousand copies were sold in a few days and many thousands afterwards. Liston from London wrote immediately in praise of chloroform, saying, " Simpson deserves all laudation." Other doctors and surgeons congratulated him; the general public got to hear of chloroform quickly, for on November 27 the Duchess of Argyll sent congratulations from herself and the Duke, and in December Lord Blantyre wrote asking for some to give to the local doctor. Six years later the use of chloroform was greatly helped by its employment by the Queen. Simpson received a letter from Sir James Clark, one of her physicians, saying:

The Queen had chloroform exhibited to her during her late confinement. . . . It acted admirably. It was not at any time given so strongly as to render the Queen insensible, and an ounce of chloroform was scarcely consumed during the whole time. Her Majesty was greatly pleased with the effect, and she certainly never has had a better recovery.

Of course opposition arose to anæsthesia in general and chloroform in particular. People who will attack any innovation, however true and beneficent it may be, always have existed and always will exist. I know of Englishmen who believe the world to be flat. Some of the loudest detractors were those who, taking their stand on Genesis iii. 16, " I will greatly multiply thy sorrow and thy conception; in sorrow thou shalt bring forth children," proclaimed that it was immoral to use anything to relieve the pains of childbirth. I have met such people in my own lifetime. Simpson rushed into print at once to show their folly, pointing out that a deep sleep fell upon Adam before the rib was taken out of his side and quoting texts against them. He made several excursions into the lay press, for example, a man died after chloroform, the coroner's verdict was that death was due to this. Simpson immediately wrote to the newspaper to show that it was not. He was opposed by some of his own profession, but he quickly got together statistics which indicated that the mortality of amputation of the thigh was halved by the use of chloroform, indeed the advantage of anæsthesia for operations was so obvious that the professional objections were merely silly. Simpson was one of those who really seemed to enjoy a fight. Directly anyone opposed anæsthesia Simpson pounced on him like a terrier on a rat. All this pungent and prolonged controversy meant publicity for anæsthesia, those who attacked it promoted its adoption.

It was nearly fifty years before any better way of inducing anæsthesia than by chloroform was discovered. During this time, because of chloroform, surgery advanced enormously; operations not previously feasible were undertaken and all surgery was rendered painless. The two who have made modern surgery possible are Lister and Simpson. The last has also relieved the pain of childbirth.

He recounted, before the Medico-Chirurgical Society of Edinburgh in 1848, some experiments made to try to discover a local anæsthetic; he used chloroform and various gases including carbonic acid gas, and although some numbing was produced, it was quite insufficient for use in operations.

Messrs. Duncan and Flockhart have kindly given me the following account of their sales of Chloroform—the figure after each year is pounds of chloroform: 1859, 13,901; 1862, 28,307; 1867, 36,000; 1895, 121,212; 1905, 148,122; 1915, 267,500. Two facts are of interest: firstly the continuous advance in the sale of chloroform; secondly the large amount sold in 1915 owing to the War, for, from the first, it was maintained that chloroform was particularly suited to military surgery in war time.

Since the beginning of medicine surgeons have been greatly troubled by the difficulty of stopping bleeding from wounds, including those due to operations. Even when it seemed arrested, dangerous and often fatal secondary hæmorrhage might take place. In Simpson's day local styptic drugs, the cautery, torsion and ligatures were all used and all were unsatisfactory. He made many trials of various ligatures particularly those of wire, but finally hit upon the original and ingenious plan of passing a needle through the tissues across the artery, which was thus compressed by the needle above it and the tissues below it. This he called acupressure, which in a paper read before the Royal Society of Edinburgh on December 19, 1859, he described as a new hæmostatic process founded on the temporary metallic compression of arteries. Later, in 1864, he published a book on the subject. It is certainly an efficient method; for a time it it was much used, but, as improvements in ligatures came along, it was gradually discarded. The word acupressure is now often absent from text-books on surgery. Syme was furious with him for trespassing into surgery. He came into the operating theatre with a copy of Simpson's original paper, called for an operating knife, cut the pamphlet to shreds before the assembled students, threw the remains into the sawdust, saying: "there, gentlemen, is what acupressure is worth."

This was not Simpson's only trespass into surgery. For the last twenty years of his life he repeatedly called attention to the terribly high mortality after operations in hospitals; he diligently collected statistics and showed that the mortality after limb amputations was four times as high in hospitals as in private practice. As he truly said the man on a hospital operating table was exposed to a greater chance of death than was a soldier on the field of Waterloo. Therefore he advocated new airy hospitals, if possible in the country. It was left to Lister to show the reason of the high hospital mortality, but Simpson's powerful advocacy was of help in hospital reform.

Thompson resigned the chair of Pathology in 1842. Syme and others tried to get it abolished. Simpson threw himself into the argument with his usual vigour; he thought it should be retained. The Crown referred the question to the Town Council, who decided to retain it, and Willian Henderson received the chair. It was an unfortunate choice, because not long after he became a homœopathist. This raised another fierce storm in Edinburgh. Henderson resigned his post of physician to the infirmary. At the first meeting of the Medico-Chirurgical Society for the session 1851-2, Syme moved that the public profession of homœopathy should disqualify from becoming a member or remaining a member of the Society. Simpson seconded in a long speech. On many other occasions during the quarrel he wrote and spoke, finally publishing a book against Homœopathy which reached its third edition in 1862. It was dedicated to Stokes of Dublin. Its compilation must have cost the author much time, for it teems with references, many of them quaint and out of the way.

Simpson took an interest in the spread of cholera, suggesting it was by the water supply. He wrote to propose the stamping out of small pox by (1) notification, (2) isolation in hospital of all notified cases till their power of infection has passed, (3) patients only to be attended by those who, having had the disease or having been vaccinated against it, cannot have it, (4) proper purification and disinfection during and after the disease by water, chlorine, carbolic acid or suphurous acid, of rooms, beds, and clothes used by the sick and the attendants. The same method he says might be applied to other diseases. His mention of chlorine and carbolic acid is noteworthy when we remember the part they were soon to play in surgery.

He was a voluminous writer. His many contributions to the literature of gynæcology were of value for their excellent teaching, the result of unusually large experience; he was ingenious in his improvement of instruments. The chief of his medical works were published in three large volumes after his death under the editorship of Dr. Watt Black, Sir Walter Simpson his son, and Alexander Simpson his nephew, who succeeded him in the chair of midwifery.

Outside his profession, his pastime was the study of archæology. He was President of the Society of Antiquaries of Scotland and a member of several Archæological societies. The chief of his archæological papers were published in two handsome volumes in 1872 under the editorship of John Stuart. Those of most interest to doctors were " on Leprosy and Leper Hospitals in Scotland and England," " Was the Roman army provided with medical officers," and " Antiquarian notices of Syphilis in Scotland." Here again the reader must be astonished at the very many references showing wide research.

His fame spread far. The King of Denmark, hearing the word Edinburgh, remarked that was the place where Simpson lived. He was made an honorary member of an immense number of foreign and British medical societies; he was President of the Edinburgh College of Physicians and of the Edinburgh Medico-Chirurgical Society; he was foreign Associate of the Imperial Academy of Medicine of France, his name was not on the list of candidates submitted, nevertheless the members insisted on his election; he received the honorary D.C.L. of Oxford and in 1866 he was created a baronet, having twice before refused a title; ten years earlier he was awarded the Monthyon prize of two thousand francs for " the most important benefits done to humanity." Towards the end of his life he received the Freedom of the City of Edinburgh, he was a candidate for, but did not obtain, the post of Principal of the University.

On February 12, 1870, he went to London to give evidence in a divorce case; finding the trial postponed for four days he came back to Edinburgh to see patients in the country, then took train to London and gave his evidence. Between York and Edinburgh, on his return, he was so ill that he had to lie on the floor of the carriage. A few days later he was called to a patient in Perth; this journey fatigued him greatly and when he came home he took to his bed. Patients were not to be denied, many were seen in his sick-room, some even being carried there. Gradually he failed and death came on May 6, 1870. Burial in Westminster Abbey was offered but declined by the family; his grave is in Warriston Cemetery, and there is a bust of him in the east aisle of the north transept of Westminster Abbey. It is next to the statue of Mrs. Siddons. No work was done in Edinburgh on the afternoon of May 13, the University and Stock Exchange were closed, all flags were at half mast, for on that day the funeral took place in the presence of thirty thousand people, nearly two thousand followed the hearse. Next Sunday references to Simpson were made from nearly all Edinburgh pulpits and a special densely crowded service was held in the Free Church Assembly Hall. The Queen wrote to express her sorrow. Scores of obituary notices appeared and numerous public bodies sent letters of condolence.

Simpson's talents were entirely practical. He was not a thinker, which is as well, for he gave himself little time for thought; he was always rushing. His home practice was a rush, tearing about the country to see patients was a rush, he rushed into print, he rushed his scanty holidays, calling them scampers; if there was time after a country consultation he rushed off to see ancient stones and buildings, and he rushed into controversy in which he excelled and which he continued till he was victorious. Edinburgh was a quarrelsome place. Simpson was only twenty-eight when he had an unimportant quarrel with Dr. Lewins which nearly ended in a duel. Syme was often in angry dispute, and when he applied to be surgeon to the Royal Infirmary he was not appointed lest Liston and he should quarrel openly in the hospital. He strongly opposed Simpson's appointment to the chair of midwifery; he took an opposite side to him on the question of the continuance of the chair of pathology; he attacked Simpson's professional competence. All this led to replies from Simpson. In 1850 he got a poisoned wound in the finger, an abscess in the armpit followed; Syme was called in and for a time their antipathies were healed. But this led to another feud because Professor Miller thought he should have been consulted and an enormous battle between him and Simpson ensued. Two years late Simpson entered another controversy to defend Syme, who had been attacked at the annual meeting of the British Medical Association for performing the operation of urethrotomy. Simpson wrote many letters calling the attack " groundless vituperation." We have seen that he joined Syme in the crusade against homœopathy, and also that, alas, the quarrel between these two broke out again violently over acupressure and led to more contentious writing and even a large book. These were but a fraction of Simpson's many controversies; the time and fighting energy he spent on them was extraordinary. It is doubtful whether he was ever defeated.

Not only his face but his whole appearance helped to his fortune. From the crown of a large head untidy curly hair hung down, framing a refined and kindly countenance. The forehead was both high and broad, the loquacious, penetrating eyes looked at you with tenderness, sympathy and humour, the upper lip was delicate, although firm, both lips were usually expressing a friendly smile. He was of nearly average height, with a broad massive frame. There was nothing remarkable about his hands except that his sense of touch was singularly delicate. After looking at his portrait you feel that, if you had seen him, you would have noticed him at once as a remarkable man.

SIR JAMES PAGET

No one in the nineteenth century occupied a more leading position in the medical profession than Sir James Paget. Surgeons, scientists and the general public all looked upon him in reverent admiration, for his work, his writing, his speaking and his character. He had no enemies; nobody was jealous of him.

Happily he wrote his own memoirs, which were edited and amplified by that charming writer, his son Stephen. Samuel Paget, James's father, born at Yarmouth in 1774, was an active, handsome, refined, honest man with much busy energy. After leaving school he became a clerk in the office of Mr. Kerridge, a merchant in the town, who contracted for the supply of provisions to His Majesty's ships, of which there were usually several off Yarmouth. This Kerridge died suddenly. Young Samuel, although only 17 years old, immediately posted to London and interviewed the authorities at the Admiralty so favourably that he was allowed to continue the contracts, to do which he had to borrow money. He was successful; Lord Duncan, after the battle of Camperdown, said, at a banquet held in Yarmouth, that the victory was due to Samuel Paget, to whom a gold medal was given. Wealth followed, a large house was built, a carriage was kept, much expensive hospitality was dispensed and he was made Mayor of Yarmouth. After a while the business went downhill, he and his family became poor, all their fine trappings were sold. Samuel, however, lived on till he died at 82 of old age, that most rare of all causes of death.

His wife, whom he married in 1799, was Miss Tolver, an accomplished, handsome lady, who played her part in her husband's life well, keeping his large house, assisting at his hospitality and taking an interest in local affairs. She was a woman of wonderful industry; she knitted a bed quilt six feet square all in one piece; she collected everything—autographs, seals, caricatures, shells, corals, agates, china, glass and curiosities of all kinds. Each separate collection was arranged in order and labelled by herself. She studied painting under old Crome, learning to imitate his style so well that her pictures could be sold as his. Of this marriage there were seventeen children, of whom nine—seven boys and two girls—grew up to full age. She was an excellent mother to them all, putting aside everything, when necessary, for them; if they were away she punctually wrote to them in her beautiful handwriting. The last two years of her life she was speechless and partially paralysed, but she never complained either then or when the family fortune declined.

The three elder of the seven brothers, Frederick, Arthur and George, went to Charterhouse, having Thackeray among their friends there. Arthur Pendennis is said to be drawn from Arthur Paget. George, who went to Cambridge, was bracketed eighth wrangler, obtained a medical Fellowship at Caius and was ultimately Regius Professor of Medicine at Cambridge. "In all the family there was not one who did not show power and strong will for work; not one who was ever unfair, stupid or dishonest."

James was born on January 11, 1814. Like all his brothers he went to a school in Yarmouth kept by a Mr. Bowles who had been an actor and was then a Unitarian minister. The best to be said of the education he received was that it was fair for what it cost—eight guineas a year. He learned enough Latin and Greek for commonplace understanding, but never acquired anything that could be called classical knowledge. By the time he was thirteen his father had begun to lose money, therefore James could not go to a public school. At his own wish it was decided that he should go into the Navy and he studied for this purpose, but, at the last moment, although some of the uniform had been bought, the intention was given up, upon the urgent entreaties of his mother. This was fortunate, for no one could be more unfitted for the Navy than James Paget.

On March 9, 1830, he, after the payment of a premium of 100 guineas, became, for four and a half years, the apprentice of Mr. Charles Costerton, an active, energetic, well-educated practitioner in Yarmouth. His time was chiefly occupied in dispensing, seeing a few out-patients, in receiving messages and, at Christmas, making out bills. It is interesting to read of the charges. An ounce draught cost a shilling, a pint of mixture five shillings, leeches sixpence, bleeding five shillings or half a guinea. Paget had ample leisure, Costerton and a young surgeon named Randall helped him to learn about bones, he dissected amputated limbs and, at the end of his four and a half years, had learned about as much anatomy as a hospital student would acquire in a year. He read many medical books and taught himself French, but he was always of opinion that four and a half years was too long for apprenticeship. Outside professional subjects he drew, and drew well; he used to tell of such a beautiful drawing he made of an ulcerated bowel that the widow of the patient begged for a copy of it. His chief recreation was botanizing. Hours and hours were spent roaming about the country collecting plants and correctly naming them; fortunately there was, in his father's library, Smith and Sowerby's great English Botany in thirty-six volumes. Dawson Turner, the botanist, got to know of him, and spoke well of him to Hooker, the famous botanist, who wrote to Paget suggesting that they should exchange specimens. Charles Paget was at this time studying the insects of the neighbourhood. He and James published in 1834 *A Sketch of the Natural History of Yarmouth and its Neighbourhood.* The book contained the names of 766 insects, 729 flowering plants and 456 non-flowering plants. The introduction, written by James, consists of thirty-two pages and shows his industry, method, observation and thoroughness. He considered this botanical training to have been of great value for his future profession, not only as regards facts, but also as regards method.

In October 1834 he entered as a medical student at St. Bartholomew's and lodged at 9 Charlotte Street, Bloomsbury, with his brother George; George went to live at Cambridge in December, and James then took lodgings with his friend Johnstone at 12 Thavies Inn. George, having a rich fellowship, advanced money to James for his fees, because their father's affairs were now in such a bad way that he could not pay them. George was also able to give James introductions to Cambridge men who came to St. Bartholomew's. In his Memoirs there is an excellent critical account of the medical school of this hospital at this time. " Work was very little helped by either the teachers or the means of study." Paget thinks this was for his good, as it made him work diligently on his own account. Certainly he did this; he rarely went out because he read hard every evening; at the instigation of his friend Johnstone, he taught himself German in order to study anatomical and physiological books in this language. He says: " I cannot overstate the advantage I thus gained, not only in knowledge but in reputation." So rare was a knowledge of German then that he was asked by Marshall Hall to call on him so that he might translate to him what Müller had just published about reflex action. He laboured strenuously in the dissecting-room and dead-house; at the end of his first year he was first in the examinations in Medicine, Surgery, Chemistry and Botany, and he was fortunate, thus early, to make an original discovery. The little specks sometimes seen in human muscle, and before Paget's time called bony spicules, were examined by him with some trouble, for there was not a microscope in the hospital. With a letter of introduction from his friend Dawson Turner, he went to the head of the Natural History Department of the British Museum who also had not a microscope, but sent him on to the head of the botany department who had. He lent it to Paget and thus enabled him to see that each of these specks was a little worm (trichina spiralis) curled up and surrounded by a capsule.

In his second year at the hospital his natural industry, his want of money and his complete lack of interest in games or sport made it easy for him to continue to be the industrious apprentice. At the end of the year he was first in the examinations in Anatomy and Physiology, Clinical Medicine, and Medical Jurisprudence, which last he only crammed up four or five days before the examination. The qualification of M.R.C.S. was obtained in 1836. One of his examiners was Sir Astley Cooper, who, being a Yarmouth man, asked young Paget to breakfast.

The question of what to do now arose. Nothing was settled, he " drifted " back from Yarmouth, where he had gone for a holiday, to London in October 1836, to try to maintain himself, if he could. In this very month the seemingly imprudent act of engaging himself to Miss Lydia North, the youngest daughter of the Rev. Henry North, was committed. But, says he, " No human wisdom could have devised a step so wise as was this rash engagement" for, during the more than seven years before he could marry, it gave him "help and hope enough to make even the heaviest work seem light." A pupil was taken at £10 a month, but the youth's idleness so wearied Paget that he dismissed him and went to Paris with £10 which his father gave him. Returning to London he tried coaching without success. Things looked black until he got a place on the staff of the *Medical Gazette*, of which he was sub-editor from 1837 to 1842. He wrote leaders, reviewed books, translated—for this he learned Dutch and Italian—and reported lectures. The pay was only £50 to £70 a year. Journalistic work of the same kind was done for the *Quarterly Review* and many articles were written in the *Penny Cyclopædia* and the *Biographical Dictionary*. Only those who have done it can know the grim drudgery of this hack writing; it used to take him to between one and two in the morning, if he had an evening off he wrote till three the next night. For several years during his long waiting period he was Curator of the Museum at St. Bartholomew's, earning thereby £40 a year: "Probably I would not have taken the place but for the need of money." It was dreadfully underpaid, the hours 12 to 4 except on Saturdays. He speaks of the weariness of the occupation, putting up specimens, preparing diagrams for surgery lectures, getting bodies for dissection and many other pieces of jobwork. In 1839 he was made Demonstrator of Morbid Anatomy; soon after, at the request of the students, he lectured on the subject, introducing the method of lecturing on actual specimens from the post-mortem room. These lectures were popular, but all this morbid anatomy teaching was unpaid, he only got a handsome silver tea-service, an address and a good dinner. His practice was minute, from £3 to £14 a year. Two bitter disappointments came close together. He was promised a Demonstratorship of Anatomy, regarded as a sure road to an Assistant Surgeoncy, this promise led to a row, for the custom was that apprentices who were articled to surgeons at a fee of 500 guineas had a prior claim. The Governors upheld their claim, consequently the offer to Paget was withdrawn. He began to write a book on General Anatomy. He submitted the early chapters to publishers, who declined the proposed volume. These were seven dreary years, average income £170, of which fifty guineas went in rent for his rooms in Searle Street, no opportunity of learning surgery, except that in 1841 he was elected to the small post of Surgeon to the Finsbury Dispensary, which he resigned in 1843. " Nothing but what might be called thoughtlessness—a happy state of mind which, to many who are healthy and rather over-worked, is better than patience—would have held me in my place."

The first small sign of better things was in 1842, when he was appointed to assist Stanley in cataloguing the specimens at the College of Surgeons' Museum, this enabled him to give up the *Medical Gazette* which " had long stunk in his nostrils." The catalogue occupied some hours daily for seven years. He described every specimen as he saw it before him, putting down nothing but what could be then and there seen, this being the only way to make a scientific catalogue. He now also began to write annual reports on physiology for the *British and Foreign Medical Review*. These, as Michael Foster says, show how admirably he kept himself abreast of the latest knowledge.

His Memoirs often tell of the low ebb to which the Medical School of St. Bartholomew's fell about a century ago. The authorities determined on extensive reorganization. A separate lectureship on physiology was founded; Paget, in May 1843, obtained the post. His voice was good, his lectures were extempore, great trouble and wide reading went to the preparation of them. They were well attended and must have reached an audience of many thousands, for they supplied nearly all the material of the first edition of that famous book Kirkes' *Physiology*. He became so well known as an excellent speaker and lecturer that it is of interest to read his advice, which is, that if you are born with the gift of fluent extempore speech, as he was, do not let it run away with you so that you speak too often, studiously prepare every speech, even to learning by heart the important passages, and be careful, as in writing, always to choose just the right word.

The Governors of St. Bartholomew's Hospital, in the same year, started a students' residential college, on the lines of a college at Oxford or Cambridge. Paget was appointed War-den. This made a complete change from the lonely life of the previous seven years, when he had dined by himself in a chop house, or in his rooms off a joint which lasted many days. Now he dined in the company of twenty or more students with varied food and much talk. Journalism was discarded. Gradually the general supervision of all students came to him; he was soon the treasurer of the school, in which, now and onwards, the numbers of students increased greatly. He was in this year selected as one of the three hundred original Fellows of the College of Surgeons.

The long engagement ended in May 1844 when he and Miss North were married. One day sufficed for a honeymoon, after which the pair came to rooms in the college and soon to a small adjacent house, called the Warden's House, where they remained for another seven years. It was a very happy marriage. Paget in the evening always worked in the family room with his wife, children and visitors all talking or playing music. He says, " I have never once had to leave my family or any quiet party of friends in order to work alone and undisturbed."

At the age of 33 Paget was made Assistant Surgeon to St. Bartholomew's on the ground, according to him, that he was useful to the school and ready to work hard at anything. " This same year I was elected, to my great surprise, Professor of Anatomy and Surgery to the Royal College of Surgeons." It was a great and rare honour. The lectures given were on *General Pathology.* They were largely attended, printed as given in the *Medical Times and Gazette,* and finally published as his famous *Lectures on Surgical Pathology.* The Pathological Catalogue of the College of Surgeons, containing just such a description as a catalogue should give of 3,520 specimens, was finished in 1849. Three years previously he had published his *Records of Harvey,* which not only show his skill in writing, but his great love for his hospital which he liked to describe as the oldest, the largest, the richest and the best hospital in London. His affection for it was deep and endured to the end of his life. Everyone knows the tale that once when Abernethy, the Bartholomew's surgeon, entered the lecture theatre at the beginning of a new session, he looked at the students and exclaimed, " Good God, what is to become of you all ? " Paget, with the help of Callender and Thomas Smith, tried to answer the question by laboriously tracing a thousand students. The statistical results may be found in the *St. Bartholomew's Hospital*

Reports for 1869. The essay ends with this conclusion, characteristic of Paget: "Nothing appears more certain than that the personal character, the very nature, the will of each student has far greater force in determining his career than any helps or hindrances whatever." In 1850 a paper by him *On the Freezing of the Albumen of Eggs* appeared in the *Philosophical Transactions*, and the year after he was elected to the Fellowship of the Royal Society.

Paget had by his industry, his excellent teaching, his admirable writing and by the fact that under his wardenship the number of students at St. Bartholomew's had doubled itself, attained the fine position of being "the first man of his day." Nevertheless it was clear that a change must be made, for he was exhausted by overwork—no bed before one, breakfast finished by eight—and he could not bring up a family on the five or six hundred a year he was earning. So he started practice in 24 Henrietta Street, Cavendish Square, at the age of 38. In the beginning it was difficult to make ends meet, but, except for setbacks owing to illness, all went well; by 1878 he was earning over £10,000 a year. He then gave up operating, restricting himself to consultations. Such was the eminence he had attained that it was quite common for a patient, about to be operated upon by another surgeon, to ask that Paget might be present so that he could be consulted if unforeseen difficulties should arise during the operation. The first fee I earned was in 1879, when I went with Sir Henry Howse, to whom I was dresser, to assist him at a lithotomy on a patient in a London suburb. Sir James Paget was present. He says his practice was not due to self-advertisement, sheer impudence, unfairness or greediness, but to the good opinion of his fellow practitioners; this, as he truly writes, is the finest kind of consulting practice, incomparably superior to that due to public notoriety.

In 1858 he moved to Harewood Place, it was a risk, but it succeeded. Life, with any consultant, is a series of risks. If Paget had died at 47 his family would have been left in extreme poverty, and if he had died before 60 they would have been poor. He took his full share of gratuitous patients, and of professional duties such as committees and societies; the hospital occupied two hours daily. An average working day was sixteen hours long, much to do on Sundays, and from 5,000 to 8,000 miles to be travelled in a year. He acquired the knack of writing in the train. Four times, during active practice, he had pneumonia, but fear of losing fees forbade a holiday. " I am on every ground of interest that I can see, utterly averse from leaving home, and I shall fight against the prescription to the last." His first holiday was in 1861, the year in which he became full surgeon at St. Bartholomew's ; the family did not go away together till 1868. The reason for this demoniac slavery was that, not only had he to keep his family and pay off debts incurred on his own behalf, but in addition he, in association with his brothers, was determined to pay with full interest the heavy debts left by his father ; the last instalment of these was paid in 1862.

His deep knowledge of pathology led to his being consulted about rare diseases and those difficult of diagnosis. The feeling existed that you could not have a better opinion than that of Paget, nor could you go to a wiser man. Hence his enormous practice, hence, too, his appointments to Queen Victoria for forty-one years, and to the Prince of Wales for thirty-six years. The natural charm he possessed led to his being a friend of the Royal family ; he went abroad with the Prince and Princess and stayed with them in this country ; they came round St. Bartholomew's with him ; the Prince attended Paget's Hunterian oration, the attachment lasted, for his wife notes that in 1880 he went to dine with the Prince and he and the Princess visited him in the last year of his life. His Memoirs are dedicated, by permission, to Queen Alexandra.

Many doctors have died as a direct result of their occupation ; Paget nearly did. In February 1871 he, his surgical registrar and his house surgeon made a post-mortem examination at the hospital. Young, the house surgeon, cut his hand ; Paget insisted that he should wash in hot water and suck the wound ; he did and was not taken ill. Paget and Bloxam, the registrar, continued the examination. Neither was cut nor scratched, yet both nearly died of blood-poisoning. After his recovery he gave a clinical lecture on his own case, unique, he said, because although he had been attended by ten doctors he recovered. Such a severe illness suggested the wisdom of giving up active hospital duties. He did this and was made consulting surgeon, a baronetcy was conferred upon him, and his friends gave him the beautiful portrait which Millais had painted.

Strenuous practice continued: "A very full day's work; then at the Medico-Chirurgical from 7.30 to near 11; then some food and start at midnight for Bradford." Professional posts occupied him: he was President of the College of Surgeons and of the Medico-Chirurgical Society, a member of the General Medical Council (this he disliked as he had little faith in it) and a member of the Senate of the London University. Time was found for original work such as the publication of his lectures and his paper on osteitis deformans, and also for good annual holidays.

The highest of all his honours was that he was President of the International Medical Congress in 1881, when it met in London, the most successful of its meetings. The committee which arranged it sat for two years previous to it. Paget did not miss a single meeting of this committee. On the opening day, before an audience of three thousand, one third from abroad, he gave his address. There were present the Prince of Wales, the Crown Prince of Germany, Pasteur, Virchow, Koch, Charcot and hosts of other distinguished persons. Sir James and Lady Paget kept open house all the week, three times a day they entertained members of the Congress. To one luncheon-party the two Princes came, also Darwin, Pasteur, Virchow, Huxley and Tyndall. Their host was now 67 years old, no wonder his health again broke down and compelled him to take a holiday in the South of France.

Back again, work again. He read a further paper on osteitis deformans before the Medico-Chirurgical Society, attended the meeting of the British Medical Association at Worcester, and gave the first Bradshaw lecture *On Some New and Rare Diseases.* The year after (1883) he gave an address on Collective Investigation. He was appointed Vice-Chancellor of the University of London. In 1884 he delivered an elaborate lecture on the relation between National Health and National Work, and, in the autumn, attended the International Medical Congress at Copenhagen, where he made speeches and went to dinners and luncheons with Royalties. Incredible as it may seem, he had contrived during the last seven years to prepare, with the help of Goodhart and Doran, a new catalogue of the College of

Surgeons' Museum. The three met at two o'clock on Saturday afternoons, Paget did by far the larger part of it and corrected the proof. This new catalogue was published in 1885; the event was commemorated by the Council of the College placing on the staircase a very fine bust of Sir James by Boehm. He was Chairman of the Commission appointed to investigate the Pasteur treatment of rabies, writing the report himself at the age of 73 and receiving from Pasteur a letter of thanks for it. This report enabled Mr. Long to stamp out hydrophobia in this country. At the same age he was President of the Pathological Society and one of the trustees of Queen Victoria's Jubilee Fund, and therefore he was partly responsible for that great present-day Institution, The Queen's Institute of District Nursing. Next year he actually accepted an invitation to be Chairman of the Commission on Vaccination which sat for seven years and held thirty-nine meetings. In 1890 he attended the International Medical Congress in Berlin; on the occasion of Virchow's seventieth birthday he was Chairman of the Virchow Testimonial Fund. Constant requests for addresses came to him; he must have yielded to most, for he gave so many. All were full of interest—to give one example, speaking of the power of science to satisfy the love of novelty and of wonders, he says he observed that Janotha played 5,995 notes in four minutes and three seconds or rather more than 24 per second; then follows a delightful account of what this must mean. He refused to speak at the Church Congress on vivisection, for he thought it an error for one profession to discuss what it considered the wrong-doings of another, such discussion, he said, would be nonsenical and mischievous.

In 1894 he moved to 4 Park Square West, not putting up a plate. His wife died next year. Very slowly old age overtook him; he died in December 30, 1899, within a few days of being 86 years old. The funeral service was in Westminster Abbey.

More than thirty learned bodies conferred distinctions upon him, perhaps the two he valued most were the Honorary Gold Medal of the Royal College of Surgeons of England, the highest honour the College could give, and his election as a Corresponding Member of the Académie des Sciences. " Charcot telegraphed this to me yesterday; it is, I think, the highest distinction of its kind, the 'blue riband' of science; far more honourable than anything I should have thought that I had fairly earned. I must try to be harmlessly proud of it." He was proposed by Pasteur, who sent him an affectionate letter of congratulation.

Wherever you saw James Paget, you said, there is an outstanding man; his tall thin figure, his beautiful, sensitive, intellectual face commanded your attention, which was still further attracted by the beauty of his voice and diction, by the clearness of his statements, his right choice of words and by the compactness of his speech. He was a really great orator. Bunsen heard his Croonian Lecture—spoken, not read—and said after it, "I never heard eloquence till now." Among his audience for the Hunterian Oration were the Prince of Wales, Mr. Gladstone, the Duke of Argyll, the Duke of Westminster, Dean Stanley, Lord Acton, Mr. Huxley, Mr. Tyndall, Lord Ripon and many other distinguished people. Gladstone divided mankind into two sets: the happy ones who heard the oration and the to-be-pitied ones who had not; he considered it a unique work of art, a miracle of compression. Paget spoke at a particularly brilliant Royal Academy dinner; his and Lowell's speeches were thought the best. At an Alpine Club dinner he explained that he did not know the Alps. "Ah, but," he continued, "there are beauties on the Norfolk broads." These he described so wonderfully that the listeners hung upon his words and, after a pause of surprise, overwhelmed him with applause.

Added to the gifts of face and speech were those of the mind; his clarity of thought, his industry, his freedom from envy, hatred, malice and all uncharitableness, his inability to quarrel, his determination to think of things, not persons, his infinite courtesy, his hospitality, his generosity and his chivalrous disregard of his own health. All these traits contributed to make him the best exponent of the medical profession to the public that there has ever been; they raised the medical school at St. Bartholomew's and endeared him to the students. He never allowed his private engagements to interfere with those at the hospital; one of his last dressers says no student ever missed his lectures on surgery—"he never had a note . . . and every word he said was sweet to listen to." The same qualities which

made the students love him, endeared him to a multitude outside the profession; patients were all ears to listen to him and
anxiously interpreted even his looks. An obstinate woman in
the hospital at first refused to do as he advised, but on seeing
his expression cried out " Oh, Sir, only don't look at me like
that, and I will do whatever you like."

In the earlier part of his professional life he rarely went out,
partly because he had no inclination to do so, but also because
he had to study every evening and he was very poor. Later
he much enjoyed good society; he belonged to Grillion's, the
Club, the Literary Society, the Philosophical Club, Nobody's
and his hospital club. His popularity was due to his qualities
and also to the fact that he never pretended to be anything but
a surgeon; he did not make the common, foolish mistake of
thinking that because he was pre-eminent in his profession,
it followed that his opinion on matters outside it was of importance. Among his friends were Lord Acton, Gladstone, New-
man, Pusey, Ruskin, Tennyson, Browning, George Eliot,
Lowell, Dean Church, Lord Herschell, Holman Hunt, George
Richmond, Romanes, Tyndall, Huxley, Flower, Pasteur, Darwin, Florence Nightingale, Marshall Hall, Bowman, Sharpey,
Virchow, Vrolek, Kolleker and Rokitansky. They met him
either at his clubs, in society or at dinner at his own house.
We find Gladstone and Virchow dining there with him;
another time it was Pasteur, Tyndall, Lord Avebury, Sir George
Buchanan, Lord Reay and Sir Andrew Clark; another, it
was Romanes and Browning, who told the tale that someone
had asked him for an old tie to help to make a patchwork
quilt of the ties of great men. Tennyson would come to read
his poems. George Eliot and Pasteur were especial friends.
Paget was pall-bearer at the funerals of Tennyson and Browning
and was asked to be at that of Darwin, but was prevented from
accepting.

He wrote as he spoke; no higher praise can be given. His
style was like that of Lamb or of Cobbett in his quiet moods.
The *Lectures on Surgical Pathology,* delivered before the Royal
College of Surgeons, were published in 1853; several subsequent editions appeared. This book has become classical, as I
know to my cost, for more than eighty years later when I applied
at the library for the last edition it was out, someone was reading

it. The fame of these Lectures depends upon the accuracy of the descriptions, the frequent appeal to the microscope, the wide reading on the author's part revealed by them, his constant appeal to actual specimens or patients and upon the beauty of the writing which makes them good to read even now. I let the book fall open where it would and found in front of me this description of granulation tissue:

Cells upon cells, such as I have already described, are heaped up together in a layer from half a line to two lines, or, rarely, more in thickness, without apparent order, and connected by very little intermediate substance. Singly they are colourless, but in clusters they are ruddy even independent of the blood-vessels. In granulations that are making healthy progress—in such as, after three or four days' growth, are florid, moist, level, scarcely raised above the surrounding tissues, uniformly granular, or like a surface of minute papillæ—one can conveniently trace the cells in various stages, according to the position they occupy. The deeper-seated ones are always most advanced, and often much elongated and fusiform; while the superficial ones are still in a rudimental state, or, near the edges of the granulating surface, are acquiring the character of epithelial cells.

Is it not a pleasure to read ? Those anxious to hear these lectures were so many that extra seats had to be placed in the theatre. They were published in the *Medical Times and Gazette* as they were delivered, and helped, as much as anything else, to the great advances in morbid anatomy which were made in the last half of the nineteenth century.

He was a supreme clinical lecturer and, what is more, his clinical lectures are admirable to read. They were published in 1875 with the title *Clinical Lectures and Essays* and, being translated into French, won high praise from Pasteur. I have just reread them with enjoyment, some, e.g. those on strangulated hernia and pyæmia, have not the same importance now as then; others should be read to-day, especially those on nervous mimicry and constitutional diseases. Speaking to students, he says, " The reasons for liking to see operations are so many and strong and, for the most part, so bad, that it is useless to argue against them." At the end of the lecture on the Calamities of Surgery we find:

Men constantly say, " These things have happened to better men . . . so I need not be surprised at having them." There is no more miserable or false plea than this. Why, if you know that another man has fallen into a fault, the

blame to you for falling into the same ought to be much greater, not less. . . .
But there are some people who seem to have the happy art of forgetting all their
failures, and remembering nothing but their successes, and, as I have watched
such men in professional life, years have always made them worse instead of
better surgeons. . . . They make their brains like sieves, and they run all the
little things through, and retain all the big ones which they suppose to be their
successes; and a very mischievous heap of rubbish it is that they retain.

Again, at the end of another lecture:

It is among the first necessities for success in practice that, in the total phenomena
of a disease observed in any patient, you should be able to estimate what belongs
to the disease and what to the man. A farmer may as well expect success if
he sows his fields without regard to their soils or to the weeds that may " of themselves " come up in them, as one of us may expect it if we treat diseases without
exactly studying the constitutions of those in whom they occur.

Paget's only original experiment in physiology is recorded
in the *Philosophical Transactions* for 1850 under the title of
Observations on the Freezing of the Albumen of Eggs. Hunter
observed that a living hen's egg may be lowered in temperature
many degrees below 32° F. without freezing, one that was not
living froze at 32° F. He asserted that what prevented the
living egg from freezing was vitality: he was a vitalist. Paget
ingeniously passed a fine probe through a small hole in the
shell of a living egg so as to detach the albumen from the shell,
such an egg froze at 32° F., but nevertheless a living chick
developed. Its vitality clearly was not abolished by freezing;
hence Hunter was wrong and another blow was delivered to
vitalism. Why a living egg did not freeze at 32° F. obviously
depended in some way upon the albumen or its relation to the
shell. This resistance of a living egg to the effect of cold is
remarkable. Paget submitted one egg to a temperature below
5° F. for an hour; nevertheless a perfect chick came out on
incubation.

He gave the Croonian Lecture before the Royal Society in 1857,
On the Cause of the Rhythmic Motion of the Heart, putting forward
the fruitful suggestion that " the time-regulated rhythmic action,
whether of the nervous centre or of the independent contractile
walls is due to their nutrition being rhythmic." Hughlings
Jackson seized this illuminating idea to explain the periodicity
of epilepsy. Paget lectured before the Royal Institution in 1859,
on the same subject, under the title of *The Chronometry of Life,*

and thirty years later he wrote in his *Studies of Old Case Books* an essay on *Errors in the Chronometry of Life*. I have already spoken of the value of Paget's lectures and reviews of physiological literature. He, like Bowman, received the rare honour of being elected an Honorary Member of the Physiological Society.

Two diseases are named after Sir James. In an article, of only three pages, in the *St. Bartholomew's Reports* for 1874 headed *On Disease of the Mammary Areola preceding Cancer of the Mammary Gland,* he describes fifteen cases, in all of which the well-known " Paget's Disease " of the nipple was present, all were followed by cancer, always beginning in the substance of the mammary gland beneath, and not far under the skin disease. He was the first to observe this disease of the nipple which has since been extensively investigated, but its relationship to cancer remains obscure. Two years later he read a paper before the Royal Medico-Chirurgical Society *On a Form of Chronic Inflammation of the Bones* (osteitis deformans). He reminds us that Wilks had shown a case in point twelve years earlier before the Pathological Society, but to Paget must be given the credit of recognizing a new disease, describing it accurately and naming it. He gave an account of seven further cases before the same Society in 1882. Sometimes it is called Paget's Disease of the bones. Descriptions of it, and of Paget's Disease of the nipple, occur in numerous text-books. He was much interested in symmetry. As early as 1841 he read a paper before the Royal Medico-Chirurgical Society on *The Relation between Symmetry and Disease of the Body*, and said that, when uninfluenced by disturbing causes, all general or constitutional diseases affect equally and similarly the corresponding parts on the two sides of the body. This he called the law of symmetry. He returned to the subject in 1880, pointing out that when a leaf takes on an autumnal tint, the change is symmetrical in the two halves of the leaf, and, ten years after this, he was still pondering on the matter.

In his old age, Paget, like most of us, regretted that so little use can be made of Old Case Books, but he did better than others, for when 78 years old he published his last work *Studies of Old Case Books*. It is still read for the clinical wisdom in it. Perhaps the most attractive chapters are those on *Spines suspected of Deformity,* on *Diseases of Structure due to Disturbance of Nerve Force* and that on *Use of the Will for Health.* Girls nowadays are allowed healthy physical development, not so in Paget's time. He was constantly consulted by mothers about their daughters' spines, never their sons'. The boys were allowed to sit as they liked and to take exercise,

prudent things as in the daughters would be deemed shameful. Thus boys spines grow straight; the muscles helping to support them are not overtired, or, when they are, they can be rested in any comfortable posture. But in girls the postures deemed graceful must be maintained till some deformity is discovered or suspected, and then the poor girls must be made miserable by the treatment deemed necessary for its cure.

Every doctor saw numbers of these girls, and it is largely owing to Paget's teaching that girls owe their emancipation from the then fashionable disorder known as a weak spine.

Bound in the same volume are his reflections on what he called the chronometry of life, a subject to which I have already alluded as being of constant interest to him. The observance of time, he says, is characteristic of life, depending essentially on properties inherent in the living bodies themselves, and not on conditions external to them. We have a natural span of years; we do not, in health, die because of change in external conditions of living, we grow, maintain bodily perfection, then degenerate and die. We see the same observance of time in the varying rate of eruption of our different teeth which shows well the punctuality of time. With birds' eggs it is the same, if the eggs of a number of different species be hatched simultaneously in an incubator, each will hatch at its own time. Turtles lay their eggs in the sand, go away, but return at the time the young are hatched. Sleeping and waking are time phenomena and many other instances are given. Paget believes that in the study of pathology we do not sufficiently consider how much of disease or of its variations may be due to disturbance of time rate. He suggests that errors of chronometry, that is to say the unpunctualities of life, may be seen in the fact that some people look older, some younger than their years, in some the hair goes grey early, often the teeth grow faster than the jaws so that they are crowded; sometimes the teeth are delayed, the wisdom teeth may not appear till middle age or later. We meet with old people perfectly healthy except that their digestion has worn out more rapidly than the other bodily functions, or we see tottering old men whose muscles have worn out while their digestion is perfect, and so with other functions. Many of the so-called diseases of old age are, Paget would say, errors in the chronometry of life.

SIR WILLIAM BOWMAN

This distinguished man was remarkable because he obtained great renown in two departments of medicine, and had, by the age of 25, become a famous histologist.

His father, John Eddowes Bowman, a banker at Nantwich, was a botanist and geologist of considerable attainments and a Fellow of the Linnean Society. His mother, Elizabeth, the daughter of William Eddowes of Shrewsbury, was a good draughtswoman and painter of flowers; from both parents therefore he may have inherited his power of accurate observation and execution. William, their third son, was born at Nantwich on July 20, 1816. He and his two brothers were educated at Hazelwood School, near Birmingham. This extraordinary institution was founded at Hill Top by a disciple of Priestley, Thomas Wright Hill, said to have been endowed with every sense except commonsense. By the time Bowman entered it, Rowland Hill, of penny-postage fame, Edwin Hill and two other brothers were assisting their father Thomas. Rowland entirely rebuilt the new school at Hazelwood, being his own architect and clerk of the works. The principle of the school was that the boys were to govern themselves. A constitution and a code of laws were both drawn up by a committee of boys, the last filled a hundred pages. The laws, which demanded rigid punctuality, were strictly enforced. Bad marks could be cleared off by useful work done in play hours. A court of justice was established, with boys for magistrates, jury and constables. This educational system is described in a book by Matthew, Rowland's brother, which was widely reviewed. The surprising thing happened, the school became successful and famous. When he inspected it, Jeremy Bentham threw aside all he had done himself in the way of educational reform. Boys from all over the world, many of them sons of distinguished men, came to it. William Bowman went there at the age of ten years; reports written by Mr. Hill indicate that he thought very highly of the lad, who won many prizes, printed the school magazine and showed himself to be deft with his fingers. Such a school must have had some influence upon him.

The story is told that while there his hand was injured by the explosion of gunpowder with which he was experimenting ; the healing of the wound so interested him that he determined to be a doctor. Be that as it may, when he left school at the age of 16, he was apprenticed to Mr. Joseph Hodgson, a Quaker surgeon, well known in the Midlands, the author of a book famous in its day, *On Wounds and Diseases of the Arteries and Veins,* who became President of the Royal College of Surgeons and a Fellow of the Royal Society. He was surgeon to the General Hospital, Birmingham. Bowman studied anatomy and physiology ; also clinical medicine in the hospital, giving much time to the last. Throughout the whole of his life he was insistent upon the great importance of seeing as much as possible of actual clinical practice and post-mortem examinations. He learnt to express himself well, as we see in his earliest writings. There is a note by him on the influenza outbreak at Birmingham in 1833, which shows the disease to have been then pretty much what it is now ; in 1834 he read a paper on *Hæmorrhage from External Injury* before the Birmingham Medical Students' Society, and in 1835 one on *Spinal Paraplegia.* Both are admirable students' essays ; he was clearly well read and observant, and it is interesting to see that he was not wedded to bleeding. His ability to draw is shown in four beautiful coloured plates, illustrating disease of the larynx, which he prepared for Mr. Ryland, Surgeon to the Town Infirmary, Birmingham, who used them for his book on the subject published in 1837. He also made a series of measurements of the orifices of the heart for Dr. Blakiston who, in recognition of his industry, gave him a fine microscope which he kept to his dying day. It is clear that during his home life, his schooldays, and his student days he lived in an intellectual atmosphere in which he learned to work hard, therefore he left Birmingham with bright prospects.

On arrival in London in 1837, he, in October of that year, joined the Medical Department of King's College, as an advanced student working under John Simon, who was then beginning his own fifth year of studentship and had just been made Prosector to Todd for the physiology lectures. F. T. McDougall was Demonstrator of Anatomy. Young Bowman was again fortunate in his companions, for John Simon, of exactly the same age, was a man of very wide interests in pathology, surgery, public health and the fine arts. It must be exceptional in the history of physiology to find, as here, a pair of student demonstrators, one of whom became a fellow of the Royal Society at 25, the other at 29. McDougall gave up medicine in 1839, went to Oxford, rowed in the winning University eight, married the sister of the lady who married Bishop Colenso, and became the famous Bishop of Labuan and Sarawak who brought medical aid to the natives, fought the pirates, founded an exceedingly successful mission and made translations into the Malay language. By the time he was 21, Bowman was or had been in close association with seven persons who are chronicled in the *Dictionary of National Biography,* where he also appears.

He visited the hospitals of Holland, Germany and Vienna in 1838. Simon in that year became Demonstrator of Anatomy as a colleague of McDougall, Bowman becoming Physiology Prosector to Todd; this began the intimate association with Todd which had so great an influence on Bowman's life, as will be seen when we come to consider their joint work. Next year Bowman moved to the junior demonstratorship of Anatomy, in 1840 he passed his examination at the College of Surgeons and in 1844 he became a Fellow.

King's College Hospital, an adapted old workhouse in a depressing neighbourhood, just south of Lincoln's Inn, was opened in 1840. Partridge and Fergusson were appointed surgeons, with Simon and Bowman their respective assistant surgeons; eight years later Simon moved to St. Thomas's Hospital. Bowman thereupon became senior assistant surgeon at King's, attaining full surgeoncy in 1856, soon after which date he resigned, because his private practice did not leave him time for his duties at King's, where he had also lectured on physiology, for the most part jointly with Todd, from 1847 to 1855. He was made an Honorary Fellow in 1855, a member of the Council in 1879, and for some time was Chairman of the Medical Committee. The high position he occupied in professional estimation is shown by the fact that ten years after he had ceased to practise as a surgeon, he was chosen to give

" The Address in Surgery " before the annual meeting of the British Medical Association. In 1846 he was appointed surgeon to the Ophthalmic Hospital in Moorfields, becoming full surgeon in 1851 and retiring under the age limit in 1876.

Sir William Fergusson was an able, original surgeon, who did so large a private practice that there was little left for his surgical colleagues at King's, consequently, after Bowman joined the Ophthalmic Hospital, he gradually became more and more identified with ophthalmology, and, after the the death of John Dalrymple in 1852, he took the position of the leading ophthalmologist in London. He regretted this trend in his affairs and for years protested that he was a surgeon. His only contribution to surgery was an article on this subject in the *Encyclopædia Metropolitana*. In 1842 he wrote a short article in the *Lancet* in which he demonstrated that in a fatty liver the fat is deposited in the hepatic cells.

Bowman was a refined man, of slender build, with pallid delicate features and dreamy eyes, fond of the country and of his tranquil home at Hampstead, where he was surrounded by choice books and works of art. Abstemious in food, he rarely took alcohol and did not smoke. He was never robust, although hardly ever ill; Sir James Paget regretted that he had not felt able to take an active part in the official and public work of his profession, but he sedulously attended meetings of learned societies and for a term he was honorary secretary to the Royal Institution. He was an excellent man of business and made a good chairman, with quite exceptional powers of persuading others to take his view. The want of good nursing at King's College Hospital led to the formation of a Committee. It advised that the nursing should be undertaken by the St. John's House Sisterhood; this did much to improve the hospital nursing. Bowman helped in this and also in sending nurses to Miss Nightingale in the Crimea, and he was a member of the Nightingale Fund till his death. In 1842 he married Miss Harriet Paget; they had seven children. His addresses in London were in order: Norfolk Street, Strand; Craven Street; Golden Square ; and then, in 1850, 5 Clifford Street. From 1857 to 1871 he had a house at North End, Hampstead, where he used to rise early and do a little gardening before going to his consulting-rooms in town. Disliking late hours, he rarely went into Society. After 1887 he gradually gave up practice and lived mostly at Joldwynds, near Dorking, a beautiful house built for him by Philip Webb—a picture of it may be seen in *Philip Webb and his Work*, by Lethaby, published in 1935; here Bowman died of pneumonia on March 29, 1892, at the age of 76. He was buried at Holmbury St. Mary.

As a teacher he was painstaking and thorough, lecturing slowly in order that the students might take notes; by no means eloquent, he spoke well and he wrote well. As an ophthalmic surgeon he was a fine operator of great manual dexterity, his thin delicate artistic fingers, absolutely devoid of the slightest tremor, seemed made for operations on the eye; people came from all over the world to his Tuesday and Friday clinics at Moorfields. This skill led to a very large practice, whilst the fundamental importance of his contributions to ophthalmic surgery gave him an outstanding position among his professional brethren. Hence he was the President of the Ophthalmological Section of the Seventh International Medical Congress in 1881, and also was the first president of the Ophthalmological Society when it was formed, largely by him, in 1880; this Society founded the Bowman lecture in honour of him. The first lecture was given by Sir Jonathan Hutchinson, a later one was delivered by his old clinical assistant, T. Pridgin Teale, who spoke of Bowman's absolute truth, his single-mindedness and his extraordinary operative skill. The books dealing with the eye form the "Bowman Ophthalmological Library" in the Royal Society of Medicine. He was the close friend of both Von Graefe and Donders. Henry Power writes, "It will be long before the world will see three such men, all possessing unusual ability and exceptional attainments, all intensely earnest in their work, and all glowing with the interest that is excited by the discovery of a new and unexplored country, meet together in such amity and love." Bowman wrote a particularly graceful and affectionate obituary notice of Donders in the *Proceedings of the Royal Society* for 1891, which anyone wishing to know of Donders must read. The awarding of a baronetcy to him indicates the professional position which Bowman attained.

Scientific honours fell to him; he became a Fellow of the Royal Society at the age of 25, and at the age of 26 he received the Royal Medal of the Society for his work on the kidney and on muscle. The Physiological Society was founded in 1876. Bowman was a guest at the inaugural meeting and later was elected an Honorary member. He was then past 60, and this recognition of his work of long ago pleased him greatly. Sir Edward Sharpey-Schafer, in his *History of the Physiological Society*, speaks of Bowman's epoch-making observations on the structure of striated muscle, on the intrinsic muscles of the eye, especially the ciliary muscle, and on the structure of the kidney, and also of his gentle and modest disposition and of the respect which he inspired.

The crowning honour paid to him was that, on his retirement from practice, the Bowman Testimonial Fund was inaugurated in July 1888, at a meeting held at Sir George Johnson's house. Its design was to make to Sir William Bowman some acknowledgment of the appreciation in which he was held on account of his high character and his professional and scientific attainments. Four hundred and forty-six persons subscribed, among them were ninety Fellows of the Royal Society, many persons outside the world of science and many foreigners. Both the Ophthalmological and Physiological Societies contributed. The money collected was spent partly on having his portrait painted by Ouless—it was exhibited at the Royal Academy in 1889, where a beautiful portrait of him by Watts had been shown in 1865—and also on a handsome reprint, in two volumes, of his publications, revised by himself and edited by Professor Burdon-Sanderson and Mr. Hulke. Even then there was a considerable balance which was used to diminish the cost of the volumes to the subscribers. The first volume had a reproduction of the portrait by Watts, the second one of that by Ouless.

In June 1847 he gave four lectures at Moorfields on *The Parts concerned in the Operations on the Eye and on the Structure of the Retina*. They make excellent reading, being precise and clear; all through nothing is told on hearsay, the author has investigated for himself and described what he has found. Illustrations from Comparative Anatomy abound. He dedicated them to his old master Joseph Hodgson and published them in the *London Medical Gazette*. They received the great distinction of being translated into French in the *Annales d'Oculistique*. The *Lancet*, in its obituary notice of Bowman in 1892, said they are " still read by every man who pretends to know anything of the literature of the subject." They were republished as a book ; some of the original matter in them was also published in April 1847 in Todd and Bowman's *Physiological Anatomy and Physiology of Man* (Pt. III, Chap. XVII, of Vision) and some of it in a paper *On some points in the Anatomy of the Eye, chiefly in reference to the power of Adjustment* read before the British Association in 1847. Power says "this paper has become classical from the novelty and value of the facts recorded."

Bowman's fame was partly owing to the peculiarly skilful delicacy of his fingers, as shown in his ophthalmological work, his histology and his drawings, some of which still illustrate the text-books of to-day.

We must remember that, in his day, histology was in its infancy. Microscopes had not reached their present excellence, microtomes, modern staining and embedding were unknown, sections were cut by hand. Yet such was his tactile delicacy and skill that he was able, we might almost say, to found histology, books on which still describe Bowman's sarcous elements, Bowman's capsule and Bowman's membrane. In his four lectures given in 1847 many original observations are to be found, for example, the erroneous description of the insertion of the recti into the sclerotic is corrected, the structure of the cornea as observed by himself is described, with special attention to the corneal tubes and the anterior elastic lamina. The famous discovery is announced that the structure, previously known as the ciliary circle, is an unstriped muscle which Bowman called the ciliary muscle. This discovery was made simultaneously by Bruecke, but Bowman knew nothing of this. He also tells us that "we need not hesitate to admit the muscularity of the unstriped fibres of the mammalian iris."

His originality is shown in many other papers on ophthalmological subjects. In one, published in 1851, on a new method of treating certain cases of epiphora he remarks that the object of meibomian glands is not to prevent agglutination of the lids, but, by maintaining a greasy surface, to prevent tears from escaping over the cheek and he describes a method of slitting up the lachrymal canal which has become one of the common methods of treatment. In 1857 he gave a description of the treatment of lachrymal obstruction by the passage of probes downwards into the nose. This was entirely original. It is interesting to note that he " constantly kept in view the analogy of these obstructions with those of the urinary passages." His paper on the use of two needles at once in operations for capsular cataract, and that on the operation for conical cornea, were novel and are well known to ophthalmic surgeons. In 1864 he gave an account of how by puncturing with two needles in cases of detached retina he had been able in some cases to improve sight.

Bowman had a great advantage over many, in that as he grew in age his mind retained its youthful willingness to receive new ideas. Helmholtz devised the ophthalmoscope in 1851. Bowman was immediately profoundly interested, and was one of the first to become expert in its use. The discovery was made by Von Graefe, in 1857, that iridectomy was an effective remedy for acute glaucoma. Bowman translated and published here Von Graefe's paper, and adopted the operation, which he performed for the first time in 1857. He and other leading ophthalmic surgeons were quickly convinced of its value; Bowman especially did much for his profession and for the sufferers, by the emphatic way in which he advocated the new treatment, and by the severe trouncing he gave the obstinate diehards who were opposed to it. Again, it was he and Critchett who brought before their colleagues in this country the method of extraction of cataract by a traction instrument with iridectomy, which method came from Berlin, and Pridgin Teale tells how when he suggested that the probes for obstructed ducts should have a bulb at the end, Bowman immediately adopted the suggestion. But the open-mindedness with which he considered novel suggestions was tempered by a most excellent critical judgment, quite free from the common failing shown in a willingness to adopt any proposition just because it is new.

We will now turn to his original histological work. The long paper *On the Minute Structure and Movements of Voluntary Muscle* begins with a critical account of the many discordant views on the structure of muscle. Then the author unfolds his own theory, which made him famous. The amount of work in the paper is prodigious; muscle fibres from man, ten other species of mammals, six of birds, seven of reptiles, ten of fish and six of insects were laboriously examined microscopically. A primitive fasciculus consists, he says, of primitive fibrillæ which are composed of elongated polygonal masses of sarcous elements.

This name is new; "Bowman's sarcous elements" has become a common phrase in books on histology. They, he tells us, are united together, endways and sideways, so as to constitute, in these directions respectively, fibrillæ and disks. The dark longitudinal striæ are shadows between fibrillæ, the dark transverse striæ shadows between disks. Every primitive fasciculus is invested by a highly delicate, transparent and probably elastic membrane, the sarcolemma; this discovery is new, so is the name which has passed into general use. Eighty-five delicate drawings by Bowman illustrate his paper, as I have already said, some are still reproduced in modern histological books. Those of the sarcolemma are particularly good. There is one in which Trichinæ have completely destroyed the sarcous elements, but are surrounded by the sarcolemma. The nuclei of the cells from which muscle is formed are described. The ends of the fasciculi in tendons do not taper, but are obliquely or transversely truncated, a new observation at variance with the teaching of the day. The histological study of muscle is very difficult, other interpretations of its structure have been suggested, but Bowman's were entirely original and reasonable, and it is everywhere agreed that he made a great step forward.

Less than two years after the communication on muscle had been brought before the Royal Society, Bowman read before the same Society his still more celebrated paper *On the Structure and Use of the Malpighian Bodies of the Kidney*. Previous knowledge was obscure and unsatisfactory. He, with wonderful clarity of expression, made the subject plain. This paper describes the renal tubes as consisting of a basement membrane—a term used for the first time by the author—lined by epithelium which is continued over the Malpighian bodies. All the blood of the renal artery (with the exception of a small quantity distributed to the capsule and fat) enters the capillary tufts of the Malpighian bodies; thence it passes into the capillary plexus surrounding the uriniferous tubes, leaving the kidney by the renal vein. The Malpighian bodies and the origin of the renal tubes from around them are clearly described. There are two perfectly distinct systems of capillary vessels, that of the Malpighian bodies which may be termed the portal system of the kidney, and that of the capillary plexus surrounding the tubes. This view is confirmed by examining the kidney of the boa. The function of the capillaries of the Malpighian bodies is the excretion of water and salts, the function of the epithelium of the tubes is the secretion of the other constituents of the urine from the capillaries around them. All this is now so completely the common knowledge of every first year's medical student that we rarely stop to reflect upon the greatness of Bowman's discovery, which was not only one in histology, but one in physiology, made by deduction from microscopical structure. No wonder Michael Foster called him the father of the kidney.

The remainder of his work to be noticed was done in association with R. B. Todd, an able Irishman, a pupil of Graves, who, after taking his degree at Trinity College, Dublin, came to London in 1831, being then 22. He lectured at the Aldersgate Medical School, took the degree of Doctor of Medicine at Oxford, and in 1836 was appointed to the chair of physiology at King's College, where later on he became physician. He had much energy; Willoughby Lyle says, "It was Bentley Todd who actually resuscitated the Medical Department of the College," of which he was the first Dean. He also succeeded in his ambition to be a physiological physician. Hughlings Jackson constantly said that he adopted Todd and Robertson's hypothesis that local paralysis after an epileptic seizure was due to exhaustion. As a lecturer on physiology Todd was accurate and clear, and encouraged scientific investigation among his pupils, many of whom became distinguished. He was a fine clinical teacher and a voluminous writer; his practice was very large. In Thackeray's Roundabout Paper *On Letts's Diary* is the touching story of the death of "a famous doctor, into whose consulting-room crowds came daily, so that they might be healed." It is said that this doctor was Todd. He died in 1860, being only 51 years old, but few have had a greater influence for good in both scientific and clinical medicine than he. His fame is not yet dead, for, in his Harveian oration for 1934, Dr. James Collier said: "Dr. Todd, who was by far the greatest clinical neurologist Great Britain has produced until the time of Hughlings Jackson, was the first to begin the breaking up of the spinal diseases, at that time all classed as paraplegia, by his discovery of locomotor ataxy as a distinct disease."

Todd and Bowman became great friends directly Bowman went to King's; together they visited continental hospitals in

1838. Bowman speaks of his colleague as "my loved and honoured friend and workfellow." For eight years they were joint lecturers on physiology at King's College; under their joint names the first volume of the *Anatomy and Physiology of Man* appeared in 1846, the second volume in 1856. The authors were determined to write an original book, for, in the preface they say, "The reader will find opinions expressed more or less at variance with those generally received. To these the authors have been led during their anxious attempts to render their descriptions direct and faithful transcripts from nature." The publication of this book was an epoch in physiology; it was the first in which the histology of the various organs and tissues was given; it is clearly written, easy to read, and a very large number of the excellent woodcuts are from drawings, often direct on to the wood, made by Bowman, from his own specimens.

In 1832 Todd, being then just 24, began the preparation of the *Cyclopædia of Anatomy and Physiology*, visiting Paris next year to arrange for foreign contributors. The five volumes appeared between 1836 and 1859. Their six thousand pages were edited solely by him, they contain contributions from him, and many distinguished men, e.g. Bowman, Paget, Richard Owen and Simon. This Cyclopædia did as much to encourage and advance the study of physiology and of comparative and microscopic anatomy as any book ever published, and it is still valuable for the number and variety of its original articles. Bowman's contributions were those on "Mucous Membrane," "Muscle," "Muscular Motion," and "Paccinian Bodies"; the best solely by him in the *Anatomy and Physiology of Man* were those on "Ossification," "Muscle," "Nervous Tissue," "Skin, Nails and Hair," "Taste," "The Olfactory Region," and "The Cochlea." All these are original in the sense that Bowman describes and figures what he himself has observed. If anyone wants to see him at his best in description, the article "Mucous Membrane" should be read, always remembering that microscopic research was then in its infancy and that consequently the histology of mucous membranes was especially difficult. He begins by telling us that "The skin is the outer tegument of the body; the mucous membranes form its internal investment, and are continuous with the skin." Ducts with their glands are merely prolongations of the same tissue which everywhere consists of basement membrane with superimposed epithelium. Both these are described in microscopic detail, then follows an account of the blood-vessels, nerves, lymphatics and areolar tissue of this great system and a description of its difference in different places. Finally there is a general outline of the functions of the mucous system, which are four : the reception of impressions from without, the defence of the body from external injurious influences, the absorption of foreign particles and the separation of such as are for any reason to be eliminated.

The originality of Bowman's studies in both ophthalmology and histological physiology was so exceptional that he became celebrated as an ophthalmologist and also as a physiological histologist. His additions to our knowledge in either of these departments of learning would have made him illustrious ; he, however, is doubly distinguished.

SIR JOHN SIMON

This versatile man, surgeon, pathologist and sanitarian, was partly of French extraction, for both his grandfathers were Frenchmen who emigrated to England; both married Englishwomen. His paternal grandfather, Louis Antoine Simon, kept a hatter's shop in Vere Street, London, where Marshall & Snelgrove's shop now stands; he died suddenly while fencing at the French Embassy in 1803; his wife, an Englishwoman, died in 1837. They had one child, Louis Michael Simon, who married a Miss Nonnet, daughter of Nonnet, a jeweller of Bath, who had married an Englishwoman. Louis Michael was in early life a shipbroker, then a member of the Stock Exchange and on the committee of it for many years; he died on December 7, 1879, aged 97 years; his wife died in 1882, aged 95 years. They had fourteen children.

One of these, John, the subject of this notice, was born October 10, 1816, in London and christened at Pepys's church, St. Olave's, Hart Street. Soon after, the family went to live at 1 Park Terrace, Blackheath, moving in 1823 to 10 The Paragon, Blackheath. Young John was sent to a preparatory school at Pentonville and afterwards for seven and a half years to Dr. Burney's celebrated school at Greenwich, where he had John Birkett, the well-known surgeon, as a schoolfellow. After a year at Hohensolms, in Rhenish Prussia, he was, in 1833, apprenticed to Joseph Henry Green, at a fee of 500 guineas. Green was surgeon to St. Thomas's Hospital, and had been appointed Professor of Surgery at the recently founded King's College, then without a hospital. Simon went for dissections and lectures to King's and for clinical surgery to St. Thomas's. On August 14, 1838, he passed his examination at the College of Surgeons, and was immediately appointed Demonstrator of Anatomy at King's, having as a colleague Francis Thomas McDougall who is described in the account of Sir William Bowman. In 1840 King's College Hospital was opened. The surgeons were Partridge and Fergusson, the assistant surgeons Simon and Bowman. Simon refers in his *Personal Recollections* to the help and stimulus he always derived from Bowman. He held the post of Demonstrator of Anatomy at King's for nine years, that of assistant surgeon for seven years, and he was the first doctor to be made a Fellow of King's College. In 1847 he was appointed Lecturer on Pathology at St. Thomas's and was given a few surgical beds there; he became assistant surgeon in 1853 when he left King's for good.

To begin with, in his student days, he had lived at Blackheath, starting at 7 a.m. to walk the 8 miles to his lectures, on three nights a week he did not get home till 11 p.m., for Green lectured from 8 to 9 p.m. This was too exhausting, so he took lodgings in Arundel Street; he afterwards lived at other lodgings, but mostly in Wellington Street, Strand, from 1833 to 1847. During these years he wrote an article on the Neck for the *Cyclopædia of Anatomy and Physiology,* he won the Astley Cooper Prize in 1844 with an essay on the Thymus, he brought before the Royal Society a paper on the Thyroid which secured his election as F.R.S. in 1845 and, in 1848, he read a paper on " Subacute Inflammation of the Kidney " before the Royal Medico-Chirurgical Society. He filled up his spare time with holidays abroad and with wide reading, studying oriental languages and metaphysics. This is reflected in the first lecture he gave on Pathology in 1847, for its title was "Aims and Philosophic Method of Pathological Research."

He fell in love with Miss Jane O'Meara, and they became engaged in 1843; marriage was then impossible, for he only received £25 a year for all the work he did at King's, but as the pay for the Pathological Lectureship at St. Thomas's was £200 a year he, with financial help from his father, was married to Miss O'Meara in 1848. They did not have any children. After a honeymoon in Devonshire, he and his wife returned to live at Lancaster Place, moving in 1853 to 37A Upper Grosvenor Street. They came to know many interesting people such as Mowbray Morris, manager of *The Times,* Edwin Chadwick, G. H. Lewis, Woolner, Charles Henry Kingsley, Arthur Helps, Burne-Jones and Ruskin, and they often entertained distinguished visitors from abroad; Simon's facility in speaking French and German made this easy.

Liverpool had the honour, in 1847, of being the first town to appoint a Medical Officer of Health, next year the City of London decided to do the same. Immediately after returning from his honeymoon, Simon received this post, the salary being £500 a year, rising to £800.

The *Personal Recollections* by Simon omit to say why he took the appointment of Medical Officer of Health to the City of London. It was a strange thing to do, because he had always wished to practise surgery and only a year before he had been made Lecturer on Pathology at, and had been put on the Surgical staff of, St. Thomas's. Possibly the certain income attracted the young couple. Anyhow, it led to his becoming famous, for his fame does not rest on either pathology or surgery but on sanitary science. From 1848 to 1876 when he retired, almost all his energies were spent on this. The result is to be seen in the Reports which he issued.

The fact that the City created such an office directed public attention to the medical aspects of sanitary science. Simon's duty was to medically advise the City Commissioners of Sewers as to the best means of abating the local conditions of unwholesomeness. This he was to do by inspection and report. He began with causes of death and, with the help of the Registrar-General, obtained mortality returns for presentation to the Commissioners at their weekly meeting. Adequate sickness returns were not available, compulsory notification not being in force, but many doctors soon voluntarily sent him notice of cases of fever. He, accompanied by Nuisance Inspectors, made weekly inspections with regard to overcrowding, ventilation, cleanliness, drainage, water supply, dust removal and the like. At the end of each year he presented an annual report written so forcefully as to demand attention. For example, speaking of the obstructiveness of landlords who will not improve drainage after receiving instructions to do so, Simon would abolish the difference between a " notice " and a " peremptory notice " and advises that on the very day the period of grace has expired, " the work, if undone, should be given over for completion by the Commissioners " as the Act directs. He points out that London sewage ought not to be poured into a tidal river ; he completely abolished cesspools. The Commissioners had to give ear to an officer who writes :

In inspecting the courts and alleys of the City, one constantly sees butts, for the reception of water, either public, or in the open yards of houses, or sometimes in their cellars; and these butts, dirty mouldering, and coverless; receiving soot and all other impurities from the air; absorbing stench from the adjacent cesspool; inviting filth from insects, vermin, sparrows, cats and children; their contents often augmented through a rain water pipe by washings from the roof.

Naturally, he considers the system of intermittent water supply bad, for it stints the use of water and prohibits the flushing of drains. Thousands of people had no water supply in their houses (when present it was intermittent) and were solely dependent on fetching it in a pail from a stopcock only turned on for a short while daily.

He writes thus of the condition of the poor:

Men and women, boys and girls, in scores of each, using jointly one single common privy; grown persons of both sexes sleeping in common with their married parents; a woman suffering in travail in the midst of the males and females of three several families of fellow-lodgers in a single room; an adult, sharing his mother's bed during her confinement; such are instances within my knowledge of the degree and of the manner in which a people may relapse into the habits of a savage life, when their domestic condition is neglected and when they are suffered to habituate themselves to the uttermost depths of physical obscenity and degradation.

Again:

Courts and alleys with low, dark, filthy tenements, hemmed in on all sides by higher buildings, having no possibility of any current of air, and (worst of all) sometimes so constructed, back to back, as to forbid the advantage of double windows or back doors, and thus to render the house as perfect a *cul de sac* out of the court as the court is a *cul de sac* out of the next thoroughfare. . . . It is no uncommon thing in a room 12 feet square or less, to find three or four families styed together (perhaps with infectious disease among them), filling the same space night and day—men, women and children in the promiscuous intimacy of cattle. . . . Whatever is morally hideous and savage in the scene—whatever contrast it offers to the superficial magnificence of the metropolis—whatever profligacy it implies and continues—whatever recklessness and obscene brutality arises from it—whatever deep injury it inflicts on the community—whatever debasement or abolition of God's image in men's hearts is tokened by it—these matters belong not to my office. Only because of the physical suffering am I entitled to speak; only because pestilence is for ever within the circle; only because Death so largely comforts these poor orphans of civilization. . . . In the few houses of Seven Step Alley and its two offsets, there occurred last year 163 parochial cases of fever; in Prince's Place and Prince's Square, 176 cases—think, gentlemen, if this had occurred in Southamptom Place and Russell Square!

Under the heading of Offensive Trades, Simon tells us that within the City there are 138 slaughter-houses, and in 58 of these the slaughtering occurs in vaults and cellars. This in itself is filthy and disgusting, but near these slaughter houses the trades of gut spinning, tripe dressing, bone boiling, tallow melting and paunch cooking flourish. There is the smoke nuisance:

Soon after daybreak, the great factory shafts beside the river begin to discharge immense volumes of smoke; their clouds soon become confluent; the sky is overcast with a dingy veil; the house chimneys presently add their contributions, and by ten o'clock one may observe the total result of this gigantic nuisance hanging over the City like a pall. Thus people resign themselves to dirt and the windows are kept shut.

With regard to burials:

There are, indeed, few of the older burial grounds within the City where the soil does not rise many feet above its original level, testifying to the large amount of animal matter which rots below the surface. The vaults beneath churches are, in many instance, similarly overloaded with materials of putrefaction.

A horrible account is given of how coffins in vaults, after a time, burst.

His report on cholera, issued in 1854, is an eloquent appeal for a better sewage system and for a continuous water supply. Apparently the stopcocks were not available on Sundays because he says, " I trust it is no heathen's part to urge that the Christian Sabbath suffers more desecration in the filth and preventable unwholesomeness of many thousand households, than in the honest industry of a dozen turncocks."

Those few extracts will, I trust, show how Simon's Reports differ from most. They are something more, namely literary essays of high merit which compel attention. I have not given his remedies for the evils he brilliantly makes alive to us, for they have been adopted by the City. He never lets himself rant, never can critics say here is a man with a bee in his bonnet. His writing is far too impressive and dignified for this. The Corporation listened to him, for he appealed to its pride to put its great City in order as far as it legally could. His Reports received the honour of being reprinted as a separate volume in 1854. Simon took the opportunity of writing a preface, because " national prevalence of sanitary neglect is a very grievous fact." This preface would move a heart of stone by its pleading for better health for all, especially the poor. I wish I could reprint it, but I must restrict myself to one quotation:

If there be citizens so destitute, that they can afford to live only where they must straightway die—renting the twentieth straw-heap in some lightless fever-bin, or squatting among rotten soakage, or breathing from the cesspool and the sewer; so destitute that they can buy no water—that milk and bread must be impoverished to meet their means of purchase—that the drugs sold them for sickness must be rubbish or poison; surely no civilized community dare avert itself from the care of this abject orphanage.

The remedy suggested is what amounts to a Ministry of Health to look after health matters of every kind, including adulteration of food and drugs. For the minister " What a career ! It would be idleness to speak of the blessings he could diffuse, the anguish he could relieve, the gratitude and glory he could earn."

These Reports, which were constantly quoted in the daily press, attracted the favourable attention of so many people, and appealed so deeply to them, that the Government, in 1855, invited Simon to become Medical Officer to the General Board of Health with Dr. Sutherland and Dr. Milroy under him. After much hesitation he accepted, gave up private practice, but remained surgeon to St. Thomas's Hospital till 1876. He moved to a smaller house, 44 Great Cumberland Place, then he tried living at Blackheath, but finding this too far from town he came to 40 Kensington Square in 1867, where he lived till he died.

His position at the Board was not happy; he considered it humiliating. The Board only existed provisionally and did nothing more than a limited amount of routine business, while Parliament made up its mind what it would do about Public Health. Simon, however, could not remain idle, and, on May 13, 1856, presented a report *On the last two Cholera Epidemics of London as affected by the Consumption of Impure Water*. Two water companies supplied the south of London, the Lambeth and the Southwark and Vauxhall, side by side in the whole area. In the 1848-9 epidemic, both supplied sewage-polluted water from the Thames, that of the Lambeth company being the worse, the mortality from cholera among its customers was 125 per 10,000, that among those of the Southwark and Vauxhall was 118. In the epidemic of 1853-4, the Lambeth, having a much purer supply from a new intake higher up the river, had a mortality of 37; the Southwark and Vauxhall had fouler water than ever, its mortality was 130. Thus the public learnt of the danger of sewage-contaminated water.

Sanitary Science progressed considerably during Simon's seven years of office in the City; other districts of the metropolis appointed medical officers of health, and it is remarkable what distinguished persons held these posts, e.g. Bristowe, Buchanan, Odling, Pavy, Burdon-Sanderson and Thomas Stevenson. They formed themselves into an Association, Simon being its first President.

An important event in the history of Public Health was that, in 1853, Parliament made vaccination compulsory. This led to opposition and criticism. Simon, in his official capacity, had to report, which he did in a volume of 280 pages laid before Parliament in 1857. Although still a dread disease in the East, small-pox in this country is now rare and mild, consequently few are interested in it, but it was not always negligible; in 1819 out of 215 unprotected persons exposed to infection, 200 got small-pox, of whom 46 died. Simon's celebrated essay is so closely reasoned that it is impossible to condense it; the literature of vaccination and small-pox is enormous, but this classic contribution to it is outstanding; no one working at the subject can neglect this medical masterpiece.

Acting on the advice of Simon, his colleagues at the medical school of St. Thomas's Hospital instituted a course of lectures on public heath—the first of their kind in the country; Dr. Greenhow was the lecturer. The Registrar-General's Reports only gave the general death-rate; Greenhow worked out the different death-rate from various diseases in different localities. Simon considered the results valuable and, prefacing them with an introduction of his own, presented them as a Report in 1858, pointing out that particular diseases favoured particular districts, in which, therefore, the cause for this increased mortality must exist and ought to be eradicated. This report was a step forward in Sanitary Science.

In this year the Medical Act, which created the General Medical Council, was passed. Simon helped by preparing a memorandum for the Government and therefore contributed to the legal formation of the medical profession. The General Board of Health promoted several bills for improved Sanitary Law and also that under which the Metropolitan Board of Works—superseded in 1888 by the London County Council— came into being. But the year 1858 also saw the end of the General Board of Health, its medical duties being transferred to the Privy Council, to which Simon became the Medical Officer.

It was the medical duty of the Privy Council to be responsible for public vaccination, during epidemics to issue orders and regulations, to superintend quarantine, to see that the Medical Act was properly obeyed, and to inquire and report on health matters. Simon, now 42 years old, entered upon these tasks with enthusiasm. Inspectors were appointed, numerous experts were consulted, vaccination throughout the country was surveyed, public vaccinators were required to have been properly taught how to vaccinate, the supply of lymph was regulated, vaccination inspectorships were instituted, and a bill to improve vaccination was passed.

Simon's Report for 1858 drew attention to the need to establish a scientific basis for Sanitary law and administration; one section of it dealt with the distribution of diarrhœal diseases, another with that of diphtheria; in the year 1860 his Report tells us of the distribution of pulmonary disease, it shows a mortality in mining and certain manufacturing districts nearly double that in agricultural districts and directs attention as to the way to prevent this. The Sixth Report was of importance; we learn how the poor are underfed and often shockingly housed, that they are employed, without precautions, in poisonous trades, such as those using lead and mercury, and he describes how home work, such as straw plaiting, leads to pulmonary disease; other Reports dealt with the same matters. Cholera, scurvy, cerebro-spinal meningitis, yellow fever, cattle plague, typhus, typhoid, scarlet fever, infantile marasmus and other diseases were all the subject of Reports. Sometimes, as for cerebro-spinal meningitis, medical inspectors were sent abroad to obtain information.

The dwellings of the poorer classes throughout the country were investigated, as were nuisances, quarantine, dangerous industries, venereal diseases, prostitution, adulteration of drugs and poisoning. The Registrar-General's returns were amplified so as greatly to increase their utility.

All this activity roused the Government to pass the great Sanitary Act of 1866, which laid down the principle that it is the duty of Sanitary Authorities to provide for the health of those in their charge, and other smaller helpful acts were passed. But, said Simon, good as was the Act of 1866, further improve-

ments were needed, therefore he tried " to keep well in public
eye the defects for which further legislation was required."

The Vaccination Select Committee was appointed in 1871,
Simon gave evidence. Its Report is celebrated and still worth
reading. In this year he met the menace of a cholera epidemic
by the admirable institution at ports of local hospitals to which
cases could be taken on arrival, and thus prevent the dissemination
of the scourge through the country. Also in this year the Government, at his instigation, agreed to spend £2,000 a year on Medical
Research. He always spoke with gratitude for the help given
to him by Robert Lowe, afterwards Viscount Sherbrooke, when
he was his chief at the Privy Council.

This is a condensed account of only a small portion of Simon's
activities during the fourteen years he was Medical Officer to the
Privy Council; by far the most important effects of his work
were that he taught the public that there was such a thing as
Sanitary Science and that obedience to it led to health, and that
he convinced statesmen that it was their duty to guard the health
of the nation.

The advance of Sanitary Science had been accompanied by
piecemeal legislation which resulted in legislative chaos, to
inquire into which a Royal Sanitary Commission was appointed;
Simon gave evidence. The Commission reported in 1871 that
sanitary legislation should be consolidated, that sanitary law
should be uniform, universal and imperative, that health matters
should be dealt with by local authorities assisted by a superior
authority, which, by the Act of Parliament passed in 1871, was
enacted to be, instead of the Privy Council, the Local Government Board which itself came into existence that year. Several
other Acts of Parliament arose out of this Report which received
almost unanimous approval; and for details of these the reader
should consult Simon's *English Sanitary Institutions*.

He was appointed Medical Officer to the new Local
Government Board. This had absorbed the Poor Law Board, an
inefficient body which had no medical experience and which had
been scathingly criticized. Stansfeld was the first President of
the Local Government Board and he made it, as regards Public
Health, merely the old Poor Law Board writ large. *The Times*
said: " Apart from any question of the incapacity of the Poor
Law Officials to adjust themselves to the wider environment of

their new positions, the influence of their chief seems to have been steadily exercised in the direction of placing difficulties in the way of sanitary reform." It was even suggested that he had been given the post in order to do this, because supporters of the Government made pecuniary profit out of insanitary conditions which sacrificed the lives of the poor. In *The Times Literary Supplement* for December 13, 1934, we read " there was the opposition of Whigs and Radicals to factory legislation; the *Economist* even opposed the Public Health Act of 1848." Against this condition of things Simon raged furiously but in vain. The quarrel is remindful of *An Enemy of the People*. In 1874 Stansfeld left the Presidency to be succeeded by Mr. Sclater-Booth. A brighter era seemed to be in view; the Sale of Drugs Act and the Pollution of Rivers Act were passed. " But the machinery established by Mr. Stansfeld had mainly consisted of elaborate contrivances for the hindrance of effective action and Simon was weary. In the early part of 1876 he resigned his office, and was succeeded by his old friend and colleague Dr. Seaton," who could not bring much effectiveness into his very circumscribed office; he too resigned three and a half years after his appointment and died a month later. On Simon's resignation he received an annual allowance of £1,333 6s. 8d., and a C.B. He had been so immersed in Sanitary Science for twenty-eight years that, beyond his duties as Surgeon to St. Thomas's Hospital, he had done little professional work outside Sanitary Science.

Simon and his wife had become close friends of Ruskin, whom they met by chance in Savoy in 1856. The two men, of about the same age, appealed to one another, both were ardent reformers, both wrote beautiful prose. Ruskin always addressed Simon as " dear brother John," and describes him as one of his dearest and closest friends. Simon's wife became to Ruskin " My dear P.R.S." (Pre-Raphaelite Sister) or " My dear Sibyl" often shortened to " My dear S." She was, in the old age of Ruskin's mother, " her most deeply trusted friend." Lady Burne-Jones had a great admiration for her. Many letters passed to and fro between Ruskin and Simon and his wife. A selection is given in the large edition of Ruskin's works. Sometimes he asked Simon's medical advice, not to much purpose, for he took neither physic nor advice. In one letter he writes, " You know you really are to teach me some medicine one of these days. I begin to think it's almost the only thing in the world worth knowing. History one can't know and other things one needn't—but to know how to stop pain would be wonderful." I will give one short letter to show how close the friendship was:

DENMARK HILL,
Dec. 31, 1870.

MY DEAR BROTHER JOHN,—

You will get this to-morrow morning (perhaps to-night); whenever it does reach you, I trust it may give you some pleasure in my acknowledgment, with the deepest thankfulness, of the great love you bear me, and the noble example you set me in all things. I begin this next year in the fixed purpose of executing —at least beginning the fulfilment of—many designs, long in my mind, up to such a point as I may. I trust that, except in times of illness, I shall not be a burden to you any more by complaint or despondency, that sometimes I may amuse you a little, sometimes gravely please you, and always be thought of by you in a very true and deep way, though frost-bitten in soul as well as body, winter and summer, and in New Year as Old.

Love to Jane also, and in deep gratitude.

Ever yours,

J. RUSKIN.

For centuries St. Thomas's Hospital had stood in the Borough, the entrance was in the High Street, the building extended east, as far as opposite the present main entrance to Guy's Hospital. The advent of London Bridge Railway Station made it necessary to pull down St. Thomas's. There was much controversy as to where it should go; some wanted the country. Simon by his letters to *The Times* and by his drawing up of statements from the staff was largely the cause of the building of the hospital (1868–71) on its present site opposite the Houses of Parliament. After his retirement from the post of surgeon to St. Thomas's in 1876, he was made Consulting Surgeon and a Governor.

Directly he resigned from the Local Government Board he was nominated as a Crown Representative on the General Medical Council, a post which he held till 1895. It was clear that the Medical Act of 1858 constituting the Council required revision, in 1870 this was attempted but the bill was withdrawn. Similar bills in 1877 and 1878 had the same fate. In 1879 the matter was referred to a select Committee of the House of Commons; Simon gave evidence, and also before a Royal Commission in 1880–81. A Medical Acts Amendment Bill, in which he was greatly interested, became an Act in 1886. As it was essential that it should not rouse opposition, it was almost colourless, but it gave the General Medical Council the right to inspect examinations, and provided that it should contain some members elected by the general vote of the medical profession. He was helpful in insisting on a high standard of qualification for sanitary work.

Simon was President of the Royal College of Surgeons, 1878-9, President of the State Medicine Section of the International Medical Congress held in London in 1881; the title of his address was *Experiment as a Basis of Preventive Medicine.* He received the first award of two medals given for eminence in Sanitary Science, the Harben Medal of the Royal Institute of Public Health (1896) and the Buchanan Medal of the Royal Society (1897). He was mainly responsible for the establishment of the Grocers' Company's scholarships for Sanitary Science. Many honorary titles fell to him—D.C.L. Oxon (1868), LL.D. Cantab. (1880), LL.D. Edin. (1882), M.D. Dub. (1887), an honorary degree in medicine and surgery at Munich (1872) and the K.C.B. in 1887. He was Vice-President of the Royal Society and President of the Pathological Society.

In 1896 he lost the sight of one eye, slowly old age overtook him and the end came in his eighty-eighth year, on July 23, 1904, at his house in Kensington Square. He was buried in Lewisham Cemetery, Ladywell. A bust of him made in 1876 by his friend Woolner is in the Royal College of Surgeons.

Simon is outstanding because he was a great teacher of the masses and their Governments. Not all that he fought for was attained in his lifetime, but much, the fulfilment of which he did not see, has come to pass since his death. If he could behold our Ministry of Health, the London School of Hygiene and Tropical Medicine, and the present extensive sanitary administration he would feel that ultimate victory lay with him. The obituary notice in *The Times* has this of him:

The master of sanitary science, the organizer, and for years the official head of a system of public health preservation which is without equal in the world, the philosopher whose teaching has saved the lives of hundreds of thousands of our people, whose name is a household word wherever preventive medicine is studied, and whose writings form the classical literature of the subject to which much of his life has been devoted.

English Sanitary Institutions is not a title to attract the ordinary reader, which is a pity, for Sir John Simon's book having that name is exceedingly interesting. An immense amount of study and care have been spent on it, its excellent prose carries the reader along easily.

Part one is a learned history from the earliest times to the reigns of the Tudors; Rome receives much attention; most of us will feel with the author in his affection for St. Francis of Assisi, who he says " considered in his relation to the suffering poor, is almost one of the Fathers of Medicine." The second part deals with England under the Tudors and Stuarts. The Tudors were the first monarchs who really considered the health of the people. Henry the Eighth founded the Royal College of Physicians, among its duties was that of inspecting druggists' shops to see that pure drugs were sold, and he granted a charter to the Barbers and Surgeons, as is well known because of Holbein's well-known picture of the ceremony. In 1532 Commissions of Sewers were, by Act of Parliament, instituted in all parts of the Kingdom, wide powers were given to them, they had to curb " the outrageous flowing surges and course of the sea" and also the "outrageous springs." In 1585 an act was passed which enabled Sir Francis Drake to supply Plymouth with water from Dartmoor and, thirty years later, Sir Thomas Myddelton brought water to London by the celebrated New River. The succour of the destitute had been a duty of the Monasteries and other religious bodies; some neglected it. After their dissolution, the Tudors passed several Acts of Parliament dealing with the poor. Sturdy beggars and rogues, who shirked work, were regarded as traitors to the community, therefore they were punished severely, and, according to modern notions, brutally, but the helpless poor had to be provided for in each parish by the parishioners of adequate means. The famous Poor Laws of Queen Elizabeth gave power to levy rates for this purpose. Overseers were appointed to do this, they also had to look after destitute children and had power to erect buildings for the acommodation of the poor. Overcrowding was extreme, Elizabeth tried to deal with it by prohibiting building for a radius of three miles outside the city walls, and by forbidding the cutting up of large houses into tenements. The sanitary state of large towns was dreadful; Simon gives a good account of that of London. Quarantine was found to be useless against the plague. Most opportunely the Great Fire burnt down the filthy city of London and stopped the plague.

In the eighteenth century, there awoke, in the mind of the nation, a consciousness that it was the duty of individuals as well as of the State to succour the poor and distressed. Simon, adopting the name from Green the historian, calls this belief the New Humanity. Thomas Guy, who died in 1725, gave or bequeathed to the poor considerably over half a million pounds. The two Wesleys and Charles Whitfield greatly helped the New Humanity which was the cause of reform of the prisons. John Howard, whom Simon classes with St. Francis, had by his writings revealed the hideous state of these; the jailer, having no salary, was left to make a living by exactions from the prisoners; overcrowding and consequent typhus or jail fever followed; the prisons were in such a state of disrepair that prisoners were chained to prevent escape, this being cheaper than mending the prisons. In 1807, thanks chiefly to Wilberforce, trading in slaves was abolished in the British Dominions, and in 1833 Parliament voted twenty million pounds to buy the freedom of those who were slaves. The cholera epidemic of 1831-2 helped to teach the public, on whom the leaven of the New Humanity had worked, that it was the duty of the State to protect the health of the people.

Simon now introduces us to four pioneers in the cause of public health. The first of these is Sir Edwin Chadwick, born in 1800, barrister, journalist and close friend of Jeremy Bentham, who left him a legacy and part of his library. In 1828 he was interested in actuarial calculations on the expectation of life; this called his attention to preventable causes of death and thus he became a sanitary reformer. In 1832 he was appointed assistant commissioner on the Poor Law Commission, quickly he collected a vast array of facts and showed such ability in suggesting remedies for the evils disclosed, that, next year, he was made full commissioner, and a member of the Commission on Factory Children which led to the passing of the Ten Hours' Act and to half-time education. In 1834 he was appointed secretary to the new administrative Poor Law Commission, which in 1838 addressed a letter to Lord John Russell, then Home Secretary, demonstrating the filthy conditions under which the poor of London lived, whereby they were exposed to contagious disease and ill health. This brought them upon the rates, yet the authorities had no power by which they could prevent this preventable illness. Two appendices disclosing the facts on which the letter was based accompanied it, one from Dr. Neil Arnott and Dr. J. P. Kay, the other from Dr. Southwood Smith. The directing hand that wrote the letter was Chadwick's and to him therefore belongs the credit of beginning Sanitary Reform. Simon points out that publication of the letter and its appendices in 1838 is memorable in history, because of the tone now first taken by a department of state with regard to the prevention of disease, and because three doctors had been asked to report on the condition of the London poor. The letter led the House of Lords to call for a report on England, Scotland and Wales which was presented in 1842.

The report was very long, but Chadwick prepared a synoptical volume which was widely read, 10,000 copies being distributed. It was entitled *General Report on the Sanitary Condition of the Labouring Population of Great Britain*. In this he disclosed that the state of affairs was as dreadful throughout the country as in London, he put forward remedies, and it is of interest to observe that Medical Officers of Health were suggested. Such a report naturally led to a Royal Commission, and this entirely confirmed Chadwick's account of existing evils and approved in substance of the remedies he advised. Legislation followed, in 1848 the Public Health Act was passed, it authorized the establishment of a new executive department, the General Board of Health. Before this some smaller acts had been passed, so that authorities could appoint Medical Officers of Health, abate nuisances prejudicial to health, provide free baths and wash-houses, give gratuitous vaccination and compel registration of births, deaths and marriages.

There were many defects in the constitution and powers of the General Board of Health, at first there was no doctor on it, but soon Dr. Southwood Smith was appointed. It was somewhat overwhelmed by the cholera epidemic, its most notable activity was its campaign against uncleanliness, particularly by the establishment of proper sewage works and by the use of glazed pipes for drains. It did not do as much as was hoped and it aroused great opposition, directed chiefly against Chadwick, its

most able and active member, who, Simon says, bore the reformer's crown of laurel, in that he was one of the best abused men
of his time. The Board was only appointed for five years, at the
end of which parliament refused to renew it in 1854. Chadwick
retired on a pension of £1,000 a year. During the Crimean
War he did much to improve army sanitation, later he gave
the Government valuable help on drainage questions. His work
for Sanitary Science was known all over the world and he
received many distinctions in connection with it. He died
July 6, 1890. His fame still lives. In *The Times* for July 17,
1935, we read:

> The improvement in public health activity which began with the passing of
> the first Public Health Act in 1848 was mainly due to the strenuous efforts of
> Edwin Chadwick as secretary to the Poor Law Commission. In a series of
> memorable reports Chadwick exposed the appalling insanitary conditions which
> existed and the tremendous burden of avoidable sickness and destitution which
> they caused. It is impossible to over-estimate the value of the 1840 report of
> the Select Committee on the Health of Towns, or the still more famous 1844–5
> report of the Royal Commission on the State of Towns. They were not merely
> State papers, but great civilizing documents.

Dr. Neil Arnott, born in 1788, was a ship's surgeon to the
East India Company; he settled in London, did a large
practice and became a member of the Senate of the London
University. He was a genuine philanthropist, a notable sanitarian and a distinguished physicist, who became an F.R.S.
When he was fifty years old he and Kay issued their appendix
to the letter of 1838. He died in 1874.

Dr. James Phillips Kay (afterwards Sir J. P. Kay-Shuttle-
worth) was an assistant Poor Law Commissioner and later
secretary to the committee of the Council of Education.

Dr. Southwood Smith, born 1788, at first a nonconformist
minister, graduated M.D. at Edinburgh. He did a large
practice, was for many years physician to the Fever Hospital,
was one of the promoters of the Anatomy Act and published
the *Philosophy of Health*. This book, many editions of which
sold largely, had great influence in directing public attention
to national health, for which cause its author worked day
and night. In 1833–4 he was on a Commission to collect
information as to children in factories; from 1839 to 1854 he
was Chadwick's chief medical associate and all that is strictly

medical in the reports of the General Board of Health was his.
Jeremy Bentham appointed him to dissect his dead body which
he did at Grainger's Webb Street School. He died in 1861.

These four sanitary reformers were greatly aided by the labours
of that statistical genius, William Farr, born in 1807 of poor
parents, but helped to become a doctor by the benevolence of
Mr. Pryce. Farr wrote an article on vital statistics in 1837
which was the foundation of a new science and caused him to be
appointed compiler of abstracts in the Registrar-General's office.
This led to the annual publication of his renowned letters on
the causes of death in England which show a mastery in the
marshalling of facts and in the science of statistics, and form an
eloquent and philosophical statistical history of the people. A
committee of the Statistical Society published a selection of his
works under the title of *Vital Statistics*. He wrote much, was
very popular, had great industry, was a wide reader, an excellent
linguist and a prominent member of the Statistical Society, of
which he was President. He received many honours, was an
F.R.S., a D.C.L. of Oxford and a C.B. Before his death in
1883 a large fund was raised to provide for his unmarried
daughters, and at his death the Government gave £400 to it.
Simon tells us that it was Chadwick who first recognized Farr's
genius and secured for him the post of compiler of abstracts.
There is no doubt of the immense service he rendered to Sanitary
Science by promoting the use of exact numerical standards in
place of the former vague adjectives.

Simon became Medical Officer to the General Board of Health
in 1855, and the account of "English Sanitary Institutions"
from then till 1876 when he left the Local Government Board
has already been given, consequently my abstract of his book
is nearly finished. There is in it an admirable criticism of
Stansfeld's futile policy and of the few medical clauses in
the Act of 1888 conferring on each county, for prescribed purposes, the right of self-government. There are also suggestions
for considerably increasing the efficacy of Medical Officers of
Health. A thoughtful essay on the "Politics of Poverty" and
one called "Conclusion" finish the book which was published
in 1890. A second edition appeared in 1897, it contained an
appendix on "Charitable Bequests forbidden by Law" and
another on "The Ethical Relations of Early Man."

The Council of the Sanitary Institute were of opinion that "Mr. Simon by his magnificent labours pointed out the way to effect an enormous saving of life in our great cities, among our manufacturing people, as well as in our rural districts." As, however, his works were entombed in a mass of blue books and reports, not easy of access, the members of the Council decided to do him the honour of publishing, by subscription in his lifetime, abstracts of his works. This was done by a committee, with Dr. Seaton as editor, and two volumes, entitled *Public Health Reports* by John Simon, were published in 1887.

Simon's lectures on Pathology were printed, in 1850, as a book entitled *General Pathology*. It certainly would not be of much use to a student desiring facts for an examination, but it would be welcome to him if he wished to be taught to think. It introduced to the reader the work of continental pathologists and it foreshadowed bacteria, for the author attributed to "contagia" two characteristic endowments: (*a*) that they produce their characteristic results in the smallest conceivable doses, (*b*) that they undergo, in the body on which they act, a striking and singular increase, which increase, if recovered from, confers immunity. The book is dedicated to Green with the grateful and affectionate homage of a pupil to his master.

Joseph Henry Green, Professor of Surgery at King's College Hospital, Surgeon to St. Thomas's Hospital for many years, twice President of the Royal College of Surgeons, is remembered not so much as a surgeon as from the fact that he was a philosophic disciple of, and a great friend of, Coleridge. He left behind him the manuscript of his book *Spiritual Philosophy founded on the Teaching of the late Samuel Taylor Coleridge*. Mrs. Green asked Simon to see it through the press. This he did and he supplied as an introduction an admirable " Memoir " of the author's life. When and how Green and Coleridge became acquainted is not known, but they were close friends from about 1817 till Coleridge's death in 1834, spending hours together every day even when Green was most busy professionally. The titles of his two Hunterian orations indicate his bent, one was on Vital Dynamics, the other on Mental Dynamics. Inheriting money from his father, he retired from practice in 1836, and, having been made trustee for Coleridge's children, and having received the bequest of a large part of his library, " as being the friend most intimate with my intellectual labours and aspirations," Green devoted most of his time, during the rest of his life, to acting as Coleridge's literary executor, to studying his philosophy and to seeing through the press two of his philosophic works, to one of which he contributed a long philosophic preface. In 1863 he died the death of a philosopher, for Simon writes " he in silence set his finger to his wrist, and visibly noted to himself the successive feeble pulses which were but just between him and death. Presently he said ' stopped.' And this was the very end."

Simon's Astley Cooper Prize Essay on the thymus gland is a laborious piece of work. The first twenty pages are historical, next comes the development of the gland studied mostly in swine and oxen, then its size and structure are discussed, finally there is an elaborate account of its comparative anatomy, well illustrated with good pictures. His paper on the " Comparative Anatomy of the Thyroid," read before the Royal Society, June 20, 1844, is a brief account of the subject. Both these essays are of value chiefly from the point of view of Comparative Anatomy.

He contributed the article on contagium to Quain's *Dictionary of Medicine* published in 1876. Remembering this date we see Simon to be in front of his time, for he writes " contagium must either be, or must essentially include a specific living organism able to multiply its kind." He prophesies that septic infections, typhoid, cholera, diphtheria and small-pox will be found " to have, as their contagia, microphytes respectively specific to them."

SIR WILLIAM WITHEY GULL

When Gull was a child he could hardly have dreamed that he would be given the opportunity that came to him of entering a profession which suited him so exactly and which he adorned so well.

He was born at Colchester on December 31, 1816, the youngest of a family of eight children. His father, John Gull, was a barge owner and wharfinger, who moved to Thorpe-le-Soken, in Essex, four years after William's birth. He died of cholera in 1827, leaving his wife, Elizabeth Gull, to bring up her large family on very slender means. She was a woman of character who devoted herself to her children, instilling in them the proverb "Whatever is worth doing is worth doing well." Her youngest child often said that his real education had been given him by his mother. First he went with his sisters to a day school, then to a day school for boys till he was fifteen, when he became a boarder there for two years. Next he was for two years a pupil teacher in a school at Lewes kept by Mr. Abbott, with whose family he lived. Here he fell in with Mr. Joseph Woods, the botanist, and, to the end of his life, remained fond of looking for unusual plants.

He returned home to Beaumont, the parish adjoining Thorpe, his mother having moved there in 1832. He was now nineteen, had studied with application, knew some Latin and Greek, but felt unsettled, not knowing what to do. He thought of going to sea, but his mother would not consent. Mr. Harrison, the rector of Beaumont, kindly asked the boy to come to him for classical tuition three days a week; on the other days he looked for plants and rare things on the seashore of the Hamford Estuary. This continued for a year, during which Gull decided that he would like to be a doctor, which however seemed impossible for want of money. The rector chanced to mention Gull's desire to Benjamin Harrison, the Treasurer of Guy's, who had come to stay with his nephew, no doubt partly because the parish of Beaumont was the property of Guy's Hospital. The nephew took his uncle to Mrs. Gull's house. The same singular gift for seeing great merit, which had made Benjamin Harrison help Bright, and bring Addison on the staff of Guy's Hospital, now made him, at once, offer to take Gull as a student at Guy's. He promised him two rooms in the hospital, £50 a year and every opportunity for study, saying " I will help you if you will help yourself." On these conditions Gull came to Guy's in September 1837. He certainly carried out his share of the bargain.

During the first year Harrison made him copy out in a fair hand the catalogue of the museum drawn up by Hodgkin. In his spare time he worked for the Matriculation Examination at the University of London, passing in 1838. The Treasurer thereupon, at a meeting of the staff, proposed that Gull should be a perpetual student, free of payment. This was agreed to and his teachers welcomed him cordially. Gull used often to speak of their kindness, especially of that of Dr. Guy Babington. He took his M.B. in 1841 with honours in four subjects, he obtained the M.D. in 1846, with a gold medal, and he carried off many hospital prizes.

In 1842 he was appointed to teach Materia Medica, being given therefore £100 a year and a small house close to the hospital in King Street—now Newcomen Street; later on he was provided with a larger one in St. Thomas's Street. Next year he lectured on Natural Philosophy, and from 1846 to 1856 he was lecturer on Physiology at Guy's and Professor of the same subject at the Royal Institution for two years, 1847–9. Here he met Faraday and the two became friends. Gull was put in charge of the wards for lunatics at Guy's, long ago abolished; he was also for a time Medical Tutor and, being given residence in the hospital, was appointed assistant to the second Mr. Stocker, the resident apothecary, whose duty it was to look after patients in the absence of the staff. Stocker and he were excellent companions; Gull, holding these appointments, was enabled to live, and, being close to or in the hospital, had, during his junior years, a vast clinical experience, which his industry and natural gift of observation enabled him to utilize to the utmost. Frederick Denison Maurice was resident chaplain from 1836 to 1846. He was " delighted with the establishment" and lectured to the students on philosophy. Kingsley called him " the most beautiful human soul " he had known. Gull became a friend of his and must have been influenced by such a man.

In 1848 Gull was elected a Fellow of the Royal College of Physicians; in the same year he married Susan Ann, daughter of Colonel Lacy of Carlisle. Soon after this he left his rooms in Guy's, going to live at 8 Finsbury Square, where he rapidly became popular as a physician. Few can have embarked on practice with a wider knowledge of clinical medicine. In 1851 he was appointed assistant physician and in 1858 full physician. In 1856 he gave up lecturing in physiology in order to join Dr. Owen Rees as lecturer on medicine. Two years later he was elected a Fellow of the Royal Society and afterwards served on its council; honorary degrees from Oxford, Cambridge and Edinburgh were awarded to him. He conscientiously did his share of professional public work, for he was on the General Medical Council during many years, and on the Senate of the University of London for thirty-three; he did much to promote the foundation of the Brown Institute; he was President of the Clinical Society; he helped to form the Association for the Advancement of Medicine by research; he went to Copenhagen to a meeting to promote Collective Investigation and he made himself helpful in many directions.

In 1862 he moved to 74 Brook Street; his practice grew so rapidly that in 1866 when between 49 and 50 he resigned his physiciancy to Guy's Hospital. In 1871 he was appointed consulting physician and later on a Governor of the Hospital. Apart from an attack of typhoid fever, his health was good until 1887 when, while at his house in Scotland, he was seized with hemiplegia and aphasia due to a cerebral hæmorrhage, of which the only warning had been unexplained hæmoptysis not long before. After a few weeks he recovered sufficiently to return to London. He remarked characteristically " One arrow had missed its mark, but there are more in the quiver." The next two years he lived in London, Brighton and Reigate; during this period there were several more cerebral hæmorrhages, the fatal arrow causing coma struck him in January 1890 and led to his death on the 28th of that month. Happily his mind was hardly clouded during these two years; he liked to talk of Guy's Hospital, to which he said he owed everything. He was buried,

next to his father and mother, at Thorpe-le-Soken, on the third
of February, a beautiful, warm sunshiny day. A multitude
attended, the heads of his profession, colleagues, pupils, friends,
patients and servants.

Gull would have come to the front rank of almost any
profession. His figure was an asset, he was tall and erect, his
dark hair fell over his brow, beneath which shone his expressive
eyes and below were his firmly closed lips. He looked as though
born to command, his appearance was compared to that of
Napoleon. He was much amused one day when he was
spoken to in St. Thomas's Street as Mr. Spurgeon. They were
not alike except that both men appeared wise and domina
and also looked as though they knew it. Seeing Gull in a cro
you were compelled to ask who is that man. When he ta
you still felt the domination. He never said a foolish thir
spoke authoritatively and epigrammatically; at his own
table he would command the attention of the whole co   ;
a lady declared that a conversation with him was "   ost
striking event of her life." Occasionally he enforced   nion
egotistically and arrogantly and this led to a few   ttable
quarrels with other doctors, but directly he saw h   take he
was truly sorry. His strong sense of duty mad   do his
share of committee work, but from what has be   d it is not
surprising that he did not excel in this, althou   s judgment
was sound. When it was being discussed wh   the Apothe-
caries Company should be allowed to give   dical qualification, he said, "The road to medical know   e is through the
Hunterian Museum, and not through an   othecary's shop."
Hardly the best way to placate the Ap   aries Company.

It is natural that such a man should   uire great popularity
with his patients; many fashionabl   octors have possessed
to some degree the personal power of Gull, without any pretence
to much medical learning, but he had, by indefatigable
industry, acquired a profound knowledge of all branches of
medicine, he had a scientific mind, he had to a high degree
the gift to observe, he reasoned accurately, he knew the relative
importance of facts and lastly he had excellent judgment in the
art of applying his knowledge to a particular patient. Therefore
in him were combined an arresting personality and the possession,
to an exceptional degree, of a knowledge of the art and science

of medicine. No wonder he carried all before him and, as his colleague, Wilks, said, " he remains one of the foremost men of mark of his time." In the nineteenth century no doctors were so well known to the world as Astley Cooper, Paget and Gull.

Luckily Gull, like Napoleon, had the power of almost instantaneous sleep. During his hardest professional life he slept ten hours nightly. His capacity for work was immense, recreation, with him, meant a change to the study of something outside his profession, mostly books. He was always punctual and never in a hurry. He rose at eight and breakfasted at nine-fifteen. Between these times he studied his favourite authors. He read each in his own language, for he knew Latin, Greek, German and Italian. His excellent memory enabled him to quote felicitously, which he did with obvious pleasure. Love of good poetry was natural to him and this liking was cultivated by his friendship with Maurice ; George Herbert was perhaps his favourite poet. He really grew to know his author, for a book was studied, pondered over, digested and absorbed, passages which impressed him being committed to memory on the spot. After books, the recreation he loved was the country. In later years his holidays were almost entirely passed among the mountains of Scotland. He did not care for sport, but observing the skies, the hills, the flowers, and the animals gave him great pleasure. There was hardly a walk but that some insect or plant was brought home for observation.

It is true that he became rich, this was not his fault ; patients would see him. The obituary notice in the *Proceedings of the Royal Society* says : " Few men have practised a lucrative profession with less eagerness to grasp at its pecuniary rewards. He kept up the honourable standard of generosity to poor patients." Further he often helped considerably the younger men of his own profession.

Gull was undoubtedly a really great physician. Wilks, who knew him well, speaks of " his extensive and thorough acquaintance with every subject in medicine, gained by his indefatigable industry when a young man, aided by his natural acumen, which gave him wonderful powers of penetration." All this is undoubtedly true. His marvellous memory enabled him always to have at his disposal a vast fund of knowledge from many books, not only on medicine but on sciences allied to it and on philosophy; further by this same memory he drew upon the recollections of his extensive experience. Then he was thorough in his examination of a patient, nothing escaped him; rightly he was contemptuous of those who were not thorough, as he said " What can you know of a man's constitution unless you have examined his urine ?" He was not one of those who neglect the story of the patient's illness, a favourite piece of advice to his students was "never disregard what the mother says." One day he turned this teaching amusingly against his ward clerk S——, whose duty it was to give the history of a child in the ward who had a rash. Gull said it had measles. Shortly after he left, it became evident that the child had small-pox and it was sent away. Many went round the wards with Gull next day to see how he would deal with his mistake, one which has been made many times and by the best observers. Gull said quietly,

You know, gentlemen, that I have over and over again pointed out that the diagnosis between measles, scarlet fever and small-pox could be made from a correct history of the development of the symptoms; in the case of this child I trusted to S——; I thought I could trust him, but I was mistaken. I am sorry.

He always held his clinical flair in subjection to his reason, he poured scorn on those, so common in medicine, who draw conclusions from insufficient data. He was never afraid to say " he did not know." He had no sympathy with doctors, who, when they do not know what to do, say we must do something. Said he, in such circumstances, give nature a chance, for many patients will get well without any drugs. A favourite saying of his was " Medicines do most good when there is a tendency to recovery without them," which, taken in its sarcastic sense, is correct. He published a paper on the mint-water treatment of rheumatic fever. The object of this was to show that patients, with this disease, improved just as well on no medicine as on the many drugs then employed, for the salicylates had not then come into use. The mint water was given merely as a placebo. So ready were doctors then to give drugs, that many quite failed to see Gull's point, consequently mint-water treatment became fashionable for rheumatic fever. His scientific mind made him protest so loudly against the prevailing habit of giving drugs without any evidence of their benefit, that some of the profession took a dislike to this part of his teaching. But time has fully vindicated him; hosts of drugs given in his day have disappeared from the pharmacopœa as being useless. Gull could use with admirable skill, on appropriate occasions, drugs such as mercury, opium, quinine and digitalis, the efficacy of which was beyond doubt. It is certain that his teaching did great good in promoting rational treatment in medicine, in which he was a pioneer and for which he deserves great credit. To appreciate the difficulty of his crusade, we must remember the unquestioning faith in bleeding, blistering, purging and physicking which held sway in his day. After his retirement he said, "One thing I am thankful that Jenner and I have together succeeded in doing. We have disabused the public of the belief that doctoring consists in drenching them with nauseous drugs." He was perfectly honest in all things; this reforming attitude, which was wrongly regarded as a kind of therapeutic nihilism, was carried out both in hospital and private practice. He congratulated one of his hospital patients, to whom drugs had not been given, on recovery from a severe attack of typhoid. The man replied, "Yes and no thanks to you either." He went to a consultation two hundred miles into the country and, to the dissatisfaction of the doctor whom he met, he refused to write a prescription, because he said the patient only required the encouragement of being convinced that he did not need drugs for his recovery. He often refused to repeat a visit on the ground that he wished the sufferer to feel that it was unnecessary. At another consultation, in which he saw, with the local doctor, a patient suffering from rheumatic fever, he did not tell the patient's friends that he had detected a pericardial rub, but he did tell the doctor who said, "Dr. Gull, it was very good of you not to let them see I had made a dreadful mistake. I cannot think how I can possibly have failed to detect the pericarditis." "Never mind," said Gull, "it is just as well, for if you had detected it perhaps you might have treated it." Let no one run away with the impression that, because Gull did not give unnecessary drugs, he did not treat his patients. He gave drugs when necessary, and nobody could have been more solicitous in helping nature in every way. A comfortable bed, opium to relieve pain and attract sleep, aperients if needed, a fire to make the room cheerful, something to relieve the thirst and dry mouth of fever were all attended to in the greatest detail.

This leads to another point in his teaching. So many regarded the patient as a case, gave what they thought, often wrongly, was an appropriate remedy, and there was an end of the matter. Gull raised his voice emphatically against this and his protest did much to improve clinical medicine. He always said with truth that in every case we had to treat a disease in a particular man. He used the phrases "a typhoid man," "a pneumonic man" and taught that he had to treat the disease as it affected a particular person, so that when he saw a patient he not only tried to find out what was the disease from which he suffered but what kind of man he was. This is all self-evident, but many doctors did not act as though it were, and even at the present day some fail in this respect.

Like all competent physicians, he followed his fatal cases to a post-mortem examination. He says his attention was for years "much given" to examination after death. A patient of his left the hospital; one Saturday afternoon, Gull heard that this patient had died, at his home, twenty miles from London. Gull at once sent a note to his house physician at Guy's asking him to breakfast on Sunday and telling him to bring tools to make a post-mortem examination. This he did, the two drove to the patient's house and, after much opposition, which Gull overcame, the post-mortem examination was made and the diagnosis established.

He greatly disliked writing, his addresses make now rather dull reading; nevertheless, as he was an eloquent speaker they were, when spoken, admirable. In them we see the reforming zeal by which he tried to awaken the public and the profession to a higher and more efficient practice of medicine. He preached that the prevention of disease should be our first aim. "There is a belief," he said, "amongst the poor that disease comes by Providence and is cured by drugs," adding, "whilst you put up a public house at one end of your street and a provident dispensary at the other, how can you expect your people to be healthy?" In his Harveian oration we find him saying, "I ought to urge upon the profession the most strenuous and united exertion for limiting the spread of these diseases if it be not possible to altogether stamp them out." His address to the Clinical Society illustrates his clarity of thought; for example, he says, "It seems probable that, in a good deal of our clinical pathology, we have mistaken the end for the beginning; and being impressed chiefly by the more prominent, or more easily demonstrable lesion, have regarded it as a cause, when it was but a part of another and antecedent state." He goes on to urge that the beginnings of disease are to be learnt in private practice, a view re-enunciated a few years ago as though it were new. He characteristically concludes by reminding his audience that the two special objects of medicine are to do good and not to do harm. Throughout all his addresses we see the width of view that characterizes a great mind; this naturally made him dislike specialism. He was optimistic enough to hope for increase of knowledge by the collective investigation of disease, although he derided drawing conclusions from data which were not comparable with each other. Time has shown that this is precisely where collective investigation fails.

From his juniors, Wilks and Pye-Smith, we learn of the excellence of his teaching in the hospital. The students adored him and hung upon the compact, trite, short sentences into which so much instruction was compressed. His saying, " However clever you are, there are three diseases you are sure to overlook. They are phthisis, syphilis and itch," was handed down and repeated to many generations of students and must have saved hundreds of mistakes. He compelled his pupils to observe for themselves and drummed into them the necessity of thoroughness in clinical examinations. Like other physicians in those days he went round the wards on Sunday morning, teaching the senior students. An old disciple writes:

As a lecturer Gull was careful, instructive and interesting, full of impressive aphorisms, and ripe conclusions, using apt and striking metaphors, but only sparingly, and enforcing what he taught by a dignified, slow, and careful reiteration, which never wearied, and which required more than average carelessness to forget. His lectures on medicine were accurate and full of information. . . . Not many years ago, we heard an old student of Guy's descant on his beautiful lectures, and especially those on fever. On being questioned as to what Gull said which most struck him, he said he could not remember anything in particular, but he would come to London any day to hear Gull reiterate the words in very slow measure " Now typhoid, gentlemen."

In 1874 he gave the Introductory Lecture at Guy's on October 1. It was announced that he would lecture in the Anatomy Theatre which could seat a large audience. So many came that hundreds could not get in and all tramped off to the ballroom of the Bridge House Hotel which was packed and there the lecture was given.

Gull did an enormous private practice, for there was no physician better skilled or with larger experience and, in addition, he had a way of dealing with patients that was unsurpassed. The term "fashionable physician" is not one that the best in the profession care to have applied to them, because many ignorant doctors have been so designated. Gull therefore when these two words were said of him rightly replied "No, the physician in fashion" which exactly expressed what he was.

He was already famous, but was made more so by the illness of the Prince of Wales at Sandringham. On November 13, 1871, he first felt out of sorts. His medical attendants, Dr. Lowe of King's Lynn and Dr. Oscar Clayton, for a few days thought his lassitude and fever to be due to a sore on a finger, but the fever continuing they on November 20 diagnosed typhoid fever. Gull was sent for the next day, and Sir William Jenner arrived on the 23rd. It turned out to be a severe attack complicated by bronchitis, and for many days the Prince was in great danger. Queen Victoria went to Sandringham to be with him. For a month everything except the Prince's illness was forgotten, the only news that interested the people was that in the bulletins issued from Sandringham, which were posted at the police stations throughout the country. I was a lad then and my father sent me every evening to the police station to get the latest news. It was not until just before Christmas that bulletins were issued only once a day. After the Prince's recovery, a thanksgiving service, which Queen Victoria attended, was held in St. Paul's. Gull was made a baronet and his practice became larger than ever. He left a fortune of £344,000.

His reputation, his impressive figure, his fine wise features, and short authoritative sentences gave him an extraordinary hold over his numerous patients. Wilks, his colleague, says: "When Gull left the bedside of his patient and said in measured tones 'You will get well,' it was like a message from above." He used words ingeniously when dealing with patients. A man with a countenance which suggested intemperate habits was rejected by an insurance company; he was very angry, saying he would get a report from Sir William Gull, who wrote:

Life good, but might be injuriously affected by the use of stimulants, if his habits should become or continue intemperate. . . . I beg to state that I this day made a medical examination of Mr. A. C. and excepting a disordered condition of the stomach and liver, which may be corrected and its recurrence prevented by a strictly abstemious regimen, Mr. C. is free from disease.

Many were his clever sayings, especially to patients who fancied themselves ill. They usually did good, for they really indicated to the unhappy sufferer that there was nothing the matter with him.

Gull would have made a good actor and from time to time his histrionic talent peeped out. He was once called to a consultation about a young lady, and it chanced that he passed her open bedroom door on his way to meet her mother and the doctor in another room. He walked straight up to the mother, saying, "Madam, I congratulate you; your daughter will get quite well." She, taken aback, replied, "But you have not seen her." He replied, "Madam, I saw her through the open door of her bedroom, that was quite enough." He had been told the patient had typhoid, he saw her sitting up in bed. Any sufferer from typhoid who sits up in bed must be doing well.

All that has so far been said shows Gull as an exponent of the science and art of clinical medicine; he did so much to raise these that he deserves to be remembered for that only, but in addition he made first-class additions to our knowledge. There are ninety-four articles mentioned in the bibliography of his writings. Considering that it was irksome to him to put his pen to paper, this represents much hard work, and work which is always that of a student of nature; nowhere is there anything addressed to the public to attract attention to himself. Throughout he shows an extensive acquaintance with the literature of his subject. Many of his papers, after his death, were edited and reprinted as a book by his son-in-law, Theodore Acland.

That, early in his career, his ability received attention beyond his own hospital is shown by his being appointed, three years before he became assistant physician to Guy's, namely in 1848, to deliver the Gulstonian Lectures before the Royal College of Physicians, he having been made a Fellow in that year. Like so many young physicians he was attracted by the nervous system: these lectures dealt with this. When we read them now, we must remember that the work of Marshall Hall and Brodie had hardly become general knowledge and that ignorance about the nervous system was widespread. Therefore it was not unimportant for Gull to insist that in paraplegia motion is affected more than sensation, and that in hemiplegia the lower extremity recovers before the upper. He was on the right track, for he attempted, after death, to find the lesion which had caused the symptoms; and he said:

One of the great causes of our little advance in the study of nervous affections seems to me to have arisen from a tacit assumption that the phenomena were too uncertain and varying to admit of any general expression. . . . My endeavour therefore to establish some general laws, if fruitless, must still, I think, be in the right direction.

For more than ten years after these lectures Gull devoted much thought and labour to a study of diseases of the spinal cord. Three papers on Paraplegia appeared in the *Guy's Hospital Reports* (1856, 1858 and 1861), and there were some others less important. He insisted that the symptoms in diseases of the spinal cord depended upon the position of the lesion. The medical profession was—and is to some extent now—cursed with a propensity to rest satisfied that it explained phenomena by calling them idiopathic, rheumatic or gouty. Gull's scientific mind made short work of this nonsense, saying, " To call them idiopathic is to satisfy ourselves with a term without meaning, and to call them rheumatic is to impose upon ourselves the fallacy of the *ignotum per ignotum*." In the first three cases, out of the sixteen which form the basis of the first paper, the paraplegia was due to a tumour of the cord, he protests against the teaching of the day that such tumours are usually malignant and he emphasizes the importance of the symptoms, pain and spastic extension. Throughout all these papers the clinical and post-mortem descriptions are admirable; further, we have, what was then unusual, a careful microscopic examination of the cord. To Gull belongs the credit of being the first to describe disease of the posterior columns of the cord in association with the symptoms of locomotor ataxy. Case 19 is that of a man aged 28 who had the characteristic pains, numbness and ataxy. The spinal cord was normal to the naked eye, but microscopic examination showed that " the posterior columns were atrophied throughout their entire length." There is an excellent plate to illustrate this. Gull remarks that the case supports the theory of Dr. Todd that the posterior columns " propagate the influence of that part of the encephalon which combines with the nerves of volition to regulate the locomotive powers." He also points out that the lesion would have been overlooked but for the microscope.

Paraplegia is often associated with inflammation of the bladder. Brown-Séquard explained this by suggesting that the condition of the bladder induced a reflex contraction of the vessels of the spinal cord and so, rendering it functionless, induced paraplegia. His authority made this view popular and " Urinary Paraplegia " was diagnosed in many cases. Gull said that these required a " winnowing criticism," which he gave : first, on clinical grounds ; secondly, on experimental, for he, Pavy and Durham performed experiments on animals which failed to show " a reflex impression " on the vessels of the cord from the bladder ; thirdly, on post-mortem grounds, for he stated that a naked-eye examination of the cord is valueless, but that microscopical examination of the cord will always show it to be diseased in these cases. This rejection of the doctrine of reflex paralysis was a great step forwards in medicine. His last paper about the spinal cord gave a naked-eye and a microscopical description of the cord in a case of syringo-myelia, or as he called it hydro-myelus. It is characteristic of his enthusiasm that when a post-mortem examination on this patient was refused and the friends took the body away, Gull followed and with great difficulty got permission to make the examination.

He wrote (*Guy's Hospital Reports,* 1857) an admirable article on " Abscess of the Brain." It would be easy to give a clinical lecture from it to-day, the clinical and post-mortem records are so clear. The points he enforces are that there is no such thing as an " idiopathic abscess," cerebral abscess is always fatal (it was then), its course is insidious, often slow, and symptoms may be absent. The usual view was that when disease of the ear causes a cerebral abscess that disease is scrofulous. Gull exposes this error, telling us that the aural disease is inflammatory. He and Sutton wrote the article on " Abscess of the Brain " in Reynold's *System of Medicine* and he and Anstey that on " Hypochondriasis." His last paper on " Nervous Diseases " in the *Guy's Hospital Reports* is a short one in 1859 on five cases of Intracranial Aneurysm.

In 1874 Gull drew the attention of the Clinical Society to the condition which he called anorexia nervosa. The appropriateness of this name, and the fact that he was then so well known, directed attention to his short paper, before which many doctors had failed to diagnose the condition and many women had consequently suffered unnecessarily. After his paper anorexia nervosa was recognized and properly treated.

Four medical articles were published under the joint authorship of Gull and Henry Gawen Sutton, who was physician to and lecturer on pathology at the London Hospital. He died in 1891. The world outside knew little of him, neither the *Lancet* nor the *British Medical Journal* gave an obituary notice of him, but those who were fortunate enough to know him recognized in him a profound, original thinker and a thorough physician, skilled at the bedside and in the post-mortem room. In 1886 he published his lectures on pathology; they did not form a text-book suitable for pushing students through examinations, but they were delightful for those who enjoy something philosophical. His admirers were ardent admirers, and directly after his death they issued a new edition of his *Lectures on Pathology*, which contain almost the whole of the original book with many other lectures added. It was revised by Wilks, of whom Sutton had written, "I ask you to allow me to acknowledge my debt to Dr. Wilks, whose labours, in this and many other subjects, have greatly advanced pathological teaching. He taught me pathology . . . it was his mind that showed me how to study morbid anatomy scientifically." The new edition was well reviewed; one reviewer said that it made the reader a better and wiser physician.

That he and Gull were great friends is shown by many references in Sutton's first book, for example, "Sir William Gull was, at Guy's Hospital, my clinical teacher; he first taught me how to examine organ by organ." We meet the two, at Gull's house, in the evening, discussing functional albuminuria and we find Sutton quoting Gull's sayings. Their minds were similar, both were accurate, thorough observers, and rigid critical reasoners.

Three of their conjoint papers were on chronic Bright's

disease, this being the subject to which Gull, next to the nervous system, gave most attention. Bright was inclined, at times, to think that the alterations in the kidney, in what became known as chronic Bright's disease, might be the cause of the numerous symptoms and post-mortem appearances which he so brilliantly described; but he did not commit himself, for, at other times, we find him wondering whether all these and the renal alterations might not have a common cause. As often happens, others rushed in where angels feared to tread, and it became a common belief that the renal alterations were the cause of all the associated symptoms and post-mortem appearances. Gull and Sutton made themselves celebrated by attacking this view. Their first paper *On the Pathology of the Morbid State commonly called Chronic Bright's Disease with Contracted Kidney (Arteriocapillary fibrosis)* was published in the *Medico-Chirurgical Transactions* for 1872. They examined microscopically the vessels of the pia mater in fifty-five cases, and gave a table of the appearances found, including hundreds of measurements of the thickness of the walls of the vessels and of the width of the vascular channel, they also examined the minute vessels of many other parts of the body. The pathological change, to which they directed attention, they called a hyaline fibroid formation in the walls of the minute arteries and a hyaline granular change in the corresponding capillaries. They found this change in cases showing (1) kidneys much contracted, heart much hypertrophied, (2) kidney little contracted, heart much hypertrophied, (3) kidneys healthy, heart much hypertrophied. Therefore they concluded that the kidney disease was but a part, and not an invariable part, of this morbid state. The hypertrophy of the heart they attributed to the vascular change. The conclusions reached at the end of this classic paper are in the writers' own words:

(1) There is a diseased state characterized by hyaline-fibroid formation in the arterioles and capillaries. (2) This morbid change is attended with atrophy of the adjacent tissues. (3) It is probable that this morbid change commonly begins in the kidney, but there is evidence of its also beginning primarily in other organs. (4) The contraction and atrophy of the kidney are but part and parcel of the general morbid change. (5) The kidneys may be but little if at all affected, when the morbid change is far advanced in other organs. (6) This morbid change in the arterioles and capillaries is the primary and essential condition of the morbid state called chronic Bright's disease with contracted kidney. (7)

The clinical history varies according to the organs primarily and chiefly affected. (8) In the present state of our knowledge we cannot refer the vascular changes to an antecedent change in the blood due to defective renal excretion. (9) The kidneys may undergo extreme degenerative changes without being attended by the cardio-vascular and other lesions characteristic of the condition known as chronic Bright's disease. (10) The morbid state under discussion is allied with the conditions of old age, and its area may be said hypothetically to correspond to the " area vasculosa." (11) The changes, although allied with senile altera-tions, are probably due to distinct causes not yet ascertained.

Finally the authors suggest " arterio-capillary fibrosis " as a name for this condition. For accurate reasoning and lucidity this paper is difficult to beat.

In 1877 they brought before the Pathological Society a com-munication entitled *On Changes in the Spinal Cord and its Vessels in Arterio-Capillary Fibrosis.* They tell us that, during the last five years, they have continued their investigations on the con-dition of the minute vessels in all the organs of the body, and have found commencing changes which might be the cause of many supposed unimportant ailments. While they have found similar changes in all parts of the body, they here only deal with the spinal cord and describe arterio-capillary fibrosis of its vessels and the effects of this, pointing out that the results in the cord are the same as those in the kidney. In some of the examples they give, it may well have been that the nervous symptoms recorded were caused by the described changes in the cord which the authors regard as, in their turn, being depend-ent upon arterio-capillary fibrosis of the spinal vessels. Both papers are illustrated with beautiful plates.

Gull and Sutton contributed a paper expressive of their views on arterio-capillary fibrosis to the International Medical Congress held in London in 1881 and Gull, by himself, read a paper on Chronic Nephritis at the International Congress held at Copenhagen in 1884, and in 1872 he gave a clinical lecture on the same subject at Guy's Hospital. His final words in this are worth quoting, they are so like him.

It is always dangerous to rest on a narrow pathology; and I believe that to be a narrow pathology which is satisfied with what you now see before me on this table. In this glass you see a much hypertrophied heart, and a very con-tracted kidney. The specimen is classical. It was, I believe, put up under Dr. Bright's own direction, and with a view of showing that the wasting of the kidney is the cause of the thickening of the heart. I cannot but look upon it with veneration, but not with conviction. I think, with all deference to so great an authority, that the systematic capillaries, and, had it been possible, the entire man, should have been included in the vase, together with the heart and kidneys; and then we should have had, I believe, a truer view of the causation of the cardiac hypertrophy and of the disease of the kidney.

The comment on this is that Bright would have said the object of the specimen was to show that the condition of the heart was associated with that of the kidney, not that it was caused by it. Bright's disease has fascinated workers at Guy's ever since his time; Wilks clarified our knowledge of its varieties; Mahomed greatly extended Gull and Sutton's conclusions in a clinical direction and now more than a century after Bright's first publication Osman is making new observations.

When many remedies are recommended for a disease, it is probable that none is efficacious, for if one did striking good, there would not be any need to enumerate the others. Eighty years ago many remedies were advised for rheumatic fever. Gull and Sutton studied cases, some from Guy's and others from the London Hospital, and read before the Medico-Chirurgical Society in 1869 a paper with the title *Remarks on the Natural History of Rheumatic Fever*. Sutton alone contributed two papers to the *Guy's Hospital Reports* in 1865 and 1866 on the treatment of rheumatic fever by a little mint water, that is to say without drugs, but both these papers represented Gull's opinions as well as Sutton's own. The authors concluded that the course of the disease was the same with mint water as with any other remedy, that its natural path was towards recovery and that this was the reason why patients recovered, their recovery was not hastened by any treatment then in vogue. Many physicians maintained that by treatment they could ward off cardiac complications. Gull and Sutton showed that, if cardiac complications occurred, they came on early, that is to say before admission to the hospital, and that treatment supposed to avert these did nothing of the sort, for the time of their onset had passed before the treatment began. A great part of medical literature is useless because writers will not remember " that it is absolutely necessary to understand the natural progress of the disease before any conclusion can be arrived at concerning the operation of remedies."

Charles Hilton Fagge, who died in 1883 at the age of 45,

was a fine original physician who had an immense knowledge of medicine. If you asked him a question about it he could usually give, off hand, a complete history of the subject. He was the last man who, single-handed, wrote a large book on medicine which is really a piece of literature, or, I should say, nearly wrote, for it was not quite finished at his death. Other text-books are either the work of several contributors, or a compressed collection of facts to be read for information, but Fagge can be read with enjoyment as well, the out-of-the-way learning, the careful criticism, the personal touch of the author's own experience and his pleasant style make what is commonly known as Fagge's *Medicine* a great book. The late Professor Starling owned a copy of the first edition which he exchanged for one of the second on its publication, but he found that the desire to make room for new facts had led to the excision of so much of the personal character of the book that the next morning he took back the second edition, recovered the first, and like everyone who owns it, kept it as a precious possession. Sporadic cretinism had been much discussed in the clinical teaching at Guy's. We owe to Fagge the discovery that it is due to atrophy of the thyroid, and in 1871 he tells us that Gull " some years ago made me acquainted with many of the principal features." Gull in 1874 read a paper before the Clinical Society *On a Cretinoid State Supervening in Adult Life in Women.* This was the first announcement of the discovery of the malady we call myxœdema. Five cases are recorded, two in great detail and yet shortly, they are perfect descriptions of what was a newly discovered disease. It was a fine piece of observation to recognize, on clinical grounds only, that in reality this and cretinism were one disease, for none of Gull's cases were fatal, and he states that " from the folds of fat about the neck I am not able to state what the exact condition of it [the thyroid] was."

In the *Guy's Hospital Reports* for 1855 Gull has a short paper entitled *Fatty Stools from Disease of the Mesenteric Glands.* He points out that it is remarkable how little the evacuations are studied; Cod Liver Oil is often given when, if the evacuations had been examined, the oil would be seen to have been passed unchanged; sometimes this is because of intestinal disease. He quotes Bright's original observation that, when fatty stools are due to pancreatic disease, the fat is separate from the general mass of the fæces, and then he makes the remark, which had not been made before, that

where the lesion is in the absorbent system, the fat being emulsified, becomes incorporated with the evacuation and is consequently not so easily recognized. If however there be, with defective absorption, an inflammatory condition of the mucous membrane and diarrhœa, the oily matters rise to the surface of the evacuations as a creamy film, and produce the pale, chalky and soapy appearance so characteristic of chronic muco-enteritis and mesenteric disease.

He describes a case of tuberculous ulceration of the bowel with tuberculous disease of the mesenteric glands to illustrate this. To him therefore we must give the merit of differentiating between the variety of fatty stools met with in pancreatic disease and that found when there is defective absorption associated with chronic muco-enteritis.

Gull's other literary contributions to medicine are interesting, but of less importance. All show that, as in the practice of his profession, so in his writings he was a close observer with good judgment, he reasoned well and correctly exposed false reasoning in others, he was always teaching us to take a wide view, he was never afraid to say he did not know, he made several original observations, he wrote well, and by what he said and wrote he greatly enhanced the position of medicine. Many of his most important publications appeared after the Prince of Wales's illness, when his practice was so large that he might easily have become merely a fashionable physician, but he showed that then, as always, he was a thinker whose desire was to advance knowledge in medicine.

SIR SAMUEL WILKS

It was a favourite saying of Samuel Wilks that what the public thought of a doctor was of little moment, but to be honoured by one's own profession was the highest good fortune which could be attained by any man. He had this good fortune.

Samuel, the second son of Joseph Barber Wilks, cashier at the East India House, was born on June 2, 1824, at Camberwell. Many of his ancestors had been in the East India House. The future physician was one of a large family, a sister married Sir Joshua Fitch, the educationalist. He first went to a dame's school and next to a boys' school, both at Camberwell. In 1835 he was sent to be taught by the Rev. Dr. Spyers at Wallop, between Andover and Salisbury. Next year, Spyers being appointed Head Master of Aldenham, Wilks followed him there, leaving in 1839 and going for one year to University College School.

In 1840 he was apprenticed to Mr. Richard Prior, the family doctor at Newington. He tells us " a sum of money was paid as usual, and soon I was able to make up medicines for private patients in the surgery, also to vaccinate, bleed, and draw teeth with a very primitive instrument called a key." While with Mr. Prior he worked as a student at Guy's Hospital, only a mile away, being a dresser to Mr. Aston Key. He must have been diligent, for, after being at Guy's a little time, he matriculated at the University of London, of which he became M.B. in 1848 and M.D., with the gold medal, in 1850. Continuing as assistant to Mr. Prior till he died in 1847, Wilks carried on the practice afterwards for a little time, and then sold it. He used to amuse us by telling of how he got rid of the doctor's horse to a man who first felt all down its legs, next waved his cap in front of the animal's eyes, then pondered a bit, after which he said, " Will you take nineteen guineas for your blind and lame old 'oss," which Wilks did.

When he was a student, Guy's Hospital consisted only of the buildings erected under the will of the founder, Wilks saw many others added and now the hospital, the medical and nursing schools make a building more than double the size of the original. Reform was in the air, he was much impressed with the increasing cleanliness; shortly before he entered wooden bedsteads had been replaced by those made of iron, so getting rid of bugs. This led to the dismissal of the bug-catcher, who was paid £40 a year. The stimulus given to medicine by Bright, Hodgkin and Addison led to the founding of the Clinical Report Society by the students, with the object of reporting cases and thus studying medicine more systematically. Soon it became obligatory to report all cases. The reports are bound and indexed at the end of each year, so that now eighty years' experience can easily be consulted. Wilks played a considerable part in the activities of this society, and drew up tables founded on the reports. He always strove to be accurate, and he says of these tables they " have all been made solely with a view to scientific accuracy."

While still a student, in 1850, he reviewed for the *Medical Times* a book on homœopathy, a subject which always interested him, so it is worth while to see what he thought about it; his opinion never changed. He did not think that its doctrine need be untrue because infinitesimal doses are used, for the smell of flowers may produce effects, although exhaled in infinitesimal quantities. He considered that the chief arguments against it were that it had failed to make headway, and could not therefore have a scientific basis, that if the law " similia similibus curantur " were really a valid law of nature, it must have been accepted, for it had been before us for so long, and lastly that the scientific way to study disease was first to learn anatomy, physiology and pathology, but homœopathists take treatment first.

In 1854 he married Mrs. Prior, the widow of the practitioner with whom he served his pupilage. She was the daughter of Henry Mockett, of Seaford, Sussex. Wilks had no children, but after his wife's death, Miss Prior, his stepdaughter, to whom he was much attached, kept house for him until her death, which took place about ten years before his. In 1853 he became physician to the Surrey Dispensary; in 1856 he was elected a Fellow of the Royal College of Physicians and also to the post of assistant physician to Guy's Hospital, becoming full physician in 1867.

Wilks gave daily demonstrations on morbid anatomy, always instructing the students. He lectured on pathology, and he was Curator of the Museum. Post-mortem examinations had been made before his time, but only because the doctor wished to find out if his view of the patient's illness had been correct. Most physicians had not studied Matthew Baillie's book, those who were conceited said why bother about a post-mortem examination, I am sure my view was right; those who were idle did not trouble about them. Wilks was the first to make post-mortem examinations on all who died in a hospital, the first to force doctors to appreciate the fundamental importance of morbid anatomy, and to show that no one could understand medicine unless he studied in the dead-house. Everyone now admits this, but it was he who, laying this foundation-stone, raised morbid anatomy to be an essential branch of the science of medicine. Since his time it has become a necessary part of every student's education. In 1859 he published *Lectures on Pathological Anatomy delivered at Guy's Hospital during the Summer Sessions 1857-1858*. A third edition appeared in 1889. Because of this book for the next twenty-five years almost all the energy for discovery in medicine was expended, and most fruitfully expended, in the study of morbid anatomy. The Pathological Society flourished. Wilks was an active member and ultimately its President. His book is a medical classic; it is a wonderful treatise, concise, accurate and well written. Over and over again it has happened that a morbid anatomist has thought he has discovered a new fact, but reference to this book has shown that Wilks had already observed it.

In 1865 he ceased lecturing on pathology, in order to become one of the two physicians giving systematic lectures on medicine, which he did for the next eighteen years. His were so full of good material that they appeared in periodicals, and were afterwards, at the insistent request of those who heard them, issued as books. The volume on the specific fevers and diseases of the chest could be obtained from the counting house at Guy's. Many students bought it, for it was far superior to any text-book then existing. Reading it now we see how medicine has changed, for Wilks says that then scarlatina was "the worst form of specific disease existing in our country," that he had recently seen many cases of malignant small-pox and that the letters F.C.R. were used to denote a bad cold, as it was called *febris catarrhalis rheumatica*.

The *Lectures on Diseases of the Nervous System* appeared separately because, he tells us, his pupils "have constantly demanded of me their reprint in a separate form." There are added, in the book, many accounts of actual patients, omitted from the lectures. The result is a fascinating volume which can, even now, be read not only with profit, but, also, with great pleasure, for it is never dull and is full of interesting quotations, speculations and clinical descriptions. It appeals especially to the general physician, because it deals fully with nervous disorders that come his way, which are often treated scantily by the professed neurologist, for example, delirium tremens, chorea, railway spine, traumatic epilepsy, lead poisoning, hysteria and apoplexy, of which there is an excellent account. In it are many original statements, among which we have, perhaps, the first description of alcoholic paraplegia. Wilks then thought this was due to disease of the cord, but a few years later it was found to be caused by peripheral neuritis.

It cannot have fallen to the lot of many lecturers to have three volumes of their lectures printed by request. Wilks was not a great speaker, he had not the pontifical incisive manner of Addison or Gull, which arrested the attention of the audience and burnt facts into the memory of the listeners. He was an excellent talker, somewhat verbose but always interesting ; nevertheless students came away from him feeling that they would learn more by reading what their teacher had said and hence they demanded to have his lectures printed. It was the same with instruction at the bedside, he would talk voluminously, the talk wandering just where fancy led. Ordinary students were too shy to stop him by questions, so, at the end of an afternoon round in the wards, they felt that, although they had heard much delightful talk, they had not learnt much. It was quite otherwise with post-graduate students, for whose sake he went round the wards on Sunday mornings ; these visits were very popular and many, e.g. Hughlings Jackson, Sutton and Donkin, from other schools, as well as Guy's men came. At these meetings there was first-rate discussion. Donkin says, "I have regarded him as the most suggestive and stimulating teacher of the science and practice of medicine I have known." There must have been something very out of the ordinary in Wilks's discourses, for Hughlings Jackson and Sutton, both great thinkers, used to come so frequently to his post-mortem demonstrations that the students nicknamed them "Wilks's Maggots."

To return to the facts of his life. Until about 1869 he had lived in St. Thomas's Street, but he then moved to 72, and shortly afterwards to 74 Grosvenor Street, where he remained till his retirement from practice in 1901. Many of his friends knew 74 well. There was a front room in which the parrot lived; this bird was the subject of an essay by Wilks entitled *Notes from the History of my Parrot in reference to the Nature of Language.* On the first floor was a back room in which he loved to gather his friends on Sunday evening, some had dropped in to supper, some afterwards. All sorts came, doctors, literary men and sometimes an actor or an artist. The air became thick with tobacco smoke; talk, which was rarely medical, flowed continuously till about midnight.

From this house he did his private practice. This was never large, and the reason for this is not quite clear. Partly it was because, if he was not much interested in the patient he let it be seen. The tale is told of his going into the country to visit a lady who fancied herself ill, Wilks, having satisfied himself that there was nothing the matter, began to take so much interest in the pictures, that the irritated husband had to remind him that the object of his visit was the lady's health. Then he would talk too much and some of his remarks gave offence, as when he said, "Age is relative, you are a worn-out old man at thirty.' On the other hand when there was real trouble, he was all thoughtfulness and kindness. I was present when he came to see, in consultation, a man with typhoid whom he thought would die, as he did. Nothing could have been better than the way in which Wilks told the young wife, who was expecting her confinement, encouraging her to bravery for the sake of the unborn child, and helping her by his kindness which I know she remembered for the rest of her life. The profession respected his opinion as much as that of anyone, consequently a great many sick doctors, their wives and children came to him. One morning he saw three; after the last, thinking aloud he said, " What a large practice I should do if it were not for doctors." Hardly a happy remark, but it was like Wilks to think aloud maladroit sayings.

During the eighteen years of his full physiciancy at Guy's Wilks was to the front in all that was going on in the medical world. He always upheld the investigator and willingly became Treasurer of the Association for the Advancement of Medicine by Research formed for defence against Antivivisectionists. He delivered the Harveian Oration when he was 55, this was an unusual honour—an older man is usually chosen—and he gave various addresses on medicine and pathology. He was President of both the Pathological and Neurological Societies, a member of the Senate of the University of London and of the General Medical Council, he was appointed Physician to the Duke of Connaught in 1879, in 1870 he became an F.R.S. and in 1884 an LL.D. of Edinburgh. All this time he faithfully played his part in the teaching at and in the administration of his Medical School. He retired from the physiciancy at Guy's in 1885; the retiring age is 60, so he should have gone the year before, but he was asked to stay an extra year, as two of the staff, Fagge and Mahomed, had recently died. Later he was made a Governor of Guy's.

For the next sixteen years he continued to live at 74 Grosvenor Street. The chief event in this period was his election in 1896 to the Presidency of the Royal College of Physicians. This he said was the greatest honour that had ever fallen to his lot, especially as he was always averse from being considered for the post. Nevertheless, in 1893 Sir Russell Reynolds had a majority of only three over him, and in 1896, Russell Reynolds having resigned, many felt that Wilks ought to be elected, for he was by far the most eminent representative, then alive, of British Scientific Medicine. But the difficulty was to persuade him to stand. One of his colleagues called on him at four o'clock one Sunday afternoon, and argued and talked with him, imploring him to stand, till ten o'clock the same evening when Wilks cut short the discussion by saying he was going to bed, he had not consented. The same colleague called at five the next afternoon. Wilks had told his servant to say " not at home," but fortunately the servant forgot and the argument was renewed.

After about half an hour's conversation, he yielded his consent and was elected by a large majority, holding office for three years. One of the President's duties is to make many after-dinner official speeches. Wilks was never tired on these occasions, of saying that he was not fitted to be President, that such an office was not in his line, but that he had been driven into it against his better judgment by the excessive importunity and unreasonable pertinacity of one of his colleagues.

He was right in his estimate of himself; he was not a remarkably good President, but most certainly he was not a bad President, and the large majority of Fellows that gave him this office felt that, by being President, he honoured the College, which naturally wished that the most intellectual physician of the day should be at its head. Everyone admitted that Wilks held this position, and his portrait appeared in *Vanity Fair* over the title " Philosophical Pathology."

In 1897 he was created a Baronet, was made Physician Extraordinary to Queen Victoria, and it was he who proposed the vote of thanks to the Prince of Wales, afterwards King Edward VII, for presiding at the banquet, in aid of Guy's Hospital, held at the Imperial Institute on June 10, 1896. He made an admirable speech, full of his well-known affection for his hospital.

This affection led to his writing, in conjunction with Mr. Bettany, the *Biographical History of Guy's Hospital*, which was published in 1892. This labour of love contains a history of the Hospital and Medical School and an account of all the members of its staff, and of all persons of note connected with it, who had died by the time the book was written; the biographies of those personally known to Wilks are especially valuable, and the book has given great pleasure to many old students. This love for his hospital was so great that I will quote what Dr. Jessop—not a Guy's man—who saw Wilks constantly, both as his friend and his doctor, during the last ten years of his life, says about it:

Undoubtedly the most prominent feature of his life was his connection with Guy's Hospital, his affection and veneration for his old school was part of his being. . . . It was as if he was a detached portion of the hospital, so closely was he identified with the place. Personally, whenever I think of Guy's I always think of Sir Samuel Wilks as emblematic of the Spirit of that Hospital, as the ideal Guy's man, and I venture to think that Guy's men themselves would point to him as the ideal representative of the best traditions of their great School.

When he had been President of the College for three years he let it be known that he did not wish to be re-elected, for he was seventy-five years old. In 1901 he left Grosvenor Street and went to live at 8 Prince Arthur Road, Hampstead, where he spent the rest of his life. For a large part of this time his stepgrandson lived with him, but he was out at his work all day. His stepdaughter had died a year or two previously, he was very fond of her; during her fatal illness, he spent night after night in his day clothes on a sofa in her room, lest she should want him. The prospect of a lonely old age now lay before him and in addition there were family troubles, but he faced the outlook with courage, knowing that he must fill up his time and occupy his mind. A small sundial and an outside thermometer were installed for meterological observation. He soon joined and became President of the Hampstead Scientific Society, a large and very much alive body; he attended the meetings regularly, always entered into the discussions and often read papers. The subjects which interested him were diverse: Keats, the orbit of the moon, Vaccination in Italy, Fahrenheit's thermometer, the eared elm of Hampstead, death from lightning, hermaphroditism, the burrowing bees of Hampstead Heath, the unluckiness of the month of May for marriage and several others occupied him while in Prince Arthur Road. Each was investigated with great perseverance, no trouble or physical inconvenience was too great to deter him from pursuing it.

At the age of 86 years he wrote a short book called *Biographical Reminiscences,* which his friend Sir Bryan Donkin kindly saw through the press, but Wilks himself, at the age of 87, corrected the proof. It contains a few facts about his life and also about the Hampstead Scientific Society, but is mostly occupied by abstracts from the Guy's Hospital Reports of papers that he thought of special interest. Also he published in 1908 a little book on vivisection called *The Relation of Man to Animals.*

Wilks soon made a large circle of friends and quickly took a prominent position in Hampstead; the inhabitants became proud of their handsome grand old man, and looked admiringly on him as he passed them in the street. Many called to talk with him, which usually meant listening to him, but they enjoyed it. The affectionate companionship of Mrs. and Miss Martelli next door on one side, and that of Dr. and Mrs. Bashford next door on the other side helped to render life pleasant for him. Some of his friends from town also came to talk. I remember going to see him one Sunday afternoon; although over 80 he was reading the *Lancet* without glasses and smoking a cigar. After about half an hour, during which the cigar had often gone out and been relit, coffee, muffins and crumpets appeared. Wilks still went on talking for about half an hour more, then he drank the cold coffee, ate the cold muffins and crumpets and relit the cigar, which by then was in a deplorable condition. When I got up to go he said, "You have told me no news, but I suppose you will say I have not given you a chance," which I could not deny.

He suffered much during the last years, there was severe appendicitis necessitating an operation, and he underwent another for an enlarged prostate, later he had a curious cerebral attack in which he was unconscious for three days, but he recovered from all, although much weakened by each. The activity of his mind was as great as ever, books were read, flowers examined, callers came to help the old man in his loneliness. From time to time he went into town, often to Guy's, sometimes to some object of special interest. If he said he would go, he went; he was President of the Physical Society at Guy's and liked to attend the opening meeting of each session, the last time he had to be taken both to and from the meeting by a friend. The final journey was to visit the returned Arctic ship, the *Nimrod*, stationed off the Thames Embankment. His tottering limbs were assisted to let him make a thorough examination; on the way back he insisted on going to the Cancer Research Laboratory, but it was a very exhausted man that returned home.

His infirmities increased, and a few days before his death, on November 8, 1911, Dr. Jessop suggested he might like to see one of his colleagues. He chose one who he said would not give him any medicine. Dr. Jessop writes :

His death-bed might form material for a picture, " The Ruling Passion strong in Death." Propped up as well as his paralysed and attenuated form could be, three good-sized books of reference he had sent for to refer to the appearance of a nutmeg in its original form lying on the bed, his feeble hand copying a drawing in one of the books. It was under these conditions that his last hour of sensibility was spent; he became unconscious with his books around him. It was at best a poor victory for Death; the mastery was not to be gained until the very seat of life itself in the brain was stricken—only by this means could his indomitable spirit be overcome.

Everything except politics and sport interested Wilks. His accurate and scientific mind was always seeking the why and the wherefore of things, during the whole of a long life his mental activity was extraordinary. It was characteristic that when he was in Switzerland, his friend Savage could not induce him to climb, he preferred inquiring into the geology and antiquities of the neighbourhood. He admired Darwin extremely; a beautiful etching of him always hung in Wilks's room. He was a considerable reader; good literature, especially poetry, gave him great pleasure, the Bible and Shakespeare were always at hand and frequently quoted; I remember in a lecture on heat-stroke he repeated the words of the story of the death of the child of the woman of Shunem. On his bedroom mantelpiece at Hampstead were photographs of Wendell Holmes, Harriet Martineau and Wordsworth. Good pictures hung in his rooms and a visit to a picture gallery with him was most enjoyable. Added to all this was a sense of humour; he used to say that the name Samuel was a handicap to him because hardly anyone with that name could attain any position, only three had done so, namely, the prophet, Dr. Johnson and Mr. Weller Junior. Sometimes he was caustic; he had been cross-examined in the law courts about epilepsy, at the end, the cross-examiner said, "You don't seem to know much about epilepsy, Dr. Wilks," instantly he replied, "No, nor would you if you had studied it for as many hours as I have years."

The many who came to him on Sunday evenings and the ease with which he, a stranger, made friends in Hampstead show how numerous were his admirers. Two other instances may be given as indications of his popularity and of the affection for him. When he was made a baronet, his old pupils gave him a complimentary dinner, upwards of three hundred attended, forty telegrams of regret were received during the dinner and twenty of his pupils, all resident in New South Wales, sent an illuminated address. Dr. Pye-Smith proposed Wilks's health, justly saying of him "all who knew him knew that he had never sought for fame, it had come to him unasked; he had never courted popularity, yet no one in his profession was more popular." A dining club called the Fifteen Club was formed, it consisted of fourteen men who loved the pleasure of dining with Wilks, there were three dinners each year and Wilks was always in the chair. When a vacancy occurred the competition to get in was keen. The Club still exists with a full membership, twenty-five years after his death, and is now known as the Wilks Fifteen Club.

An endearing nickname is always a sign of affection; among the students he was always known as Sammy. Their love for him was admirably shown in a poem published in the *Guy's Hospital Gazette*, November 18, 1905, but written the year he retired from being physician to the hospital. It might have been thought that his brusque manner, his way of saying exactly what he thought about people, and his sarcasm, would have prevented affection and popularity, but this was not so, and the reasons which inspired affection and made him popular were, first his honesty; he did his work, said what he thought, never courted popularity, never played to the gallery, never said or wrote anything which could be possibly thought to have for its object an increase of his practice, indeed he always maintained that medicine was a poor trade, but a glorious profession. Secondly, his detestation of all humbug; such detestation was usually expressed in scathing words. Thirdly, his intense loyalty to his profession and to his hospital. Fourthly, the encouragement he always gave to young men willing to work for the science of medicine. Lastly there was his beautiful and kindly face, in his old age he had shaggy white silver hair, and looked exactly the part of a grand old man. He was often photographed and painted. One of the nicknames for him was " the professional beauty."

Few diseases, if any, are of more interest to the race or to the physician than syphilis. Until 1857 almost all diseases of the outside of the body, including the mouth, were regarded as surgical. Syphilis has many external manifestations, hence it was treated by surgeons, who believing it to be an external disease, did not trouble to make post-mortem examinations on those that died from it. In the late fifties of the nineteenth century, a man in a surgical ward died after a very long illness due to syphilis.

A great part of the cranium was carious, the scalp had partly sloughed away, producing a large, partly healed sore on the head. Wilks was then in charge of the post-mortem room; he writes:

In this case no post-mortem was wished for, as the cause of death was too evident; but on my part the wish was quite the contrary, and so the body was opened. I need scarcely say that the interior of the body was a perfect revelation to me. Amongst other notable things was a gummatous mass in the liver, which I described as a fibrous material with some rays of the same substance around it. This I showed at the Pathological Society, and a drawing of it is in the *Transactions* [Syphilitic Disease of the Liver, *Trans. Path., Soc. Lond.*, 1857, viii, 240–2]. This was the first specimen of the kind exhibited in London, and was received with considerable incredulity as to its nature by many of the members.

Wilks had made the entirely original observation that syphilis can affect the interior of the body, one of astounding importance when we remember the extensive ravages that syphilis can induce' in nearly all the human organs. He immediately followed up the matter. In 1858 he showed at the Pathological Society another specimen of syphilitic disease of the liver, and *Specimens of Disease of the Lungs, Larynx and Liver supposed to be Syphilitic*. His specimen of syphilis of the lung was the first to be exhibited at any Society. In 1859 he reported to the same Society on syphilitic disease of the testis and in 1861 on syphilitic disease of the spleen and other organs. In 1862 he gave a lecture on *Syphilitic Affections of Internal Organs* which was published in the *Medical Times and Gazette*, and in 1863 there appeared in the *Guy's Hospital Reports* his famous paper *On the Syphilitic Affections of Internal Organs* in which he gathers together all he had learnt since 1857, and shows beyond doubt that syphilis affects internal organs widely. A great discovery, to which he attributed his election to the Royal Society.

He begins by saying that it is only a few years since specimens of the affection of internal organs by syphilis were received with more than incredulity, and that still scepticism prevails largely. Soon there follows the important statement that

In syphilis there is a disposition to the effusion of a low form of lymph, or fibroplastic material, in nearly every tissue of the body, occasionally modified in character to a slight extent by the organ in which it occurs. Consequently in those who have died suffering from this disease there is scarcely an organ but what may be found affected in this particular way.

When Wilks wrote great stress was laid on the classification of syphilitic symptoms into primary, secondary and tertiary. He criticizes this and would do away with these divisions, remarking that as long as certain changes occur in any of the tissues the patient has syphilis, and when the virus has been exterminated by remedies or worn itself out, the health has been so weakened that there is a liability to lardaceous disease or to fatty degeneration. Further, he teaches that so long as changes characteristic of syphilis are going on, the virus is still active, and therefore the patient is capable of communicating the disease to others. Several authorities maintained that some at least of the symptoms attributed to syphilis were really due to poisoning by the large doses of mercury which had been given. Wilks does not believe this; he points out that these symptoms are never seen in uncomplicated cases of chronic mercurial poisoning, but he considers that if so much mercury has been given as to produce anæmia the progress of a syphilitic ulceration may be accelerated. He then tells us that if a new growth, e.g. cancer or tubercle affects, say a muscle, it destroys surrounding tissue from the first, but if a syphilitic inflammation occurs, the exudation of lymph infiltrates between the structures. If appropriate treatment is given the exudate will be completely absorbed as we see frequently in the case of nodes. When the exudate has been followed by fibrous changes restoration of the part by antisyphilitic treatment is of course impossible.

The rest of the paper is occupied with a description of the effects of syphilis on individual organs. He says of the liver,

It presented generally a number of rounded nodules, placed towards the surface. . . . They were of different sizes, varying from that of a pea to that of a marble. They were for the most part hard, one or two only showing signs of softening in their centres. When old, they were more or less circumscribed, though sending out branches of fibre into the surrounding tissue. By the contraction which had taken place, a cicatriform appearance had been produced, and thus the resemblance to syphilitic affections of the skin and mucous membrane. . . . The liver in Congenital Syphilis.—The same appearance may be found in those in whom the syphilis is congenital, and of these I shall be able to give an example.

He has no evidence that perihepatitis results from acquired syphilis, he is uncertain whether it follows congenital. Twenty-three cases illustrating syphilis of the liver are described.

The spleen is not so often implicated as the liver, but five cases of syphilitic deposit in it are given. The question whether the lymphatic glands are affected independently of the part whence the vessels leading to them proceed is left un-answered. There are two examples of gummatous deposits in the lungs in adults. Whether the changes in the lungs of syphilitic infants are due to syphilis is uncertain. The appear-ance of a syphilitic larynx is distinctive, for when the activity of the disease has ceased, cicatrization takes place, leaving the affected part puckered, hard and shiny unlike any other disease. It had been thought that syphilis did not affect the trachea or bronchi, but Wilks shows this to be wrong, and gives two examples of syphilitic contraction of the trachea and one of the same thing in a bronchus. He is unable to find that syphilis affects the stomach and intestines except that it causes ulceration of the rectum, in one case syphilitic ulceration of the pharynx invaded the œsophagus. He cannot offer any case of syphilitic disease of the kidneys. He remarks on the frequency of syphilitic deposits in muscle and gives two examples in which, from the appearance, there can be no doubt that the deposits in the septum ventriculorum must have been syphilitic, both patients, as is usual, died suddenly. He has no certain cases to bring forward but nevertheless has much reason to think that blood-vessels may be affected, if they are, the change is of a fibroid character, with thickening of their coats and proportionate diminution of their calibre. Aneurysm, he suggests, may be due to syphilis; this was correct in opinion, but his scientific mind made him hesitate until he had more facts. It used to be considered that, if a sufferer from syphilis had cerebral symptoms, they were caused by direct implication of the brain from disease of the bones of the skull. He shows this not to be the case, giving examples of syphilitic deposits in the meninges of patients whose skull bones were healthy, sometimes the symptoms were due to implication of the cranial nerves, and a good example of a syphilitic tumour of the spinal cord is recorded. Syphilitic deposits in the testis are very common and characteristic. Wilks concludes this long paper by saying that many patients stated to be suffering from scrofula are really afflicted with syphilis, either acquired or congenital.

Lardaceous Disease was often overlooked and ill understood.

Wilks collected and analysed nearly a hundred examples of it (*Guy's Hospital Reports,* 1856 and 1865), described its appearances, and showed how to recognize the condition which is nearly always due to protracted caries or necrosis of bone, which has its origin in either tubercle or syphilis. Nothing noteworthy—except histological facts—has since been added to this entirely original account of the fundamentally important discovery that syphilis does affect internal organs.

While systematically examining the lymphatic glands for lardaceous disease, Wilks found that sometimes, although no lardaceous disease is present, a more or less generalized chronic enlargement of these glands exists in association with an enlargement of the spleen in which are white masses, and occasionally also smaller white masses in the liver. The enlarged glands are discrete, hard, and contain fibro-nucleated tissue, the masses in the spleen are suet-like, the patients are ill and anæmic, there is no leucocytosis. He gave it as his opinion that this was a hitherto unrecognized disease, and the medical journals thought the same when he showed specimens at the Pathological Society. Afterwards he came across a statement of Bright's that Hodgkin had described enlargement of the lymphatic glands, Wilks then found Hodgkin's original paper, considered that Hodgkin had forestalled him in the discovery of this new disease, and therefore waived all claim and named the condition Hodgkin's Disease, by which name it has been known ever since. Wilks's magnanimity was thus described by one of the physicians of St. Bartholomew's Hospital, who in speaking of Wilks's discovery wrote, " Dr. Wilks, with the generous desire to perpetuate the name of his predecessor in the office of teacher of Pathological Anatomy at Guy's Hospital, gave the name to this morbid state of Hodgkin's disease."

Thomas Hodgkin, a Quaker, studied medicine at Guy's Hospital, went to Paris, in 1822, to work under Laennec, and on his return introduced to the hospital the use of the stethoscope. The Guy's Medical School was founded, as a separate institution from that of St. Thomas's, in 1825. Hodgkin, being appointed Curator of the Museum and Lecturer on Morbid Anatomy, made an extensive Pathological Museum and took great trouble over the catalogue of it. He had a highly scientific mind, associated with the leading scientists of his day, used the microscope and published *Lectures on the Morbid Anatomy of the Serous and Mucous Membranes.* This book is really a treatise on the whole subject of Morbid Anatomy. It is an admirable work, the only objection to it is that it is too diffuse. By it and by his teaching the author did a great deal for the study of morbid anatomy. He gave an excellent clinical and pathological account of aortic valvular disease and he has not received the credit he deserves for this entirely original communication published in 1829, five years before the appearance of Corrigan's celebrated paper.

In 1832 Hodgkin wrote an article entitled *On Some Morbid Appearances of the Absorbent Glands and Spleen.* He described six cases, as though they were all the same, but, in reality, only four were examples of what we now know as Hodgkin's disease, and the case he quoted from Carswell as another example of the condition described by himself is undoubtedly one of sarcoma. There was little to attract attention to this confusing paper and so it remained unknown until Wilks disinterred it. Wilks rediscovered the disease, he gives many more cases than Hodgkin and a more perfect description, which is free from cases which are not examples in point, so that the malady ought to be called " Wilks' Disease," but owing to his advocacy the name Hodgkin's disease is firmly established. This paper and that on aortic disease contain the only two original observations made by Hodgkin, and had he not been so fortunate as to have his name attached to a disease he would not have been well known all over the world. In 1837 he failed to obtain an assistant physiciancy at Guy's, the successful candidate being Dr. Guy Babington. He then left the hospital, although remaining friends with his colleagues. For a short time he was a lecturer at St. Thomas's Hospital, but he soon gave up medicine to devote himself to philanthropy. In 1866 he died at the age of 68 at Jaffa, where he had gone to relieve poor Jews.

There was much controversy as to the classification of the diseases of the kidney known as Bright's Disease. Wilks, in 1845, gained a prize given by the Physical Society for an essay on the subject and in 1853 published a paper *Cases of Bright's Disease.* At this time the most authoritative teaching was that the small contracted granular kidney was the last stage of a long disease which had begun as an acute nephritis. Wilks denied this and showed that there were two great varieties of Bright's Disease. One began acutely, and, if recovery did not take place, slowly became a chronic tubal nephritis, generally known as a large white kidney. The other was a chronic malady associated with a hard, contracted and granular kidney. He taught that the symptoms, age incidence, and post-mortem appearances are so different in the two varieties that they should be regarded as distinct diseases. This was an original observation which constituted a great advance in our knowledge. He admitted, as we do to-day, that a few specimens are found which are difficult to classify, and he pointed out that the fatty kidney is not Bright's Disease. The description of the symptoms is admirable and the arguments are convincing. To show that I do not exaggerate I will quote from Bartel's article in Ziemssen's *Cyclopedia of Medicine*. He says :

Samuel Wilks was the first to prove, and he did so in the clearest possible manner, from the ample clinical and pathological materials at his command, that the condition of the kidney of which we are now talking and which he described as the large white kidney ought not to be regarded as the precursory stage of that atrophic process which the German pathologist had proclaimed as the ultimate stage of every diffuse inflammation of the kidneys.

The doctrine that Wilks here upset, namely that all diseases of the kidney had begun as an acute process, was widely believed of all maladies, and he did much good by teaching that this is wrong. Many diseases he said are chronic in the whole of their course, and it was much more true to say that chronic diseases terminated as acute than that acute became chronic.

Canton showed that the arcus senilis was caused by fatty degeneration of the cornea; Wilks, for two years, looked for it in every body which came into the post-mortem room and proved that it was a genuine senile change, as is the accumulation of fat which is often seen in elderly people, further he showed that when seen in younger people it indicates that they are prematurely aged.

The marks on the skin of the abdomen of women who have borne children are well known, they are called lineæ gravidarum. Similar marks may occur when the skin is distended by dropsy in any part of the body. It was always supposed that they are due to stretching of the skin. Wilks was the first to record that exactly similar marks, for which no cause can be suggested, may be found when there certainly has not been any stretching. He described a girl who was covered in various parts of the body with white lines or seams resembling the marks on the abdomen of a child-bearing woman, and a lad aged 19, who had them on both legs. The name he gave to the condition was *Linear Atrophy of the Skin*. That it exists there is no doubt, but it is rare.

He was also the first to describe *Verruca necrogenica,* a condition of skin produced by making post-mortem examinations. Generally the change is seen earliest on the knuckles and on the first joints of the fingers, it consists of a warty thickening of the epithelium, which slowly becomes dark and fissured, until a kind of ichthyotic condition is produced. There are no constitutional symptoms, but the state of the skin usually remains, even if post-mortem work is discarded.

He also called attention to the markings or furrows found on the nails as the result of illness so severe as to bring the patient near to death's door. For example, a man went to America and back. On both voyages he was so sea-sick that he was thought to be dying. The white transverse marks on the nails were easily seen; the mark nearest the tip of his nail corresponded with the illness on the outward voyage, that at the base with the sickness on the return journey.

Because Wilks could write easily and well the bibliography of his writings given in the *Guy's Hospital Gazette* (Nov. 25, 1911) is long. During the many years he was in the post-mortem room he often published papers in which he gave both the clinical symptoms and the post-mortem appearances of interesting cases. The object of many of these contributions was to put on a firm foundation the work of others which had either been neglected or received sceptically; we have seen he did this for Hodgkin. As late as 1860 several physicians doubted whether Addison's Disease really existed. Wilks set the matter at rest by a series of papers which included every case that had been at the hospital since Addison's original discovery. He also gave several examples of pernicious anæmia and so helped to establish that this is a distinct disease, a proposition that many disbelieved for many years after its discovery. In 1852 Kirkes told us that minute emboli may be carried from the diseased heart to the tissues. Wilks brought this statement to light and accurately described the symptoms and post-mortem appearances of what we call malignant endocarditis, but which he called arterial pyæmia, a name just as good. Bright taught us that, when a patient has what we now call Jacksonian epilepsy, a lesion of the cortex of the brain will be found. Wilks frequently emphasized this in his teaching, and he published cases to illustrate the point. He was much interested in diseases of the nervous system and was one of the earliest to give bromides for epilepsy. It has been mentioned that he first described what he called alcoholic paraplegia, now known as alcoholic peripheral neuritis. He instructs us clearly and admirably on the subject of adherent pericardium, about which much confusion existed, and in so doing describes what at the present day is called mediastinitis, although he did not give it a name. Among his papers will be found an instance of acromegaly and one of osteitis deformans.

His intellectual pleasure in all that was going on in the natural world around him caused him to write, often shortly, on many subjects, perhaps the best to read now are those essays —if they may be so called—on Wendell Holmes, the origin of music, hermaphrodites, phrenology, dreams and the " History of My Parrot " which appeared in the *Journal of Mental Science*.

LORD LISTER

When Lister, holiday-making in Norway, landed in Lister-land, he speculated whether this was the home of his ancestors. Be that as it may, our first certain knowledge of them is that there were many of his name near Bingley, in Yorkshire, in the sixteenth century. His great-grandfather, a Quaker, whose parents and descendants were of the same faith, came to London about 1720. The Listers were successively yeomen and tradespeople. Lord Lister's father, John Jackson Lister, a wine merchant in Loth-bury, who was well educated, particularly in French and Latin, married Isabella Harris, a reading mistress in a Quaker school at Ackworth, near Pontefract. The history of the school tells of her gentle and graceful life and of the excellence of her reading aloud.

It is notorious that Quakers succeed in business; it is difficult to say whether this is because the attitude of mind which turns to the teaching of the Friends is good for business, or whether because the tenets of this sect inculcate industry without ostentation, and forbid many expensive pastimes, the members of it live economically. John Jackson Lister was comfortably off. He took a large country house at Upton in Essex, which still stands, being now the vicarage of St. Paul's, Upton Cross, surrounded by the dismal neighbourhood of West Ham, but a hundred years ago it was well in the country and overlooked the grounds of Ham House, where Lister's friend, Samuel Gurney the banker, lived.

John Jackson Lister, the first of the family to be distinguished, was a very able man, who, leaving school at 14, went straight into business, educated himself in mathematics and optics and did original work on the making of microscopical lenses, which led to his election to the Fellowship of the Royal Society. He and his Quaker friend Dr. Hodgkin, of Guy's Hospital, together tackled the problem of the true shape of the red corpuscles of the blood. It was fortunate for his famous son that he should have had a father who took deep interest in his son's physiological and surgical work; the two wrote to each other constantly, the son telling of what he was doing, the father criticizing. Lord Lister's mother and her family were all Quakers; as far as is known he had no remarkable ancestors on her side. A sketch of her by her husband suggests that she was both wise and beautiful.

Joseph, the future Lord Lister, the fourth child and second son of John Jackson and his wife Isabella, was born on April 5, 1827, at Upton. His childhood was passed in the somewhat severe, but not unhappy, surroundings of a strict Quaker family. First he went to school at Hitchin, and then to Grove House, Tottenham, where he received an excellent education. Quite early he said he would be a surgeon; to this he always adhered, his parents making no objection. At Tottenham he was cheerful and greatly interested in natural history. Many of his school essays have been preserved; four dealt with human osteology, one, *On the Similarity of Structure between a Monkey and a Man,* was illustrated by beautiful drawings. He was fond of macerating animals and articulating their skeletons, in the holidays he wrote to his father from Upton " I got almost all the meat off; and I think all the brains out of the sheep's head." In 1844, when 17 years old, he went to University College, London, not being able to go to either of the older universities because of the religious tests then imposed. He was fortunate in never having to think seriously of money, consequently, before entering as a medical student, he took his B.A. at the University of London, after which in 1848 he had a long holiday in Ireland to recoup from an attack of small-pox.

In this year he began his medical studies at University College, and finished by obtaining the M.B. degree and the Fellowship of the Royal College of Surgeons in 1852. At first he lived with other students who were very strict Quakers, so Lister was then a rather austere young man. Luckily he got away from this stifling atmosphere when he became a hospital resident. He then participated in the Debating Society and other student activities, and also found time to write two original papers; in one he showed that the iris had both dilating and contracting involuntary muscles, in the other he demonstrated the involuntary muscles of the scalp. These papers attracted the notice of Sharpey, the well-known teacher of physiology, who suggested that Lister should go to Edinburgh to attend the practice of Syme, a great friend of Sharpey's. Meanwhile, during his student days, he spent his holidays abroad, thus learning to speak foreign languages, especially French and German.

By September 1853 he had taken lodgings in Edinburgh. On his arrival he called on Syme to present Sharpey's letter of introduction. Doing this was the beginning of his great career; Syme took to him immediately, asked him to dine, and invited him to assist him in hospital and private work. Lister could not have had better luck, for Syme was by many thought to be the most celebrated surgeon then alive, he was a great teacher, a brilliant operator, an original thinker mixing with the best of University Society and, as he was 54 years old and very busy, he welcomed Lister as an able young man whom he could thoroughly trust. He often asked him to his house at Morningside and introduced him to many distinguished visitors, both foreign and British. Two who became great friends of Lister, were Dr. John Brown, the author of that most beautiful story *Rab and his Friends*, and Christison, the well-known professor of Materia Medica.

Syme inspired enthusiasm in many, including Lister, who was much impressed by the opportunities of learning surgery under such a master at the Edinburgh Infirmary, with its 200 surgical beds, compared with the 60 surgical beds at University College Hospital. At the end of a month he was appointed supernumary clerk to Syme, which meant that he had to assist at every operation and keep notes of the cases. Syme's private practice also gave him much experience; on one occasion he was called up at 5 a.m. to help at a primary amputation of the shoulder at Dunblane; within two months of his coming to Edinburgh he read before the Edinburgh Medico-Chirurgical Society an account of an exostosis of the humerus removed by Syme from a young lady's arm, and demonstrated, probably for the first time, that the method of ossification of these growths is the same as in epiphyseal cartilage.

He was completely contented. In December he writes:

Syme's kindness continues to flow steadily and if possible increasingly. If the love of surgery is a proof of a person's being adapted for it, then I am certainly fitted to be a surgeon; for thou canst hardly conceive what a high degree of enjoyment I am from day to day experiencing in this bloody and butcherly department of the healing act.

In January 1854 he became Syme's House Surgeon and held the post for thirteen months. As such he had entire charge of all ordinary cases and it was left to him to decide which patients should be operated on by Syme himself. To be a dresser to Syme was a greatly sought appointment, so there were twelve of them under Lister, who taught and helped them with such kindness and success that he was known then and ever after as the "Chief." He also prepared for publication in the *Lancet* a series of Syme's lectures.

A young man of great promise, named Mackenzie, was then a surgeon to the Infirmary and lecturer at the College of Surgeons at Edinburgh; the news of his death from cholera in the Crimea reached Edinburgh in October 1854. It was, after consultation with Syme, agreed that Lister should give Mackenzie's lectures during the next winter session and also apply for the vacant post at the Infirmary. Accordingly he became a Fellow of the Edinburgh College of Surgeons and worked hard at preparing his lectures, going to Paris for a month to operate on the dead body and to see something of French surgery. He took lodgings in 3 Rutland Street, opposite to Syme's consulting-rooms, in order to begin private practice; the first patient had a backward dislocation of the ankle. He gave his first lecture on the "Principles and Practice of Surgery" at 4 High School Yards, on Wednesday, November 7, 1855. As usual he was behindhand; on that day he went to bed at 2 a.m., rose at 4 and the last words were written just in time to rush, in a cab, to read them to his audience. Subsequently his lectures were delivered mostly from notes, or even without them, often because he had not finished their preparation. His father writes, "But was it not running too great a risk and tempting failure in thy first lecture to delay till so late its preparation? An example of what is to be avoided hereafter?" Alas, his father's admonition had little effect, indeed his son's procrastination got worse, throughout his life lectures and addresses were rarely finished in time, being often incomplete when he entered the lecture hall, although he had been working till the last minute in a train or cab. His dressers and a few others attended this course, the fee for which was four guineas. He taught pathology more than surgery and produced the impression that he was a thinker.

During all this while he had a compelling distraction, for he became engaged to Syme's daughter, Agnes, born in 1834. She was not a Quaker, to the regret of Lister's parents. His father said "he was not without feeling the objectionable side of the connection," still he did not oppose it, but looked forward to its making for his son's happiness. When a Quaker married outside the sect either he was disowned by it, or resigned from it, as Lister did. He gave up the Quaker dress, and had his brass plate engraved Mr. Lister, instead of "Joseph Lister," which would have been correct had he remained a Friend. He became an Episcopalian, but to the end of his life his letters showed his Quaker upbringing.

Life was strenuous, he rose at five-thirty, breakfast and preparation for lecture occupied him till its delivery at ten, the afternoon was spent in the hospital or at pathological work, the evening either at home reading or in a visit to his betrothed at Millbank where his marriage took place in Scottish fashion on April 23, 1856. The newly married couple had four months' honeymoon, one month in the English lakes, and three abroad, where Lister visited many continental medical schools and got to know various distinguished foreign scientists. He was at this time attracted to ophthalmic surgery and saw what he could of it. There were no children of this entirely happy marriage. Mrs. Lister helped her husband greatly in his work, writing his scientific papers at his dictation, she "wrote seven hours one day and eight the next" and aided him much in the construction of his papers.

On their return from abroad Lister and his wife lived at 11 Rutland Street. He was elected to the vacant assistant surgeoncy at the Edinburgh Infirmary on October 13, 1856, and for the greater part of next year Syme handed over the practice and the teaching in his wards to Lister. His winter lectures were poorly attended at the first, in 1858, there was only one student and he came ten minutes late. Astley Cooper's early lectures were also unattractive because he did not make them practical enough, directly he made them so flocks of students came. Probably the fact that many of Lister's lectures were on pathological principles was the reason for his scanty audience. He also gave a summer course on surgical pathology and operative surgery in 1858; to his disappointment only seven men attended, but, to his delight, in 1859 there were twenty-four. He saw a few private patients for Syme, but his own private practice was small, his wife once referred to " poor Joseph and his one patient."

Lister resembled Astley Cooper in another way, for he was constantly investigating. At this time, while he was teaching in Edinburgh, he published a paper *On the Minute Structure of Involuntary Muscle Fibre* which contained entirely new and correct observations. Far more important—he began his life's study on injuries and repair. He investigated the effect of irritants on the vessels of the web of the frog's foot which had never been done before, he wrote an article on spontaneous gangrene and he began a series of papers on the coagulation of the blood ; he disagreed with Astley Cooper's view that coagulation is to be explained by the withdrawal of a supposed influence exerted by a healthy vessel wall to prevent coagulation. These writings all reveal in him the gift of good observation and the aptitude to devise proper experiments.

Towards the end of 1859 the Professorship of Surgery at the University of Glasgow became vacant. Syme advised Lister to apply ; he did so for the following reasons : the pay was £400 to £450 a year, he would almost certainly be also made surgeon to the Infirmary, such a position would lead to private practice as a consulting surgeon, for there was then no one in Glasgow who practised solely as a surgeon, and lastly the post would give him a claim to any other professorship of surgery if he wished to leave Glasgow. The appointment he now sought was a Regius Professorship and therefore was made by the Crown. Usually there was much wirepulling. Sometimes these appointments were made on political grounds quite irrespective of the merits of the candidates, as in the notorious case in which the distinguished philosopher Sir William Hamilton was defeated in his application for the professorship in Moral Philosophy at Edinburgh by John Wilson (Christopher North) who did not know a word about the subject. The members of parliament for Glasgow now attempted to influence the issue, this raised a storm of protest which probably helped Lister, who was elected January 28, 1860. He had been in Edinburgh nearly seven years; when he left the students gave him a silver flagon and his colleagues entertained him at dinner. It was in 1860 also that he became a Fellow of the Royal Society.

The Glasgow home of the Listers was 17 Woodside Place. Before they moved there the new Professor was, on March 9, 1860, inducted by the reading of a thesis in Latin, immediately after which he was appointed an examiner. This work of examining was extremely tedious and tiring because he took minute pains. For example one question was divided into 23 parts, each marked separately with a fixed proportion of the 15 marks allotted for the whole question. His lectures were much more successful than in Edinburgh, large numbers of students attending; he was listened to attentively, and he tried hard, without much success, to overcome his unpunctuality.

Lister was the only surgeon outside London who was asked to contribute to a work famous for many years, namely Holmes's *System of Surgery*. He was greatly pleased by the compliment. His article on amputations gave an account of original and improved ways of performing some of these: for instance he described a tourniquet he had designed for compressing the abdominal aorta in amputation at the hip, and which he had shown to be of great value in cases of ligature of the common, internal and external iliac arteries for aneurysm, and he gave an account of the bloodless method of operating after emptying the limb of blood by elevation of it and then placing a tourniquet on the artery. He also wrote the article on anæsthetics; in the discussion which then raged on the relative values of ether and chloroform he sided with the last. This article and that on bloodless operating were quite unlike the ordinary writing in Systems, for the opinions he expressed were the result of a large number of purely scientific experiments which he had performed. Many of these were executed at home. Mrs. Lister writes, "another calf was brought in on Saturday, but Joseph could not be ready to make use of it that day, so we kept it in the wash-house till Tuesday." In addition to all his pathological and physiological experimental research he, in these years, devised several new operations: for example, one for excision of the wrist and another for stricture of the urethra.

The year 1864 was full of trouble. In it his mother died; his father survived her for five years, living alone in the large house at Upton. The surgeon son tried to enliven the loneliness of these years by writing to him weekly a long letter telling of his experiments and his surgery. Also in this year the Professorship of Systemic Surgery in Edinburgh became vacant, Lister applied for the post but was not elected.

Until the later part of the nineteenth century the condition of surgery had always been deplorable. Many limbs were amputated which would now be saved and an operator plumed himself if his mortality rate after amputation was only twenty-five per cent. Healing after operation was often very tedious because abscesses formed near the suppurating wound and these had to be opened. The cause of death after operation was nearly always some form of sepsis, e.g. erysipelas or pyæmia. Sometimes the death-rate from this was so high that surgical wards had to be closed for a time ; this happened at the Glasgow Infirmary. It was even proposed to pull down a hospital, such a surgical death-trap had it become. Doctors were blind as to the cause of this awful frequency of sepsis. When Semmelweis showed that puerperal septicæmia was due to organic dirt, they either paid no attention or reviled him, although the mortality from it was so frightful that women dreaded to go into a lying-in hospital. Hands and instruments contaminated by one sore were used to examine the wound of the next patient, the surgeon's coat was encrusted with decomposing blood and discharges. When at Glasgow, as previously, Lister pondered much on this horrible state of surgical affairs. He first tried to find out why wounds suppurated. Unfortunately he did not know of Semmelweis, but he reached the conclusion, which he taught in his lectures, that suppuration was caused by putrefaction or decomposition, which was set up by exposure of the wound to the air, or by other contamination of it. It was known that sepsis rarely occurred without suppuration, therefore Lister's whole aim was to prevent suppuration, but he was, up to now, quite in the dark as to why, when, as in the case of simple fracture, the wound was not exposed to the air it did not suppurate, yet, when it was exposed, as in a compound fracture, it did. He determined to try to stop putrefaction in wounds and for this purpose chose crude carbolic acid which he knew was employed as a disinfectant of sewage. This he first used in 1865. The patient was James Greenless who had a compound fracture. Lint soaked in the acid mixed with water, or lint soaked in a solution of carbolic acid in olive oil was used as a covering for the wound. The crude acid does not dissolve well in water and so caused some sloughing of the skin, a little pus formed but the patient got quite well, and Lister was able to say: " So it may fairly be said that the result at the end of the usual time of treatment for a simple fracture was in no way affected by its being compound."

In this same year, 1865, Dr. Thomas Anderson, the Professor of Chemistry at Glasgow, called Lister's attention to Pasteur's discovery that putrefaction was due to micro-organisms in the air. This was what he wanted, for now he felt sure that if he could prevent live micro-organisms from reaching the wound by the air, or by instruments, or by the surgeon's hands, he could prevent suppuration. Henceforth he devoted himself to devising a dressing capable of destroying the micro-organisms. He replaced the crude carbolic acid by purified carbolic acid which was soluble in water. There were many difficulties in detail, but after several trials a putty made of whitening mixed with a solution of carbolic acid in olive oil was used to cover the wound. The early cases thus treated with carbolic acid were compound fractures and abscesses. In opening the last the skin was disinfected by putting over the abscess lint soaked in carbolized oil, the knife was dipped in this oil, the abscess was opened and the pus drained away through the carbolized lint. Most of these abscesses were connected with the spine, previously almost always fatal, under Lister's treatment they did well. His earliest paper on antiseptic surgery, one of the most prominent milestones in the progress of medicine, was published in several numbers of the *Lancet* between March and July 1867. It was entitled *On a New Method of Treating Compound Fracture, Abscess, etc. ; with Observations on the Conditions of Suppuration.* Eleven cases are recorded, of which only one died, a wonderful result, hitherto thought to be impossible. This was followed by an address on Antiseptic Surgery, read before the meeting of the British Medical Association in Dublin, August 1867. Watching his eleven cases Lister made three important observations, namely, that with antiseptic surgery blood clot could become organized, dead bone could become absorbed, and pus formed by an irritant, e.g. carbolic acid, produced no general infection.

In this year he first used antiseptic surgery for the wound made by an ordinary operation, it was for the removal of a tumour.

Carbolic acid is an irritant and therefore it is undesirable to apply it to a wound after the micro-organisms in it have been destroyed by the acid or by any other means, but, said Lister, as long as there is a wound a dressing must be applied which will kill micro-organisms which might approach it from the outside. He devoted much time and thought to this, making innumerable experiments. A 1 in 4 solution of carbolic acid in water was employed for all general antiseptic measures in operations; many trials of many substances were made for the dressings. In 1871 muslin gauze impregnated with carbolic acid was evolved as being a suitable material to hold carbolic acid in even distribution. This well-known "yellow gauze" is soft, light and pliable, with a pleasant smell. A fold of eight layers thick was placed over the wound, between the outermost and next layer was a thin piece of mackintosh to distribute evenly through the gauze the discharge from the wound, directly over which was laid a piece of "green protective" (which is specially prepared aseptic oiled silk) to prevent the carbolic acid in the gauze from irritating the wound. Soon it was found that, owing to volatilization of the carbolic acid, this gauze, after some time, lost its antiseptic powers, so the innumerable experiments were continued —it is really astonishing to read of the industry and time Lister devoted to finding a perfect dressing. Gauze impregnated with sal-alembroth, a double salt of bichloride of mercury and chloride of ammonium, commonly called blue gauze, as it was stained blue to distinguish it, was employed for a while, but was given up as the salt was too soluble, finally in 1889 a gauze impregnated with a double cyanide of mercury and zinc was prepared, this proved satisfactory in every way and replaced carbolic gauze as a dressing, the object of which was to prevent micro-organisms from outside reaching the wound.

After Lister learned from Pasteur that air contained organisms which caused fermentation he tried to kill micro-organisms in the atmosphere immediately surrounding an operation by directing a fine spray of 1 in 40 carbolic acid in water around the seat of operation. Many instruments were used to make the spray, the best being one which formed steam mixed with carbolic acid. The spray was very disagreeable for surgeons and assistants, my own fingers when I was a dresser were often numb for hours after an operation; moreover those who inhaled carbolic acid were liable to carbolic acid poisoning—indeed because of this some surgeons could not use the spray—nevertheless their results were as good as those who did. The explanation is that Lister was wrong in assuming that the atmospheric micro-organisms which cause fermentation also cause putrefaction in wounds; those which do this come not from the air but from dirty organic matter. After a time he saw his error and by 1890 had given up the spray as unnecessary, indeed he said he was ashamed he had ever used it, for even if it had been necessary to kill aerial micro-organisms the spray could not have done this.

In olden days bleeding vessels at an operation were usually tied with silk threads, which were left long enough to hang out of the wound and so provide drainage. This was very unsatisfactory; the silk held micro-organisms which caused suppuration around the tied vessel; if this occurred before the vessel was firmly occluded, it was reopened as the ligature got loose in the pus, and alarming " secondary " bleeding took place. To overcome the difficulty other means of closing the artery by torsion or by acupressure were devised, but they were unreliable. Lister devoted years of time and innumerable experiments to find a ligature which could be left in the wound to become absorbed so gradually that secondary hæmorrhage would not happen, and which could be made free from micro-organisms so that no suppuration could occur around it. Silk was tried, but it was not easy to render it germ free and it was absorbed with difficulty. In the Christmas holidays in 1868, at his father's house at Upton, the carotid artery of a calf was tied with catgut, which had been soaked in carbolic acid, this was completely successful, no pus formed and subsequent dissection showed that the catgut had been replaced by fibrous tissue. Catgut is a variable, ticklish material to deal with, nevertheless, after an immense amount of investigation, Lister had discovered that a catgut ligature which could be absorbed and did not lead to suppuration could be made.

Many critics completely misunderstood Lister's discovery. They thought it consisted in his finding out that carbolic acid was a good dressing. It was nothing of the sort. His discovery was that suppuration in the wound and death from septic disease after operation were due to putrefaction in the wound, this being caused by the advent of micro-organisms, which, on their arrival in the wound, grew there. Keep out the micro-organisms and destroy any which are already there, then, said Lister, you will abolish the awful septicæmia. He employed carbolic acid for these purposes, now the same end is reached differently. Micro-organisms on the skin around the site of operation are killed by painting it with iodine, those on the instruments are killed by boiling the instruments. The surgeons and his assistants wear sterilized clothes and gloves. The wound is dressed with many thicknesses of sterilized gauze. Sterilization of all these means that they have been heated to such a degree that all micro-organisms in them are killed. Nothing brought in contact with the wound has any live micro-organisms in it, and the incoming of micro-organisms from outside is prevented by the many thicknesses of sterilized gauze over the wound. It has been found that the micro-organisms which may reach the wound from the air during the short time of operation are usually not of such a kind as to cause putrefaction, and the body itself can destroy the few dangerous ones that may fall into the wound. If—as was often the case in the war—the wound by the time the surgeon sees it, has already become infected with dangerous micro-organisms, it is pared so as to cut away the parts containing micro-organisms and is then treated like an operation wound. Lister prevented micro-organisms from growing in a wound by killing them with antiseptics—usually carbolic acid—hence his method was antiseptic surgery; the modern development of this is to render everything that can come near the wound aseptic by killing the micro-organisms by heat, hence it is called aseptic surgery.

Modern surgery owes its existence to Lord Lister. By acting upon the doctrine enunciated by him the percentage of deaths from surgical septicæmia has, in civil practice, become minute and, in military practice, small. The usefulness of surgery has been vastly extended, ten times the number of operations performed in 1865 are now done every year. Many operations—especially those on joints, the abdomen, the chest and the skull—which formerly surgeons did not dare, are now performed daily with safety, amputations are infrequent, for in compound fractures the limb can usually be saved. Thousands of men wounded in the Great War owe their lives to Lord Lister. The author of *Rab and his Friends* wrote to him saying, " You will transform the whole science and practice of surgery," and he did.

Lister did not bury his discovery but announced it from the house-tops by numerous lectures, papers and addresses, because he believed it to be for the good of the people. Like the Hebrew prophets he saw the error of the ways of his countrymen, preached against them in no uncertain language and often incurred the displeasure of his fellows. It was for the good of his crusade that, although he was a militant prophet, he was always courteous and disliked controversy.

Some of his critics, including Simpson, were unfair, because they either wittingly or unwittingly shut their eyes to his doctrine and stated that he had only used a fresh dressing, namely carbolic acid, for wounds, which had been employed before as a dressing, which was true. Many said his doctrine was wrong because they had followed his directions without obtaining his successful results, but in reality the directions had been carried out imperfectly. Nunneley, a Leeds surgeon, devoted his address on surgery at the meeting of the British Medical Association at Leeds in 1869 to an attack on Lister. It was clear that he did not understand the matter, further he made such a mis-statement of facts as to call forth a sharp correcting letter from his colleague, Pridgin Teale. In London there was much opposition, notably, from Wood of King's College and Savory of St. Bartholomew's. In Glasgow a storm was aroused because Lister said that although the infirmary was unhealthy his cases treated antiseptically had done well in it. Replying to all this took much of his time and energy. It makes sad reading nowadays, and if the surgeons who opposed him can look down on the world, let us hope they do so with shame.

It is pleasanter to turn to those who helped to spread the joyful doctrine that made surgery reasonably safe. MacCormac, Croft, Berkeley Hill, Marcus Beck and Howse, all from London, went to see Lister's methods for themselves in his own wards. In 1871 he was in Manchester going round Lund's wards where antiseptic principles were enforced and there met " Mr. Cooper Forster, a surgeon of Guy's . . . he was much pleased and said he should tell everyone he saw in London that they must see the thing to understand it." Howse and Marcus Beck were undoubtedly the first to introduce rigorous Listerian antiseptic principles into London. Beck visited Lister's wards in 1868, but unfortunately had little opportunity of employing antiseptic methods, for he tells us that he seldom got charge of inpatients and his private patients were few. Still he employed Listerism and preached it whenever he could. Howse, to whom I was dresser, was more fortunate; he told me in writing that when house surgeon at Guy's in 1867 he began trying Lister's methods. In 1870 he became assistant surgeon to this hospital and at once went to Edinburgh to study under Lister; when he returned he converted the other assistant surgeon, Davies-Colley. The assistant surgeons had beds of their own in the general surgical wards and treated many patients who had been admitted under the full surgeons in holiday time or when they were not available. The assistant surgeons, in addition, had sole charge of the septic wards. Howse writes, "We could operate on these [septic] cases in the erysipelas wards with spray and antiseptic dressings as safely as we could in the general wards or even in private rooms . . . from being deadly wards [they] became almost like the other wards of the hospital." All subsequent assistant surgeons at Guy's employed Lister's method. In 1874 Howse was made full surgeon with sixty beds; henceforth the patients in these and all those of the assistant surgeons were treated rigorously by Lister's methods. There was no opposition from the other surgeons who became as cleanly as they could be without Listerism. Howse writes, these facts will "answer at any rate as far as one hospital is concerned, the assertion that London surgeons were slow to avail themselves of the advantage of Listerism."

In the provinces Mitchell Banks and Bickersteth of Liverpool, Lund of Manchester and Oliver Pemberton of Birmingham practised and taught Listerism. In 1874 Hector Cameron became surgeon to the Glasgow Infirmary. He had been Lister's house surgeon, he used rigidly his master's methods and forwarded their adoption by constantly upholding them. From what has been said about Howse, it is clearly not correct to say, as has been done, that, at this time, Lund's and Cameron's clinics were the only two in which rigid Listerism was adopted.

Thiersch, Volkmann, Stromeyer, Nussbaum, Schultze, Sax-torph, Kocher, Lucas-Championnière are the chief of those who enthusiastically preached and practised the new doctrine abroad. We must now return to the chronicle of Lister's life. In 1866 he was a candidate for a vacant surgeoncy at University College Hospital, London. John Marshall, who had been assistant surgeon for eighteen years, was elected. Lister was much disappointed. Syme resigned his Chair of Professor of Clinical Surgery at Edinburgh in 1869. An address from 127 students there begged Lister to become a candidate, he did and was elected in August 1869. Next month his father died, aged 84. Lister, leaving Glasgow, took a house—9 Charlotte Square, Edinburgh —and, as Syme died in 1870, he quickly became the leading consulting surgeon, doing a larger practice than at any period in his career. He was appointed Surgeon in Ordinary to Queen Victoria, and, as such, opened a deep abscess in her armpit, using for the first time a rubber drainage tube with attached silk threads to prevent its slipping in or out. The Queen said the operation was "a most disagreeable duty most pleasantly performed." Life was less tiring than in Glasgow, for he visited his wards at midday instead of in the early morning, and his only lectures were two a week on clinical surgery. These were extempore, the sole preparation was that he always sat still in an armchair for half an hour before a lecture. Patients were brought in, then he gave a real clinical lecture on each, never missing an opportunity of stressing the value of antiseptic surgery. Attendance was compulsory; the number of medical students was great, even 180 entered in one year, so the audience was large, especially as some, who enjoyed his teaching, took out a second course. He was as industrious and irregular as ever; we read of his coming home to lunch from the hospital at four-fifteen, of his working at experiments till 4.30 a.m. and keeping his wife up till far into the early morning to take down notes. During the tenure of his Edin-burgh Professorship he wrote ten papers on antiseptics and two on fermentation, occupying over 200 pages of his *Collected Papers*.

The events of the year 1875 showed that Lister had become famous and did much to advance antiseptic surgery. He and his wife, after a sightseeing holiday in Italy, visited many German hospitals. This part of their tour was described by the *Lancet* as a triumphal march. At Munich, von Nussbaum met him at the station and a banquet was given in his honour, at which nearly all the members of the Medical Faculty, and many members of the Government, Town Council and the Medical Society of Munich were present. He was received at Leipzig by Thiersch; here again there was a huge banquet attended by Volkmann from Halle. Lister spoke in German; songs written in honour of him were sung, one of them was entitled " Carbolsäure Tingel-Tangel." Next morning at 8.30 a.m. he went to a clinical lecture by Thiersch, which the King of Saxony, to whom Lister was introduced, attended. After Thiersch had done one operation, Lister performed another, helped by the Professor's assistants. Volkmann took him over the hospital at Halle where he saw the excellent results of the antiseptic treatment; Bardeleben, too, showed him round the Charité in Berlin, and then took him to see Langenbeck perform his first antiseptic operation. The hospitals at Magdeburg, Bonn and Heidelberg were also visited, and when he appeared in the surgical theatre at Edinburgh on his return in June he was loudly cheered by the students. The British Medical Association met at Edinburgh in the following August. Lister read a paper on Antiseptic Surgery in which he reiterated that he was working on a new principle, namely, preventing putrefaction by keeping living micro-organisms from wounds, and that carbolic acid was merely one way of doing this.

Directly on his return from abroad he received a letter from the Queen's Secretary. Her Majesty had been shocked at what she had heard about vivisection and appealed to Lister to make some public declaration in condemnation of it. He wrote a long and admirable reply in which he excused himself, for his doing so " would not promote the real good of the community, which I know to be Her Majesty's only object in the matter." He gave the reasons why he believed that vivisection is essential to progress of knowledge and relief of suffering, saying: ' I feel sure the avoidance of needless suffering may be reckoned on with entire confidence in the performance of experiments on the lower animals in Britain." This letter remains one of the best statements ever made in defence of vivisection. He gave evidence before the Royal Commission on the subject, stating that he opposed legislative interference. Having just become the representative member for Edinburgh in the General Medical Council, he again urged non-interference and when he found that the Government were determined to pass the Bill he was active in diminishing the hardships to which experimenters might have been exposed. His opposition to legislative interference was largely because he considered it to be a slur on the humaneness of the medical profession. He was an original member of the Research Defence Society, so admirably organized by Stephen Paget.

Next year he continued his evangelistic mission for antiseptic surgery by attending the International Medical Congress in Philadelphia, where he was President of the Surgical Section. He spoke for three hours; at the dinner he sat next to the President of the United States; in both Boston and New York he was received enthusiastically. This visit gave great impetus to the adoption of antiseptic surgery in America.

In 1877 Sir William Fergusson, Professor of Clinical Surgery at King's College, London, died. The appointment of his successor gave rise to controversy, much of it unpleasant, but in the end Lister was invited to take the post. Seven hundred of the Edinburgh students signed a memorial, which they bound in red morocco, begging him not to go. Two hundred and thirty of his past students presented a like memorial. Nevertheless, he accepted the offer, leaving a magnificent position in Edinburgh for one at a small hospital with few medical students in London. To many it seemed a great pity. What decided him is unknown, it may be that as he was a Londoner he wished to return to the metropolis, it may be that he desired to preach his surgical doctrines there. He had stipulated that he should bring his own helpers from Edinburgh. Watson Cheyne came as house surgeon, John Stewart as senior assistant and there were two students, all four had learned the antiseptic system in Edinburgh. Stewart has told us of Lister's depressing beginning at King's College, active opposition from the authorities, hardly any students at the lectures, few beds at his disposal with still fewer patients in them. As time went on things improved, he remained Professor until he reached the retiring age of 65 in 1892, when he was requested to keep in charge of the wards for another year; to this he consented. His private practice in

London was never large, he came too late to secure an extensive connection, his unpunctuality was against him; further he had to depend upon his own assistants for help at an operation and for dressing after, because there were few others who properly understood antiseptic surgery. He retired from both hospital and private practice at the same time. So many years had passed since he had lived in London that he returned to it almost as a stranger, but his pleasant charm and his absence of self-assertion soon made him welcome to his professional brethren, and led to his often being asked to address a medical society.

In the eighth decade of the last century fierce controversy took place between those who believed in the spontaneous generation of micro-organisms in organic tissues and fluids—that is to say that they could appear *de novo* there—and those who said this was impossible. Lister's whole system was founded on his belief of the correctness of the second view. Hence, as at the Pathological Society, he often gave a bacteriological address. Perhaps his paper on *Fractured Patella,* read before the Medical Society, advanced the cause of antiseptic surgery as much as anything, for he showed that with it the broken ends of the knee-cap could be exposed and wired together with perfect safety, although the knee joint had to be opened, which the older surgery did not dare to do, owing to fear of pyæmia. This paper read in 1883 was the beginning of all the brilliant bone surgery of to-day. At the end of it Lister said: " I feel it to be a grievous thing that patients should be hurried out of their lives, or deprived of the usefulness of limbs, simply for want of sufficient earnestness with regard to the endeavour to obtain complete exclusion of septic agencies from wounds." But the battle was now won, for after he had attended a debate of the Woolwich Military Medical Society in the following year the *Lancet* said that it was no longer a question whether antiseptics] should be used but a question of the best means of employing them.

Lister's heart was in clinical work and scientific investigation, but to his great credit he did not shirk official professional duty. He served his time on the Council of the Royal College of Surgeons of England; he was a member of the Committee of Management; he served on the Medical Council; he was President of the Clinical Society; he gave evidence before the

University of London Commission; he was Chairman of the Distribution Committee of King Edward's Hospital Fund; he served on the Council of the Royal Society, afterwards becoming its foreign secretary, and in 1895 its President for the usual period of five years.

Coming north over Chelsea Bridge, a red building faces you, this is the Lister Institute which we owe to the generosity of Lord Iveagh. It provides for research into bacteriology and allied matters, it also provides certain materials for treatment, and investigates specimens. Lister worked hard to start it, joining committees and deputations, and when the building was finished he became Chairman of the Managing Committee and later President of the Institute. Originally, at the suggestion of Lister, it was called the Jenner Institute, after Jenner the discoverer of vaccination, but this was found to be an infringement of a previous right to use the name Jenner, so it was called the Lister Institute.

All the above activities represent unremitting, somewhat uncongenial, work done as a duty. Others were more pleasant. He was a member of the Royal Commission on Hydrophobia and thus played his part in stamping out this awful disease in this country. He read a paper on Antiseptic Surgery at a meeting— described by Paget as "utter heat and confusion"—of the International Medical Congress in Berlin in 1890 where he was received with great enthusiasm; next year he read one on the same subject on receipt of the Cameron Prize at Glasgow, he wrote one on it for the *Festschrift* prepared for Virchow's seventieth birthday, and as President of the Section of Bacteriology gave an address at the International Congress of Hygiene. At the end of 1892, he, representing the Royal Societies of London and Edinburgh, attended the historic meeting held in Paris to celebrate Pasteur's seventieth birthday. The large theatre was crammed, ministers of state and distinguished representatives from all over the world were present. At half-past ten, Pasteur, leaning on the arm of the President of the Republic, came in to the music of the Republican Guard. The President made a short speech, soon after which Lister, greeted with loud applause, was called upon for his address, which he read in French. When he had finished, Pasteur, feeble from age and poor health, stood up, came forward and embraced him. It was a dramatic meeting between two friends; each had saved, and would in the future save, thousands of lives; each had mitigated, and would in the future mitigate, the suffering of tens of thousands. Pasteur was overcome, his reply was read by his son, in it was an especial allusion to his dear Lister, who, unhappily, returned to Paris in three years' time in order to be present when Pasteur was laid to rest in a beautiful tomb in the Pasteur Institute.

It would be wearisome to describe all Lister's speeches, they were so numerous; two more only shall be mentioned. In 1894 he gave an address on antiseptic surgery before the students at Glasgow; he was welcomed vociferously; at the end " Auld Lang Syne " was sung, the horse was taken out of his cab, which the students pushed by a roundabout route to Hector Cameron's house where he was staying. Two years later he gave his address as President of the British Association, in this he explained the value of Pasteur's researches to surgery and the principle upon which antiseptic surgery is founded.

The distinctions conferred upon him by universities, scientific societies and medical bodies were very many; he received the Copley Medal of the Royal Society, he became a Privy Councillor, also a Knight Grand Cross of the Danish Order of the Danebrog; he was elected an Associate of the Académie des Sciences, the highest distinction French science can bestow, he was awarded the Prussian Order of Merit which was a rare honour, and he was an original member of the English Order of Merit. In 1883 he was made a baronet and in 1897, the year of Queen Victoria's second jubilee, he was created a baron. He spoke in the House of Lords on the Contagious Diseases Act, on vaccination, and on early closing. He received the Freedom of the Cities of London, Edinburgh and Glasgow.

There remains but little to say about the facts of his life. The death of his wife when alone with him at Rapallo in 1893 was a great blow. She helped and looked after her husband as devotedly as a mother, sitting patiently for hours taking down notes at his dictation and travelling with him on his many journeys. They were completely bound up in one another.

On his eightieth birthday, many admirers, wishing to do him honour, published, with his consent, a handsome reprint in two volumes of his papers under the title of *The Collected Papers of Joseph, Baron Lister*. The day was celebrated all over the world.

In this country the daily and the medical press commemorated it. Deputations from Amsterdam, Copenhagen and the English College of Surgeons waited on him, at his house in Park Crescent, to present addresses. Flowers and telegrams poured upon him. Vienna and Berlin held meetings in praise of him. The remaining four years of his life were passed in retirement, either in his London house, where he had lived ever since he took the appointment at King's College, or in the country. During these years his health gradually failed and he died at Walmer on February 10, 1912. A funeral service was held in Westminster Abbey four days later; he was buried in Hampstead Cemetery next to his wife.

Only two portraits of him were painted in his lifetime; one —the more satisfactory—by Ouless is in the Royal College of Surgeons in London; the other by Lorimer is in the Library of the University of Edinburgh. Replicas of both are elsewhere. After his death Sir Thomas Brock made the bust in the London College of Surgeons and the medallion in the north transept of Westminster Abbey—these are excellent. In 1924 a bronze monument also by Brock was set up at the North end of Portland Place close to Lister's house, this is much less successful. There is a statue in Glasgow. Lister Memorial Lectures were founded at the Royal College of Surgeons in London and in Canada. An admirable *Life* of him was written by his nephew Sir Rickman Godlee.

Those who consider that genius consists in an infinite aptitude for taking pains, will find, in Lister, an admirable example to support their thesis. His careful industry was wonderful. In this account attention has been directed only to such of his work as bears upon surgery, but he was an investigator of the front rank in other fields. Half his *Collected Papers* are on histology, physiology, pathology or bacteriology. These alone would have given him a great scientific position, it is because of the earlier of them that he became a Fellow of the Royal Society at the early age of 33, and was President of the Section of Bacteriology at the International Congress of Hygiene. Bacteriology occupied an enormous amount of his time. The notes of the results of his experiments in this occupy four or five hundred closely written foolscap pages. They led to his memorable friendship with Pasteur, for whom he had a reverential admiration, and of whose work Lister said, "We find that a flood of light has been thrown upon this important subject (i.e. antiseptic surgery) by the philosophic writings of M. Pasteur."

As a surgeon he was thorough, careful and slow, he does not appear to have had that brilliancy—the good fortune of only a few—of being rapid and yet, like Lister, observant of every detail. Antiseptic surgery enabled him to perform with perfect safety entirely new operations of his own devising, e.g. on the knee joint, and he was ingenious in improving many instruments.

He took immense pains with his teaching and, even if it fell on the deaf ears of the dullard this mattered but little, for he was an inspiration to those who cared to learn from him. The worshipful admiration of old dressers and house surgeons is proof of this. He spoke clearly with a pleasant voice which could fill a large hall and what he said commanded the attention of his audience. He had no arts of oratory and was at times prolix both in writing and speaking, but what he meant was always perfectly clear.

Fortunately there is no need for me to try to describe Lister as a man, because he had, as a patient in the Edinburgh Infirmary, the poet Henley who wrote a beautiful sonnet entitled " The Chief " :

> His brow spreads large and placid, and his eye
> Is deep and bright, with steady looks that still.
> Soft lines of tranquil thought his face fulfill—
> His face at once benign and proud and shy.
> If envy scout, if ignorance deny,
> His faultless patience, his unyielding will,
> Beautiful gentleness and splendid skill,
> Innumerable gratitudes reply.
> His wise, rare smile is sweet with certainties,
> And seems in all his patients to compel
> Such love and faith as failure cannot quell.
> We hold him for another Herakles,
> Battling with custom, prejudice, disease,
> As once the son of Zeus with Death and Hell.

JOHN HUGHLINGS JACKSON

John Hughlings Jackson, from time to time, published in the *Lancet* a series of papers called *Neurological Fragments*. These were reprinted in book form by Dr. James Taylor, who prefaced them with a biography of Jackson which is the chief source of our knowledge of his life.

He was born at Providence Green, Green Hammerton, two or three miles north-east of York, on April 4, 1835. His father, Samuel Jackson, a yeoman, owned and farmed his own land, and was also a brewer. His mother, Sarah Hughlings, was of Welsh extraction. There were four sons and a daughter, she married Dr. Langdale. One of the sons, William, who went to New Zealand, so distinguished himself in the Maori War that the Government gave him a grant of land and he was elected to the House of Representatives. The home at Providence Green, where John was born, is a substantial plain farm-house, with the date 1790 at one corner. John always retained a great affection for it, visiting it regularly once a year; he remarked that it was not generally known that the Garden of Eden was close to Providence Green.

He attended the village school at Green Hammerton, later going to one at Tadcaster and finally to a school at Nailsworth. He always had a poor opinion of these schools, consoling himself, however, with the reflection that he had not suffered from over-education.

Hughlings Jackson was apprenticed to Mr. Anderson, a lecturer in the Medical School of ten or twelve students, which then existed in York, the same school that his Yorkshire friend, Jonathan Hutchinson, had attended seven years previously. From York he came to St. Bartholomew's Hospital, studying under Sir James Paget, whom he often quoted and for whom he had great admiration. The qualifications of M.R.C.S. and L.S.A. were taken in 1836. Returning to York as house surgeon to the Dispensary, he came under the influence of

Laycock, then lecturer on medicine at the York Medical School and later Professor of Medicine at Edinburgh. Laycock was chiefly interested in mental disease. Hughlings Jackson frequently refers to him as a brilliant and stimulating thinker, and mentions the help in morbid anatomy given to him by Dr. Shann and Mr. North of York, where there was a medical club and each member, whenever possible, obtained a post-mortem examination and invited all the others to attend. He returned to London in 1859, with an introduction to Jonathan Hutchinson, whom he had not previously known. About this time his intention was to devote his life to philosophy, but Hutchinson persuaded him not to abandon medicine. The two became lifelong friends. At the end of Jackson's life Hutchinson had misgivings about his original advice, for he then thought, greatly as medicine had gained from Hughlings Jackson, there might have been a greater gain to the world at large if his friend had been left to devote his life to philosophy.

In the year of his arrival in London Hughlings Jackson was appointed physician to the Metropolitan Free Hospital and Lecturer on Pathology at the London Hospital. Next year he took the degree of M.D. of St. Andrew's, and the member-ship of the Royal College of Physicians of London. In 1862 he became Lecturer in Physiology and assistant physician at the London Hospital, the full physiciancy was reached in 1874 and held till his retirement from the Hospital in 1894. He had the honour of delivering three sets of lectures before the Royal College of Physicians, the Gulstonian, the Croonian and the Lumleian, and of receiving the Moxon medal from it. He served on its Council and as a Censor. In 1878 the Fellowship of the Royal Society was conferred upon him, this and the D.Sc. of the Yorkshire University of Leeds, the M.D. of Bologna and the LL.D. of Edinburgh all pleased him greatly.

The nineteenth century saw such an increase in our under-standing of nervous disease that modern neurology may be said to have been born during it. Many of the best intellects in the profession devoted themselves to neurology; they were helped by the founding, in Queen Square, of the National Hospital for the paralysed and epileptic in 1859, by the formation of the Neurological Society and by the publication of *Brain*. Brown-Séquard persuaded Hughlings

Jackson to study neurology specially, and in 1862 he was appointed assistant physician to the National Hospital, where Brown-Séquard was physician; here he worked till 1906 when he became consulting physician. So greatly had he added to the good fame of the Hospital, that a marble bust of him, subscribed for by his medical and surgical colleagues at the Queen Square Hospital and a few others, was, in 1907, placed in the entrance hall of the hospital. On his retirement from the London Hospital, he was in 1894 presented with his portrait, which is now in the Royal College of Physicians, a replica being at the London Hospital. His old teacher, Sir James Paget, made the presentation, happily saying that Hughlings Jackson "had given lucidity to physiology and guidance to surgery." He had earlier received from this hospital a gold watch with an inscription recognizing his devoted work in the last great cholera epidemic.

I attended a meeting held on November 14, 1885, at Dr. de Watteville's house, 30 Welbeck Street, at which it was agreed to found the Neurological Society. Hughlings Jackson was elected the first President, giving his Inaugural Address "On the Scope and Aims of Neurology" on March 24, 1886. The Vice-Presidents were Wilks and Crichton-Browne, each becoming President in turn; Hughlings Jackson was elected an Honorary Member in 1904. The Society became the Neurological Section of the Royal Society of Medicine in 1911. In 1889 the Council of the Neurological Society stated that "The Council has by request inaugurated a lecture in honour of the discoverer of Cortical Epilepsy and its relation to Cerebral Localization, to be termed 'The Hughlings Jackson Lecture.'" The discoverer gave the first lecture on December 8, 1897; its title was "Remarks on the Relation of the Different Divisions of the Central Nervous System to one another, and to the Parts of the Body." Subsequently the lecture was given by various distinguished neurologists. Later a sum of money was collected, by subscribers from all over the world, to provide for awarding a gold medal, with an honorarium to the lecturer, who should be selected every three years, the balance to be expended on books on neurological subjects for the library of the Royal Society of Medicine. On the medal is a portrait of Hughlings Jackson.

The first number of *Brain* was published in April 1878. In 1887 it became the journal of the Neurological Society which in 1906 dedicated to Hughlings Jackson Part IV of *Brain* " as a tribute of Respect and Affection in the 50th year of his Medical Practice." His photograph formed the frontispiece to this number. Several of his papers appeared in *Brain*.

Very shortly after his arrival in London he became Clinical Assistant to Mr. Poland at Moorfields Eye Hospital. When he gave, in 1877, the annual oration before the Medical Society, he said, " I think it the luckiest thing in my medical life that I began the scientific study of my profession at an ophthalmic hospital." It was owing to Hughlings Jackson's insistence that neurologists and general physicians learnt the importance of ophthalmoscopic examination of the eye. He himself made several contributions to the Ophthalmic Journals, he gave the Bowman lecture in 1886 in which he referred to the great personal help he had received from Bowman and Hutchinson. " In fourteen years, in season and out of season," he urged that patients with what was then called optic neuritis may see quite well. This important observation we owe to him. He pointed out that vertigo associated with ocular paralysis was not the result of diplopia, but of erroneous projection; he also claimed that appreciation of the size and shape of objects depended only on the activity of the ocular muscles, and he enunciated the doctrine that, in remembering the shape and size of an object there is slight activity of central motor centres, just as much as there is slight activity of sensory centres in remembering colour. Movements of the muscles of the eye were of great interest to him as supporting his doctrine that the anatomical substratum of a word is a motor, an articulatory process. Towards the end of the Bowman lecture he tells us how we may assign the varieties of ocular paralysis to one or other of the three levels.

During his early days he joined Hutchinson in going to Societies to report meetings and to the hospitals to report interesting cases for the *Medical Times and Gazette*. Like Sutton, he went a good deal to Guy's, which we are told especially attracted him, hence the friendship for Moxon, to whom is owing his adoption of two classifications which will be described later, for he says, " I have much changed my opinions in this matter

since reading an able paper by Moxon *On Classification of Disease.*
After reading this paper, my eyes were opened to the confusion
which results from mixing the two kinds of study [of classi-
fication]." He quotes with approval Moxon's saying, " Never
trust a man for what he cannot know."

There is little to say about the non-professional side of Hughlings Jackson's life. On coming to London he first lived
at Finsbury Circus, which then housed many consulting
physicians and surgeons, two years later he moved to No. 4,
then in a year to 5 Queen Square, Bloomsbury, on his marriage
in 1865 to 28 Bedford Place, where he lived for three years,
going then to 3 Manchester Square; here he remained for
forty years till his death in 1911. The London County Council
have recently placed a tablet on this house to record that Hughlings Jackson lived in it. His accomplished wife, Elizabeth
Dade Jackson, was his first cousin, their engagement lasted
eleven years, the same period as their married life. They were
very happy together, he said, " There was nothing in the world
to compare with domestic happiness." By a strange irony she
died from cerebral thrombosis associated with fits of Jacksonian
epilepsy. After her death he was a lonely man, more shy than
ever. Sir Farquhar Buzzard in his Schorstein lecture (*Lancet,*
Oct. 27, 1934) describes how, at the Buzzard family lunch,
without any announcement Jackson would often come in, no
one took any notice, he pulled up a chair, made a few remarks,
perhaps told a humorous story, then in ten minutes he would
mumble something about an engagement and leave the room.
Nobody was allowed to get up or to see him out. Frequently he
would ask little Miss Buzzard to come for a drive, taking her to
Birch's in the city where he deposited her before a large ice; he
then drove away and returned to fetch her. Or he might take
her to the Zoo, to the Crystal Palace or to see acrobats or performing fleas. On these expeditions he rarely talked. If not
engaged on his work, or taking a holiday, he spent his life at
home. Going out to dinner or to any public function was an
abomination; it was very rare to see him at either; games and
sport had not the slightest interest for him. When reading in
an armchair by the fire, one fine winter's morning in the country,
his friend Jonathan Hutchinson suggested a walk as it was
a beautiful day; Jackson settled closer in his chair and

replied, "It's a beautiful day by the fire." He loved a fire, even in summer it was lighted on the slightest excuse; this cannot have been because he felt cold, for he rarely wore an overcoat. About eating and drinking he did not care in the least, he always hurried through his meals and turned to his easy chair and his book as quickly as possible. Even in company it was very frequent for him to rise and exclaim " Excuse me " and, without further ceremony, to turn aside to read. This was done with a special emphasis and at an earlier stage if there was a fire in the room.

Reading was everything to him, both his recreation and his work. As he disliked company, was not a scholar, played no games, was not musical, was bored by the theatre—if taken he usually came out at the end of the first act—had no taste for art, had no hobby, hardly any artistic imagination so that the pleasure of poetry and of much other literature was almost unknown to him, his reading, apart from philosophy and medicine, was only a pastime. He would read any rubbish that was handy. I have seen him drive up to Mudie's, in his open carriage, on his way from the hospital, and carry away a stack of novels. Among the multitude of these which he read he especially liked Dickens, Jane Austen and Trollope. When papers were mislaid or anything went wrong, he was accustomed to refer the misfortune to the malignant influence of Mr. Harris. He had a great admiration for Herbert Spencer, but, as Mercier rightly says, he gave Spencer far too much credit as the founder and suggestor of his own doctrines. For books as books he had no reverence. He would say, "I did not want the book, I only wanted the information that was in it." He would tear out of a book the part that appealed to him and would often send to a friend a few leaves which he knew would interest him. On one occasion he bought at a railway bookstall a yellow-back novel, he tore off both the front and back boards and threw them away, he then tore the book in half putting each half in a separate pocket. The boy at the bookstall stared in astonishment, Hughlings Jackson quietly said to him, "You think I am mad, my boy, but it's the people who don't do this that are really mad." A colleague of his bought from Hughlings Jackson's cousin his copy of the *London Hospital Reports*, thinking thereby to secure the great man's original articles therein. To his chagrin he found they had all been torn out by their author.

Both Hutchinson and Mercier thought he resembled Dr. Johnson. In so far as he was a conservative, a lover of the truth, industrious, a sayer of apt phrases, and very fond of London, he did, but he had none of Johnson's religious feeling, their philosophies were poles apart. Johnson was not a scientist but a scholar, with a fine style and the writer of real literature. Jackson was a true scientist, whose writings have no style and certainly are not good literature. Johnson enjoyed good company which Jackson did not, and it is impossible to imagine him a celebrated talker, a founder of a club and, towards the end of his life, a traveller undertaking a tour of the Hebrides.

He took holidays, although he did not enjoy them as would a lover of the country. In his youth Hutchinson and he went for Sunday walks, he did not care whither, so long as they reached a good inn at night. Later, in his more extensive holidays, he was restless, rarely remaining more than a night or two in one place and regularly breaking his vacation by returning to London once in ten days to deal with any patients who might want to see him. When away he drove about as in London, the carriage was open, if possible, for he did not seem to feel the cold. He never went abroad if he could help it. He had to go officially to the Donders Festival at Utrecht, but insisted on leaving the place as soon as the chief ceremonial was finished. His dread of being bored was extreme ; he hated anything which foretold dullness but fortunately for himself he had a keen sense of humour.

Hughlings Jackson's lectures were not well attended, for he had a weak voice, nevertheless he kept order at them. He was the quintessence of courtesy to students and fellow-doctors : when he differed from them, and they were wrong, he let them down kindly, gently and without disparagement. He was insistent on accuracy of observation and of thought as is shown throughout the whole of his work. He always wanted the truth, sometmes by giving it he displeased his patients. He never advertised himself nor did anything to attract patients. He was very retiring and never sought applause, although he valued highly the esteem in which he was held by his professional brethren. Jackson was not a man of wide ability, but there was one thing he did supremely well, hence his greatness. It was that he observed symptoms with extreme care and precision, even to the last detail, and went further than others who have done this, for he used his observations as the foundation of far-reaching doctrines which are believed in to this day. On this let me quote Sir Henry Head :

Jackson's attitude was strictly phenomenal. He never deduced his observations from his hypothesis, but any hypothesis he enunciated sprang, as it were, ready made from some clinical fact. He never experimented nor arranged a series of observations to elucidate a definite point. He stood like an observer on a bridge formulating the extent of the flood from the matter carried down by the stream. The acuteness and rapidity of the conclusions he drew from some minute indication made his slower-witted companions believe that he had produced the hypothesis from his inner consciousness; whereas, in truth, the view he enunciated was the direct outcome of some phenomenon accurately observed and carried to a strictly logical conclusion.

The nickname by which he was known was "The Sage."

I only met him three or four times. Nevertheless, from such a slight acquaintance, his kindly face, his courteous manner, the sweet reasonableness with which he listened to me and my knowledge of his master mind made me love and venerate him. I understood, at once, the devoted regard, the admiration and the reverent affection felt for him by those fortunate house physicians and colleagues who worked with him.

For the last ten years of his life his health began to fail, his deafness increased, becoming a serious trouble; the vertigo, from which he had suffered for some time, got a little better but still worried him. He then wrote little, never having the energy to even begin a book embodying his doctrines, although he wished to write it and his friends earnestly desired it. A few years before his death I called on him to try to persuade him to come with me to the suburbs to see a patient, in his charming way he asked to be excused, he was not up to it and he was sure Gowers would go. He became almost a legend before he was quickly carried off by an attack of pneumonia, at the age of 76, in his house, 3 Manchester Square, on October 7, 1911. The funeral, to which very many came, took place in the Highgate Cemetery. The fact that the obituary notice in the *British Medical Journal* filled five pages indicates the esteem felt for him by the medical profession. This is also shown by the celebration, in 1935, of the centenary of his birth by a meeting of the Hungarian Psychological Society at Budapest, at which Dr. Ladislaw Benedek, the President, read, in English, a paper on Hughlings Jackson's doctrines. The Centenary was also the occasion of a dinner, in London, of the members of the Neurological Section of the Royal Society of Medicine, at which the President, Dr. Kinnear Wilson, gave an admirable address on Hughlings Jackson, which was published in the *Lancet*.

We learn from Dr. James Taylor that, in 1901, Osler wrote, on behalf of himself, Weir Mitchell and Putnam, to Hughlings Jackson, asking him to publish a selection from his papers illustrating his views. He was much pleased by the request and suggested that there should be two volumes, the first to contain, in a methodical way, what he had done in neurology, the second, his minor contributions to it. Unhappily he was never able to carry out his intention.

That this request should have been made illustrates the difficulty of dealing with his writings. His publications are very many, somewhere between two and three hundred, they are in numerous periodicals, some of which are hard of access, most require close reading to seize the author's meaning, indeed we find able people using such phrases as " if I understand Dr. Hughlings Jackson correctly." He repeats himself very often, but generally not in the same words, so that care has to be exercised to see that his meaning is the same; he is verbose and his papers are irritatingly encumbered by long footnotes. As he hid his light under a bushel but nevertheless so greatly illuminated neurology, the guarantors of *Brain*, after his death, decided to republish some of his writings. The result is two large, closely packed volumes containing the chief of his papers and addresses, ably selected and edited by Dr. James Taylor. The size of what is only a selection indicates the amount which Hughlings Jackson wrote. My attempt to give some account of his doctrines is drawn largely from these two volumes.

The object of Hughlings Jackson's work may be summed up by saying that he, the most illustrious of clinical philosophers, desired " to develop a science of disease of the nervous system." He did not claim to be a discoverer of facts. " I am also ready to declare that the previous workers mentioned have rendered it difficult for me to put forward anything more than a sort of harmonization of their doctrines." Bright and Bell announced their discoveries in beautiful, stately books. Hughlings Jackson's desire was to preach a creed, hence by a multitude of papers and addresses he tried to reach a large audience. His sermons have so soaked into the medical mind, that most doctors, without knowing it, think as he would have had them think. Really he has done much more for the extension of thought than " the previous workers mentioned."

As his object is scientific he is constantly pleading for precision of terms, I will quote only a few examples. Function must be used in its strict sense, the function of nervous matter is to store up and to liberate a certain variety of energy. The word cause is misused, a cerebral tumour is not the cause of convulsions, their cause is the discharge of nervous energy. The phrase " a patient does not move his arm because he has lost volition over it " is meaningless. The statement that the sane man " lives in the real world," the insane " in a world of his own " is scientifically very misleading, for everybody sane or insane lives in a world of his own.

Classification, he says, is necessary and " of vast importance." We require two kinds, the empirical and the scientific. The first is, strictly speaking, only an arrangement, as when a gardener arranges his plants as they are fit for food or ornament, the last being further divided into trees, shrubs and flowers. The other classification, that of the botanist, is for the better organization of existing knowledge. Here the gardener and the botanist are distinct persons so there is no confusion; but in our profession the same person has to classify in both ways, hence often great confusion. Hughlings Jackson gives many examples: one may be quoted; there is a similar functional condition of nervous tissue in epileptic mania, epileptic aphasia and epileptic hemiplegia; in a scientific classification they are therefore in the same class, but it would be absurd to classify them together for practical purposes, and to put patients suffering from them in the same ward, because scientifically they are fundamentally alike. Scientifically and theoretically we classify diseases as they are departures from healthy states. Empirically and practically we arrange them as they approach certain types.

The following are the scientific principles or doctrines by which Hughlings Jackson sought to explain the diseases which he studied:

Evolution.—" The conclusion I have arrived at from the study of cases of disease is that the higher centres are evolved out of the lower—receiving intercalations as they ascend from the spinal cord to the cerebrum." There are three levels of evolution of the central nervous system: (1) The lowest consists of Marshall Hall's " True Spinal System," i.e. the spinal cord, medulla oblongata, pons Varolii and the nuclei for the ocular muscles. (2) The middle consists of Hitzig and Ferrier's motor centres, Schafer and Horsley's trunk centres and Ferrier's sensory region. (3) The highest consists of parts of the brain in front of the middle motor centres, namely the highest motor centres, and of parts behind the middle sensory centres, namely the highest sensory centres.

The lowest level is probably nearly the whole of the new-born infant's developed nervous system in whom the levels above this, in so far as they are not yet organized, are masses of " nervous stuff " and not centres proper; they are almost a fœtal part of the nervous system, organization in which goes on as growth proceeds. In man evolution is carried further than in the brute: man has large cerebral hemispheres; the brute, large pons and medulla. There are, in the lowest level, sensori-motor processes for very general purposes, their representation in this is re-represented in the middle and re-re-represented in the highest (popularly called the organ of the mind) which is therefore sensori-motor. Evolution from level to level is a passage from the most organized—that is centres already well organized at birth, to the highest—which are continually organizing as life proceeds. As we pass up, representation is enormously increased in complexity, in specialization, in integration, and in co-operation, so that, ultimately, all the processes of the body, motor, sensory, visceral, e.g. cardiac, are re-re-represented at the highest level in an exceedingly intricate " mix-up." Evolution is a process from the most automatic to the most voluntary, from the simple to the complex, from the general to the special. As we proceed upwards the centres have more the power of controlling the lower and are more independent of them. There is a multiplication of both fibres and cells from the lowest to the middle and highest centres. More fibres mean less paralysis from an equal-sized destruction, but, on the other hand, as there are more ganglion cells the convulsion will be the stronger from the higher centre. It will be noticed that at each level there are re-beginnings, which implies occasional stoppages, therefore, at each level, the centres may be regarded as " resistory positions." The highest level is protected by the resisting positions in the lower two, therefore its activities can go on uninterfered with by the evironment and without producing reactions. Thanks to this protection, psychically there can arise trains of thought independent of present experiences, this is internal evolution.

Dissolution.—This principle may be expressed thus : When functions are affected progressively, those first affected are the highest in evolutionary development; that is to say the first affected are the last acquired in the individual and the last to appear in the species. The next affected are those next to the highest and so on, till, finally, the lowest of all from an evolutionary point of view, that is to say the functions of respiration and circulation, are affected. Dissolution is the opposite of evolution; in dissolution there is an undevelopment from the special to the general. Hughlings Jackson believed that the principle of dissolution was confirmed by the experiments of Ferrier. In dissolution the power of the upper centres is removed; this leads to a "letting go" of the lower, which results in their excessive activity. In dissolution we have a principle for the scientific classification of diseases of the brain and of insanity which is dissolution beginning in the highest nervous processes ; the varieties of insanity would be explained by the depth of the dissolution, its rapidity, the kind of brain in which it occurred, by external circumstances and by the bodily state. Dissolution is uniform or local. An instance of the first is the effect of alcohol which flows to all parts of the nervous system, dissolution caused by it affects all the nervous centres, progressing from the highest to the lowest. Local dissolution may result from disease of part of the nervous system. Hughlings Jackson regarded evolution and dissolution as the fundamental basis of his teaching, he knew that the subject had been worked at for many years, that Bell and Anstie, without using the term dissolution, had described a reduction from the voluntary to the automatic by drugs, e.g. alcohol, but they did not appreciate the principle, nor its relation to evolution, nor its wide applicability as an explanation of nervous disorders. We owe all this to Hughlings Jackson, and we must remember that "the man who puts two old facts in new and more realistic order deserves praise as certainly as does the man who discovers a new one."

Compensation.—One convolution does not represent the entire movements of the arm, another those of the leg. Let us suppose external phenomena, e.g. muscular movements x, y, z. As we ascend in representation some units of grey matter will contain largely x less of y and z, others largely y, others largely z, at a higher level, there will be a still less individual representation of each of x, y, z in any unit, but each unit will contain more uniformly x, y and z. This explains why a small destruction of the cortical area will not completely paralyse movements x, y and z; it will weaken them all; on the other hand neighbouring areas will continue to act somewhat for each of x, y and z. Conversely stimulation of a small cortical area will cause convulsion in all of x, y and z. There is no abrupt localization in the cerebral cortex, no centre or part where, say, the hand is entirely represented. The whole cerebral cortex is conceived to be a sensori-motor seat of general representation for the whole body, including the viscera, e.g. the heart and lungs, but there are numerous areas of leading or special representation, one, say, for the hand, discharge from it will cause a spasm of the hand, but destructive lesion of it will not totally paralyse the hand, for other parts of the cortex where the hand is also represented will be able to send stimuli to it; in other words, they compensate for loss of function in the principle hand area. Hughlings Jackson gives other instances of this doctrine of compensation, saying:

I have never acceded to the opinion that speech is to be localized in any one spot, although I do believe, most firmly, that the region of Broca's convolution is, so to speak, "the yellow spot" for speech, as the macula lutea is the centre of the greatest acuteness of vision, although the whole retina sees.

Ferrier's experiments and many clinical cases support the doctrine of compensation. We must remember that differences in external conformation of animals imply differences in function of their nervous tissues, for example the cerebral centres for the tail in dogs and for the paws in cats are highly developed in these animals.

Broadbent's Doctrine.—Hughlings Jackson believed firmly in this, but carried it further than did its author, being of opinion that all movements, indeed all parts of the body, are represented in both cerebral hemispheres, but that when a movement is habitually bilateral it will be represented equally in the two, when it is unilateral it will be represented greatly in the opposite hemisphere and slightly in the hemisphere of the same side. Between these two varieties of representation there will be all degrees, according to the degree in which the movement is habitually bilateral or unilateral. It should be noted that movements, not muscles, are represented in the cortex. Ferrier's experiments and observation, e.g. the march of spasm, confirm Broadbent's doctrine, which is a particular instance of that of Compensation.

Concomitance—" The doctrine I hold is: first that states of consciousness (or, synonymously, states of mind) are utterly different from nervous states; second, that the two things occur together—that for every mental state there is a correlative nervous state; third, that, although the two occur in parallelism, there is no interference of one with the other. This may be called the doctrine of concomitance. Thus, in the case of visual perception, there is an unbroken physical circuit, complete reflex action, from sensory periphery through highest centres back to muscular periphery. The visual image, a purely mental state, occurs in parallelism with—*arises during* (not from)—the activities of the two highest links of this purely physical chain; so to speak, it ' stands outside' these links." This doctrine is at any rate convenient in the study of nervous diseases.

Hughlings Jackson gave much of his attention to the study of convulsions. These can be caused by discharges from any one of the three levels. The study of convulsions naturally led to the study of epilepsy, which he defined as the name for an occasional, sudden, excessive, rapid and local discharge from some part of the cortex which has become highly unstable. As there are different parts of the cortex so there are different epilepsies. Todd (1809–60) had concluded that epileptic attacks were due to sudden periodic discharges from the cerebrum, but his view was not widely adopted, most believed them to proceed from the medulla oblongata. Hughlings Jackson, who was aware of Todd's writings and thought highly of them, studied the whole subject so fully that the modern conception of epilepsy may be fairly said to be due to him. The following is the order in which Hughlings Jackson investigated discharges from each of the three levels.

Middle Level Discharges.—He began his investigation of convulsions by studying cases in which the fit begins by deliberate spasm on one side of the body and in which the parts of the body are affected one after another, saying that it was methodical to investigate convulsions by observing first the simplest varieties. In these we can watch the march of the spasm, for example it often begins in the index finger, next affects the hand, then the whole arm, then the face, then the leg. When, in such a case, we find post-mortem gross disease, e.g. a tumour, we can infer the seat of the discharge which produced the spasm; by doing this we learn that hemispasm and hemiplegia are, in such a case, both due to disease of the same part of the brain on the opposite side to the symptoms, hemispasm being due to instability of grey matter, palsy to destruction of fibres. Fits which begin unilaterally, most often commence in the hand, rarely in the arm; less often they begin in the lower extremity and then in the toes, rarely in the calf; they may begin in the face. That is to say the fit begins in the part which has the most varied uses, which is to be expected, for parts having most varied uses will be represented in the cerebrum by the largest number of ganglion cells, that is the largest area. The unilateral spasm above described may extend to the bilateral muscles of both sides, then to the arm, face and leg of the opposite side and probably finally to the bilateral muscles a second time. Biting of the tongue is of no value in diagnosis, as it may happen in any severe spasm. Defect of speech does not always accompany unilateral spasms, yet, if it occurs, it is most often seen when the spasm is on the right side. Spasm may stop at any stage. It does not affect the arm, then cease and next affect the face. It is a compound spasm, for instance, the face begins to be affected before the spasm of the arm ceases. Spasms of any muscles are invariably followed by paresis of the same muscles, because the grey matter, discharge from which has been over-stimulated by the gross disease, requires rest for recuperation of function; this paralysis is therefore transitory.

If the cerebral discharge spreads widely loss of consciousness ensues, sometimes, when the discharge is due to a local lesion this is so, but, most often, as Bright and others taught, absence of loss of consciousness is in favour of a local lesion. Each case must be considered thus : (1) Seat of internal lesion; as the convulsions are local, this must be local in the opposite cerebral hemisphere. At first Hughlings Jackson thought the seat was in the corpus striatum, but he was soon driven to the belief that the cortex contained the "nervous arrangements" representing movements. (2) Pathological process. Often we do not know but clinical observations will help us to decide whether the lesion is vascular or a tumour. (3) Circumstances which determine the discharge. Here we are much in the dark, but those factors which would excite discharge from healthy nervous tissue will do so the more if it be in a condition of exalted irritability.

From clinical observation of experiments made by disease Hughlings Jackson had discovered that muscular movements are locally represented on the cortex. It is true that Bright had previously described local spasm as indicating disease on the surface of the brain. Hughlings Jackson's was almost certainly an independent discovery, but in his later papers he acknowledged Bright's work, indeed he was always careful to call attention to any previous statement of his own views. He, for example, quotes Wilks as saying "the morbid conditions which we find give rise to epileptiform convulsions are remarkably uniform, they all point to presence of local irritation of the surface [of the brain]." He studied this variety of spasm so scientifically, so deeply, so brilliantly, pointing out how it illustrated his doctrines already described, that it was he who was the real introducer of the doctrine of cerebral localization. If we reflect what this doctrine has meant to medical thought we appreciate the outstanding importance of Hughlings Jackson, and can understand his delight when his teaching, reached solely by clinical observation and philosophic thought, was confirmed by the experiments of Ferrier, who says:

The proximate causes of the different epilepsies are, as Dr. Hughlings Jackson supposes, "discharging lesions" of the different centres in the cerebral hemispheres. The affection may be limited artificially to one muscle, or group of muscles or may be made to involve all muscles represented in the cerebral hemisphere, with foaming at the mouth, biting of the tongue and loss of consciousness. When induced artificially in animals, the affection, as a rule, first invades the muscles most in voluntary use in striking harmony with the clinical observations of Hughlings Jackson.

This form of epilepsy was stated by Jackson to be derived from the middle level, and it is properly known everywhere as Jacksonian epilepsy. The convulsions indicative of it are generally said to be epileptiform. Those derived from the highest level are called epileptic.

Highest Level Discharges.—The highest level is the sensori-motor seat of the re-re-representation for the whole body, including all the viscera, but there are numerous areas of " special or leading " representation, e.g. one for the movements of the hand. Discharges from this level cause what Hughlings Jackson calls genuine epilepsy, usually known as epilepsy, to distinguish it from Jacksonian epilepsy, which results from discharges arising in the middle level. The first symptom of a genuine epileptic seizure will depend upon the site on the cortex in which the discharge starts, subsequent symptoms will occur if the discharge spreads to other parts of the cortex by interconnecting nervous pathways. He thus describes what happens in a severe epileptic fit " Upon discharge of a highly unstable part of the highest centres, . . . there are secondary ' downward ' discharges of healthy middle and then tertiary discharges of healthy lowest centres. . . . All centres are involved in the order from the least to the most organized. . . ."

But, as he tells us, the process is far more complex, for there are also collateral discharges from the unstable highest centre to healthy parts around, from which there are also downward discharges to the middle and lower levels. These events illustrate the principle of dissolution. Over and over again the phenomena of epilepsy are used by him as examples of it. Because discharge leads to subsequent exhaustion of grey matter there will always be paralysis in some degree after severe epileptic convulsions; as we should expect from the doctrine of dissolution, the highest or most voluntary movements will be most paralysed. The frequent failure to observe paresis, after widespread convulsion, occurs because as all muscles are weakened paresis of them is difficult to detect.

Turning to the sensory discharges his teaching was that the highest of the three levels—that is, the sensori-motor cortex—being concerned with the highest facilities must be itself subdivided, or, as he says, have layers. If we get excessive discharge from the highest layer, this must be followed by exhaustion, which means that the normal controlling influence of this layer being taken off the next lower, the activity of this next lower is increased. So on all the way down even to the lowest of the three levels. Unconsciousness, from slight to deep coma, is due to excessive discharge leading to progressive loss of function of the layers of the highest centre. Post-epileptic mania is due to over-action of the lowest of the highest-level layers because the control of the layers above it has been taken off. Symptoms of disorder of the special senses are due to abnormal discharges from the appropriate area of the cortex.

He was much interested in the intellectual aura or, as he called it, the dreamy state. If it occurs suddenly with a warning of taste, smell or epigastric sensation, there is certainly epilepsy. Defect of consciousness, but not necessarily loss of it, is always present. These slight seizures are often misinterpreted by the patient and doctor, until the following of an undoubted epileptic seizure shows them to be genuine epilepsy. In such cases there is a discharge of this or that cortical area without any gross disease, but the occasional presence of a dreamy state with a gross lesion, e.g. tumour, reveals their pathology, as in the woman, who had a dreamy state associated with a crude sensation of smell, and in whom a tumour was found in the right temporo-sphenoidal lobe.

In epilepsy, the symptomatic condition is, as just implied, always double, i.e. due to local discharge from the upper layers of the highest level and to over-activity of the lower layers from which controlling influence has been cut off because of exhaustion following the discharge in the upper layers. This is true even if the fit consists only of a dreamy state (discharge from highest layer) for then memory is so active (activity of lower layer) that the patient is able to tell something of his dreamy state. If the discharge is extensive enough to lead to loss of consciousness and memory, but no more, then over-activity of a lower layer may cause subsequent post epileptic somnambulism, in which the patient does complicated actions unconsciously, and without recollection of them or of his unconsciousness, for example, a man drove a pair horse van from the north of London to the Elephant and Castle. He did it correctly but recollected nothing of what he had done.

The same reasoning applies to sleep with dreams, which is a double psychical condition of two opposites of the highest level;

there is loss of function of the highest layer answering to the negative part of the sleeper's mental condition, and there is the positive part which consists of increased activities of the uncontrolled lower layers which answer to the mentation of his dream. As Hughlings Jackson says, there are really two persons: A who was temporarily non-existent, B who thereupon came into existence and dreamed, but B passed away on the awakening of A. In insanity there is the same double psychical condition. There is the negative affection of consciousness from trifling confusion of thought to complete loss of it, at the same time there are positive symptoms such as illusions and delusions. The negative symptoms are often overlooked. This extremely important distinction between negative and positive symptoms must constantly be borne in mind, if we are to understand nervous diseases properly.

Jackson was, particularly in regard to epilepsy, very insistent on the difference between physiology and pathology. By the physiology of a case he meant the departure from the healthy function of nerve tissue. Obviously, in epilepsy, the nervous physiology is abnormal. How this abnormality is produced is a pathological question; he suggested that it was caused by altered nutrition, but, as late as 1882, he said our anatomical knowledge of epilepsy is only vaguely inferential. Our pathological information is nil. We have only certainty as to the physiological process.

Lowest Level Discharges.—Hughlings Jackson considered that some poisons, e.g. camphor, absinthe and the poison of uræmia act on the lowest level. The most interesting example of lowest level fits is seen in laryngismus stridulus, attacks of which occur in the young, in whom the two higher levels are not fully developed and therefore have not much restraining power on the lowest, but this is the most strongly organized, consequently, after childhood, it is difficult to upset. He says "were not the cardiac, vaso-constrictor and respiratory centres of the lowest level more strongly organized hereditarily, life would be impossible, if the centres of the highest level did not continue to be little organized and thus very modifiable, few new acquirements would be made." Rickets, it is suggested, causes laryngismus, because the rickety ribs mean imperfect respiration, which means venous blood, which acting on the lowest level centres causes convulsions. He particularly calls our attention to the fact that organized is not synonymous with complex. The highest centres are most complex, but least organized, least automatic and therefore very modifiable; the lowest are least complex, but most organized and most automatic. There are all evolutionary gradations from the lowest to the highest. A man is comatose from alcohol poisoning because his least organized (highest) centres are rendered functionless, but his most organized (lowest) centres, e.g. cardiac and respiratory, go on working, for being strongly organized they can resist the poison. Four of Hughlings Jackson's " Neurological Fragments " are devoted to the lower level.

Aphasia.—There was much confusion of opinion about this, and many theories did not fit the facts. Hughlings Jackson showed that this arose in the main from two causes. Firstly, that no distinction was drawn between a scientific and a clinical classification. Secondly, because it was not recognized that " destructive lesions never cause positive effects, but induce a negative condition which permits positive symptoms to appear." These really arise during the activity of the lower centres, which have escaped injury and from which higher control has been removed. Sir Henry Head, who has done much to make us aware of Hughling Jackson's view, puts it thus:

Every case of affection of speech exhibits, therefore, two sides—the negative and the positive; on the one hand, the patient may not be able to speak, to write, or to read, and expression by signs may be impaired. This is the negative aspect, whilst his power of writing his signature, and of swearing, or uttering other emotional expressions, form the positive symptoms and are the expression of lower mental activities.

Hughlings Jackson, in classifying affections of speech, first separates articulatory difficulties due to paresis of tongue, lips and palate, which may be accompanied by difficulty of swallowing, from true affections of speech in which there is inability to write or speak freely but swallowing is perfect. Next he says healthy language is either (1) Intellectual, that is it has the power to convey propositions by words and signs; when this is impaired, the most special, i.e. speech, is impaired most, the least special, i.e. sign-making, least or not at all. (2) Emotional, e.g. variations in voice, smiles and gestures.

It is the first which is usually disturbed in disease. Clinically there are two groups of this disturbance: the very severe, in which the patient is almost speechless and can only utter one or two unvarying words or jargon; the less severe, in which there are "plentiful movements." Head summarizes Hughlings Jackson's teaching, saying that in these less severe cases, speech suffers in proportion to the mental task the patient has to perform, in each case we must inquire "what aspect of the mind is damaged." Sign-making is the least often affected, writing usually, but then the patient can generally copy or sign his name; speech is the most often affected and in many ways, details of which are given by Hughlings Jackson. The loss of power to name an object depends upon the complexity of the task. The higher and voluntary aspects of speech suffer more than the lower, a man may have lost all speech, but he can still utter exclamations and emotional phrases such as oaths, which are automatic utterances. The "speechless man is not wordless." Writing is affected, not as a separate faculty but as a failure to propositionize in words, for, before we write anything we make—without speaking—a proposition in words which we write. There is no such thing as agraphia. The patient can copy and often sign his name, because with most people this has become automatic. Even if he cannot read aloud, he can understand what is read to him. These are all defects on the emissive side, but we also have defects on the receptive side by failure of those processes which underlie perceptual recognition. Failures of both sides may co-exist. Much discussion has taken place on "External Speech" and "Internal Speech." Jackson explained the difference thus. Take a phrase, for example "gold is yellow." Whether this is said aloud or thought, there is propositionizing. The first case is External Speech, the second Internal. If a man write, as he usually does this without uttering words, the act of writing must be preceded by Internal Speech. Behind both speaking and writing stands the proposition which when verbalized can be expressed in either speaking or writing. In the majority of cases of affections of speech mental images are unaffected.

Hughlings Jackson is constantly trying to see whether phenomena he is observing support the doctrine of dissolution. In an article on the "Duality of the Brain" he studies aphasia from this point of view. The brain is double, in most persons speech is destroyed by a lesion of it on the left side, but a lesion in the corresponding part of the right side has no effect on speech. The man with the left-sided lesion has neither external nor internal speech, he cannot propositionize. Nevertheless, he still has processes for words in his brain, because he understands a proposition, e.g. gold is yellow, stated to him, and, as the left is damaged, the right cerebrum must be that by which he receives propositions. When the statement gold is yellow is made to anyone, doing so revives in his right cerebrum similar words. A man whose left cerebrum is damaged can often utter automatic phrases such as, God bless me. This is because the right side of the cerebrum deals with both the reception of propositions and the automatic production of words, the left with the voluntary production. We must not here talk of loss of memory of words, for we are concerned solely with muscular movements. There is loss of the most special voluntary form of language (speech), without loss of the less special, that is the automatic emotional manifestations. Thus, in an ordinary case of aphasia, we have dissolution of the higher muscular speech movements governed by the left cerebrum, whilst the lower automatic, governed by the right, are intact. This is only the bare outline of the argument, which should be studied in the original paper with a constant remembrance of the difference between negative and positive symptoms.

The fame of Hughlings Jackson has grown continuously since his death. The more his writings have been considered, the more widely and firmly has the truth of his neurological and psychological doctrines become established. The year 1935, being the centenary of his birth, has seen the publication of a Hughlings Jackson Memorial Volume with a biographical foreword by Prof. Benedek, the editor. The second International Neurological Congress was held in London in August 1935. The opportunity was taken for the delivery of the Hughlings Jackson lecture, by Prof. Otfrid Foerster, before a large audience of neurologists from all over the world, which greeted the mention of Hughlings Jackson's name with great enthusiasm. The lecturer pointed out that Hughlings Jackson's entirely new conceptions had successfully withstood the test of sixty years' experience and that in the world of neurology nothing moved which was not Jacksonian.

SIR PATRICK MANSON

The Manson family had been long settled in Aberdeenshire. John Manson, a laird of Fingask and manager of the local branch of the British Linen Bank at Old Meldrum, lived just outside the town in a house called Cromlet Hill. The photograph of it, in the *Life of Patrick Manson* by Manson-Bahr and Alcock, shows it to be—for it still stands—a substantial house in pleasant old-world grounds. John married an Aberdeenshire lady, Miss Blakie, a woman having beauty, good health, good spirits, artistic talent and much resource. They had nine children.

Their second son, Patrick, was born at Cromlet Hill on October 3, 1844. The family moved into Aberdeen in 1857, for the sake of the education of their children. Patrick went to the Gymnasium and later to the West End Academy. He did not show any special promise; he was fond of carpentry and outdoor occupations. A prophetic tale is that, having shot a cat on his father's farm, he was much interested in a tapeworm he found in it on dissection. At the age of 15, he was apprenticed in the ironworks of Messrs. Blakie Brothers, where he worked just the same hours as other workmen; this was then, and is still, the usual thing for an apprentice in such works. Quite soon, however, he had spinal trouble, with loss of power in the right arm which remained all his life. He was made to lie on his back for most of the day and passed the time reading natural history; when at the end of five months the treatment was discontinued he decided to study medicine, and entered the University of Aberdeen in 1860; he also attended at Edinburgh; passing his final examination at the age of 20, he went to London to see something of the hospitals there. He obtained his M.B. and C.M. degrees at Aberdeen and soon after was appointed Assistant Medical Officer at the Durham Lunatic Asylum. There he made many post-mortem examinations and prepared his thesis on *A Peculiar Affection of the Internal Carotid*

Artery in connection with Diseases of the Brain; for this he was awarded his M.D. at Aberdeen in 1866.

Tired of Asylum work in this year he obtained the appointment to the Chinese Imperial Maritime Customs of Medical Officer for Formosa. It was in June 1866 that he arrived at Takao in Formosa. He had his official duties, which included care of patients in the mission hospital, and his private practice. This succeeded well, for in four years he was able to repay his father the £700 which his medical education had cost. It was while he was in Formosa that he first suffered from gout, which was to be a serious handicap to him in after life. Political unrest in the island led to his leaving it in 1871.

He transferred to Amoy, having the same post there as he had had in Formosa. This Chinese city, with a native population of 300,000 and about 280 foreigners, is on an island about 300 miles north of Hong-Kong. The island is only nine miles in circumference; it lies in the bay of Hiu Tau, and, having two fine harbours, open to all nations, is a very busy place, doing a large trade, for the city of Chang Chowfu is not far up the river that discharges into the bay. The native part of Amoy was filthy, but the Europeans were well housed and the climate is good. Here Manson lived for thirteen years. In addition to his official duties, he was in charge of the Mission Hospital. Those who practise western medicine in China have many difficulties to overcome. Manson found, in Amoy, persistent rumours that a poisonous pill was distributed by European doctors; this he combated, to some extent, by saying that his hospital provided the antidote. The natives did not think much of treatment which could be had for nothing; this was met by charging the wealthy, many who would not come before now came to see Manson. It was urged that native practitioners worked in the open, they would prescribe in the street, while the foreign doctor lured you into a hidden consulting-room; thereupon Manson saw and prescribed for patients in a room open to the street, this helped confidence. To obtain a post-mortem examination was almost impossible. Manson's practice was aided by the fact that his early operations did well. A young man had an enormous elephantiasis tumour, he could not work, he was a burden to his relatives who advised suicide; he tried this three times with arsenic, but took so much that each time he was at once sick and thus got rid of the poison. He consented to an operation, for he considered that, as he could not kill himself, Manson might as well do it. He completely recovered. Some successful lithotomies impressed the natives greatly, for they could be shown the stone removed.

Manson worked industriously with little help, except that for two years his brother David, also a missionary doctor, was associated with him. He enlarged the hospital, translated Curling's *Diseases of the Testicle* into Chinese, and trained a few Chinese in the ways of Western medicine. Some assisted in the hospitals, others went into practice. Manson would lend them money with which to start, and the loans were repaid.

The year 1875 was spent in England on holiday, partly in Scotland, enjoying country pursuits, especially fishing, of which he was fond. His tall, big, healthy-looking figure suggested that he was a sportsman. He married Miss Henrietta Isabella Thurburn, on December 21, 1875. They started for Amoy after the wedding. Here, except for another holiday in England, he remained until December 1883.

His activities in Amoy fall into two divisions. First, there were the duties of a medical practitioner; here he was very busy; he described himself as an indifferent surgeon, but a good carpenter. Nevertheless, in 1877 he performed 237 operations and in 1879 the number was 379. The second division of his work was original investigation. The desire to find out about diseases was very strong in him; indeed, when we consider the disadvantages he encountered it was remarkable. He went to the East very young; he had had no more scientific training than the average young medical student of those days; he had no scientific teachers with whom he could correspond; in such out-of-the-way places as Formosa and Amoy there was no one with whom he could discuss; he had no means of keeping abreast with scientific literature and he had no apparatus except a poor microscope, replaced by a better after his first holiday.

His best investigation was done in the hope that he might find out something about elephantiasis. So little did he know of scientific people and libraries that, in 1875, he actually went, of all places, to the British Museum Library to read about it. He there learnt that microscopic worms named Filaria sanguinis hominis had been found by T. Lewis, in 1872, in the blood of a patient who had chyluria. These were recognized to be embryos, the parent worm was discovered in 1876 by Joseph Bancroft of Brisbane and is now known as Filaria bancrofti. Manson correctly surmised that the cause of chyluria, lymph scrotum and elephantiasis was obstruction in the lymphatics by these worms. This is now recognized as correct, text-books contain pictures showing such obstruction on post-mortem examination. He examined very many cases and showed how commonly the embryos may be found in the blood. It is now known that in some Pacific Islands from 60 to 80 per cent. of the inhabitants are affected; the area of infection is enormous, reaching round the world in a belt of a width of about 30° both north and south of the equator. He also discovered that numbers of persons harbour these parasites in their blood, although they always seem in perfect health. He noticed that sometimes, in the blood of those who were known to be infected, the parasites could not be found; therefore he arranged for observations to be made on the blood of two patients continuously day and night for ten days and thus he learned that the parasites do not appear in the blood till evening; by midnight there may be several hundreds in a drop of blood, which means from 40 to 50 millions in the circulating blood; by 9 a.m. the blood contains none. We have since learned that if the patient sleep in the day the parasites are then in the blood, but absent at night if he is then awake, also that when they are absent from a drop of blood they have retired to the lungs to reappear in the blood when the patient sleeps. Many years later he saw in Charing Cross Hospital a man with a small tumour on the arm; it was removed, in it was found a live female Filaria bancrofti, which swam about in normal saline for twelve hours before it died. The patient committed suicide at 8.30 a.m.; there were at that time no embryos in the blood, although they had been observed there in the day-time, but at the post-mortem they were found in millions in the capillaries of the lung.

To return to Amoy, Manson rightly considered that there must be an intermediate host for the filaria, he thought the mosquito the most likely, so, in 1877, he fed mosquitos by letting them, at night, bite a man who had the embryos in his blood. He found them in the mosquito's stomach, partially traced their development there and erroneously thought that when the mosquito died in the water where it had laid its eggs, the filaria larvæ were set free in the water, and were, from that, swallowed by man or penetrated his skin by boring through it. It is now known that they are transmitted to man by the bite of the mosquito. Still Manson's was a great discovery, because he, for the first time, showed that metaxeny or change of host occurred between man and mosquitos. His researches were buried in the *Customs Reports*, but some years after he published them in a book *The Filaria Sanguinis Hominis and certain new Forms of Parasitic Diseases in India, China and Warm Countries.*

Less important work done in Amoy was that he improved the treatment of liver abscess. He saw and figured the leprosy bacillus, but did not recognize the importance of what he saw. He discovered that a form of ringworm common in Amoy was not ordinary ringworm, but was due to a fungus named by him Tinea imbricata. He fully described this fungus, and proved that it was the cause of the disease by innoculating the arms of two Chinese assistants with it. This malady is now known to be a widespread tropical disorder. He helped to popularize vaccination, and a student trained by him was appointed public vaccinator to the city of Chang Chowfu. Whilst looking for filaria embryos he found, in the blood expectorated by a patient, the eggs of what is now known as Paragonimus westermani, or the lung fluke; he traced its development and suggested that the intermediate host must be an inhabitant of fresh water; this has turned out to be correct, for the hosts are fresh-water crabs and crayfish. This form of blood-spitting is a serious disease in China, Japan and Formosa. He also accidentally found, at a post-mortem, the rare ribbon worm called Ligula mansonii, about which we know little.

Manson left Amoy for Hong-Kong because a growing family demanded a larger income. He practised there for six years from December 1883. Among his many patients was Li Hung Chang. During one of Manson's worst attacks of gout he was called, in November 1887, to go 1,800 miles by sea, to visit the great man, who was said to be suffering from cancer of the tongue. Manson had to be carried on board ship, but his gout was better on arrival at Tien-tsin; he saw his patient, found that the supposed cancer was an abscess under the tongue, and opened it. Li Hung Chang was soon well and wrote a letter of thanks to Manson, to whom he "wished an elegant time."

In Hong-Kong, Manson's organizing ability came to the front. He had much to do with the establishment of a dairy farm for the supply of pure milk; he was the main spirit in the building of the Alice Memorial Hospital, and he formed a local Medical Society of which he was the first President in 1886. In this year his own University of Aberdeen made him an Honorary LL.D., and Sir James Cantlie joined him in practice, taking on the surgical part of it. Manson now had more time, which he devoted to the founding of the Hong-Kong Medical College for the instruction of native students in Western medicine. This was a stupendous task. No education in Anatomy or Physiology is needed for Chinese medicine, which is simple oral or written tradition handed down from time immemorial; anybody can call himself a doctor. The profession of medicine is, even to-day, despised by the Chinese. It is classed with witchcraft, and many educated Chinese think that Western medicine is equally despicable. In the purely Chinese Universities the medical faculty attracts very few students. Far less than one per cent. of the native doctors practise Western medicine, nor is the demand for those who can increasing. If a Western-educated doctor treats a patient who dies, it is quite likely that he will find himself in prison on a charge of murder.

However, although the Medical College in Hong-Kong has not greatly increased the number of natives practising Western medicine, it has been of great use. The inaugural ceremony of its foundation was on October 1, 1887, the Acting Governor of the Colony was in the chair. Li Hung Chang, who was Patron, wrote a letter showing that he, at any rate, was desirous for the diffusion of Western medical and scientific thought. Manson was Dean. The project of a College of Medicine was strongly supported by Sir James Cantlie. That great political genius Sun Yat Sen became a student, and was the first to graduate—which he did with high distinction—in 1892. In a subsequent address he gave to the students he admitted that his residence in Hong-Kong and the teaching he received at the College made him a revolutionary, that is to say he wanted to reproduce in his own country what he learned while a medical student, of the purity of justice, of the incorruption and of the efficiency of the government of Hong-Kong with its effective police protection and its splendid sanitary service.

It is doubtful whether the University of Hong-Kong would have come into being had not the College of Medicine existed as a substantial nucleus. This College had no headquarters, its teaching was carried out in nine different hospitals, but here, as in Liverpool, the medical college was really the beginning of the new university, for the College authorities welcomed the suggestion that it should be a nucleus for the University when this was founded in 1912. Happily two years later the Rockefeller Foundation endowed the three principal medical chairs. Now the University of Hong-Kong is an important institution for the higher education of Chinese youths. There are faculties of arts, engineering and medicine. There are departments dealing with every aspect of the last, with Professors of Anatomy, Physiology, Pathology, Medicine, Surgery and Gynæcology; altogether there are some thirty teachers in the medical department, one being a malariologist who receives £1,230 a year. The standard of degrees is the same as in the Universities of Great Britain, and the medical degrees of Hong-Kong are recognized by the General Medical Council. The total present number of students in the University is 361, of both sexes—mostly men—of whom 280 are Chinese. There are 153 medical students, of whom 7 are women. The clinical work is done in the Government Civil Hospital and in the Tsan Yuk Hospital. So the Medical College founded by Manson and Cantlie has led to something of importance.

In 1889 Manson retired from practice in Hong-Kong, and, renting the estate of Kildrummy on Donside, became a country gentleman. Next year, owing to the depreciation of the Chinese dollar, his income became so reduced that he had to start practice again, which he did at 21 Queen Anne Street, London. It was a bold venture to undertake at the age of 46, but after a few years it was amply justified. In his house he fitted up a laboratory known as the muckroom where he worked hard at blood parasites. This room was in a state of perpetual disorder; he, however, knew his way about in it. His apparatus was a microscope and a few stains; his specimens he obtained from where he could in London and from missionary societies abroad. Once when he was examining the blood of an inmate of Hanwell Asylum the patient seized the microscope and tried to brain Manson with it, fortunately an attendant clutched the lunatic just in time. His energy was great, for he read for the M.R.C.P. examination, which he passed at the end of his first year in London, and, in 1892, he was appointed physician to the Seaman's Hospital Society, with charge of fifteen beds at the Albert Dock Hospital, a rather dreary little building in a dreary neighbourhood, a long way from Queen Anne Street. Manson put a small laboratory nearby, worked in it, often till late at night, examining the blood of the patients who came from all parts of the world. Gradually students made their way to the hospital to learn from him. In December 1893 he gave a demonstration at University College Hospital of malarial parasites in the blood; in 1894 he lectured on Tropical Medicine at the Livingstone College founded for the instruction of missionaries; later in this year he was delighted to be appointed to lecture on the same subject at Charing Cross and St. George's Hospitals; the year after he gave the Gulstonian Lectures on Malaria.

In 1896 he was a participant in one of the most extraordinary of political events. His old pupil, Sun Yat Sen, being a revolutionary of great ability, was a trouble to the Chinese Government, who placed a price on his head. He fled to London, he dined with his old teacher and a few days later, on October 11, when he was walking close to the Chinese Legation in Portland Place two Chinamen approached him, enticed him into the Legation, and acting under orders from Peking kept him prisoner. He managed, with the help of one of the English servants in the Legation, to get a note to Manson, who received it on October 17. After communicating with the Police and the Foreign Office, Manson called at the Chinese Legation and demanded to see Sun Yat Sen. The attendant denied his being there; Manson, however, found out that he was to be smuggled that night down to the docks for China, so he and Cantlie remained in a cab outside the Legation all night, thus preventing Sun Yat Sen's removal. Next day Lord Salisbury insisted on the captive's immediate release.

The appointment of Manson in 1897 to be Medical Adviser to the Colonial Office was of great importance to himself for the fine position it gave and the salary attached. But it was of much more importance to the Empire, for Manson was an admirable organizer who got on with people, was not afraid of hard work, had wide experience and was essentially progressive. Fortunately Joseph Chamberlain was then Colonial Secretary. He appreciated Manson and between them they instituted many reforms; the health of the Crown Colonies improved and the education of Colonial Medical Officers was directed specially to the work in which they would be engaged.

Manson was now an exceedingly busy man; he lectured in Tropical Diseases at the Royal Free Hospital; he founded the Section of Tropical Diseases in the British Medical Association, and in 1897 published his text-book on *Tropical Diseases,* which went through many editions, was translated into French and Spanish and was generally recognized as the standard work on its subject. A reference to the bibliography at the end of the *Life* of him shows that during the eight years he had been in London he had made very many contributions to medical literature. In 1900 he was elected a Fellow of the Royal Society. In the following year a knighthood was conferred on him, and the year after he received the Hon. D.Sc. degree from Oxford. In 1905 he delivered the Lane Lectures at San Francisco. An important date in the history of Tropical Medicine is May 1907, for then at a meeting held at the Colonial Office it was decided to form a Society of Tropical Medicine. Manson was the first President; it flourished exceedingly, attaining a membership of over a thousand. In the volume of Allbutt's *System* published this year there are more than two hundred pages by Manson.

The rest of his story is soon told, he resigned from the Colonial Office in 1912, being made a G.C.M.G. He then retired from practice, but honours still came to him; a few only need be mentioned. At the International Medical Congress of 1913, held in London, he received a gold medal presented by an International Committee, and was rightly acclaimed as the father of Tropical Medicine. Cambridge and Hong-Kong both gave him the degree of LL.D. He delivered the Huxley Lecture; he was awarded the Jenner Medal; was made a corresponding member of the Académie des Sciences and an Associate of the Académie de Médecine. He settled at " The Sheiling " on Lough Mask, County Galway, passing the time fishing and gardening. His gout greatly increased, he suffered from heart attacks, became more and more infirm and died on April 9,

1922. Three months before his death he was presented with his portrait subscribed for by his past students and friends.

Manson was a good teacher, his pupils liked him and always held him in affectionate remembrance; he wrote well, had a fluent pen and a scientific mind. His industry was prodigious, especially when we remember how often he was laid low by gout. Before his time several Englishmen in the tropics had done fine original medical work, but, although we had all India, the Dominions and the Colonies as part of the British Empire, the study of tropical medicine was completely neglected. Manson altered all this. We have seen how he enlarged the hospital and taught at Amoy, how his medical institute was the germ of the University of Hong-Kong, how with the help of Chamberlain he reformed the medical work in the Colonies, how he wrote an admirable text-book and dozens of articles, thereby keeping tropical medicine to the front, how he founded the Royal Society of Tropical Medicine, now housed in a fine building appropriately called Manson House, how he gladly lectured on Tropical Medicine, at several schools, and I shall show how energetically he urged forward the study of malaria and how he was the moving spirit in the foundation of the School of Tropical Medicine. I can remember the total absence of the teaching of tropical medicine in London. Now we have that magnificent building and hospital, the London School of Hygiene and Tropical Medicine; it, the Liverpool School of Tropical Medicine, the University of Edinburgh and the English Conjoint Board all grant diplomas in this subject. Such a diploma is essential for many medical colonial appointments, and the University of London M.D. can be taken in Tropical Medicine. All this is due to Manson; it is entirely just to call him the Father of Tropical Medicine.

Laveran in 1880 discovered the malarial parasite in the blood of patients suffering from malaria. Manson in China did not hear of this till five years later, then, when he looked for the parasite he could not find it, but he succeeded in doing so in London in 1892. Hereafter he was much interested in the subject. It was clear that the parasite must have an intermediate host and naturally with his knowledge of filaria he suggested that this host was the mosquito. He enunciated this hypothesis in a paper *On the nature and significance of the Crescentic and Flagellated*

Bodies in Malarial Blood (*Brit. Med. Jour.*, December 8, 1894) in the following words:

The Mosquito having been shown to be the agent by which the filaria is removed from the human blood-vessels, this or a similar suctorial insect must be the agent which removes from the human blood-vessels those forms of the malarial organism which are destined to continue the existence of this organism outside the body. It must, therefore, be in this or a similar suctorial insect or insects that the first stages of the extra-corporeal life of the malarial organism are passed.

He suggested that the flagella of the malarial parasites getting into the insect penetrate the cells of one of its organs. He considered it impossible to say how the parasite passes from the insect to man and commended his hypothesis to those who are in parts of the world where it can be tested. All the three Gulstonian lectures given in 1896 were devoted to malaria. The mosquito theory was reiterated, the flagellum, he said, is the first stage of the life of the malarial organism outside the human body, the suggestion was made that when the mosquito dies the malarial organism is conveyed in the dust from dried-up pools to the human body. He was wrong in this, wrong about the flagellum, which is a male sexual organ, and the suggestion that mosquitos convey the disease had been made by both King and Laveran before Manson published it, but there is every probability that he was unaware of this, so that with him the suggestion was original.

Manson certainly did, by his frequent insistence on the mosquito hypothesis, educate the profession in it and indeed in the whole subject of malaria. He told Ross of his hypothesis in November 1894. Ross replied that Laveran had made the same conjecture, but said he " was tremendously impressed with the argument and determined to test the hypothesis thoroughly on my return to India." Whether Ross would have studied the subject if this conversation had not taken place, no man can say, but it was Ross alone who discovered the life-history of the malarial parasite. During the four years his investigation took he wrote 110 letters to Manson describing its progress. Manson constantly replied, he kept people in England informed of the work of Ross, examined the specimens he sent ; wrote strong letters to the Government officials in England urging them to do all they could to enable Ross to carry on his research, saw Lord Lister and Joseph Chamberlain imploring them to press for the giving of facilities to Ross, he even got Lord Lister to come to his house to see the slides Ross had sent, and he persuaded the Royal Society to send Dr. Daniels to India to help him. The whole friendly correspondence between these two men is a credit to both. Ross, speaking of Manson's letters, called them " a noble series such as few men have received."

In order to make the general public appreciate the importance of the part played by the mosquito in malaria, Manson obtained, from malarial marshes near Rome, some live mosquitos infected with malaria. They were allowed to bite two healthy Londoners —one Manson's son; both got malaria and the parasites were found in their blood. Conversely he arranged for two English doctors to live on a very malarious marsh at the mouth of the Tiber, for three and a half months, during the malarial season; they went abroad during the day, but for the whole time they were in a mosquito-proof hut from an hour before sunset to an hour after sunrise. The malarial mosquito only bites at night, therefore these two did not get malaria, while the unprotected people round about suffered severely. This son of Manson's went later, with a fellow Guy's student, H. E. F. Durham, to study beriberi on Christmas Island, where he was killed by a gun accident.

In the course of his constant examination of the blood of patients in the Seaman's Hospital he discovered three or four new species of filariæ. The two most noteworthy are the Filaria diurna, the laval form of Filaria loa, so often found in the West African disease known as Calabar swelling. The larvæ are only met with in the blood during day-time. Manson suggested that the intermediate host was the mangrove fly, Chrysops; this has turned out to be correct. The second was the larval form of Filaria perstans; the adult stage was found some years later, the intermediate host is not known. He also did work on the anatomy of the Filaria bancrofti and of the guinea worm.

Perhaps the greatest debt which posterity owes to Manson is that arising from his founding of the London School of Tropical Medicine. We have seen that he was, in 1897, Medical Adviser to the Secretary of State for the Colonies, at that time Mr. Joseph Chamberlain. Manson told him of the importance of investigation as to the cause of tropical disease and of the necessity of educating doctors, who were going to certain Dominions, India, and the Colonies, in tropical medicine. In 1898 Chamberlain wrote to the Board of Management of the Seaman's Hospital Society requesting them to establish a school for the teaching of tropical diseases in connection with their Albert Dock Hospital. At a dinner presided over by Chamberlain £12,000 was raised for this purpose. The School was opened on October 3, 1899, in a small laboratory in the grounds of the Albert Dock Hospital. It was an immediate success; students came to it from all over the world, and it was recognized as a School in the faculty of medicine by the University of London. Enlargement became necessary and by the advocacy of Mr. Chamberlain £73,000 more was raised. Those who had had to make the long and tedious journey to the Albert Dock were delighted when, in 1920, the school and hospital were moved into a large hotel, converted to its new use, in Endsleigh Gardens. The building was generously purchased and presented by the British Red Cross Society. In 1924 the hospital and tropical school were incorporated with the London School of Hygiene, and a charter was granted to the London School of Hygiene and Tropical Medicine. By this time the public had subscribed £250,000 to the Tropical School.

The value of tropical medicine to the British Empire is so great that in 1921 the Minister of Health appointed a Committee, presided over by Lord Athlone, to inquire into the teaching —especially postgraduate—of tropical medicine and public health. The committee recommended a central institution for all branches of tropical and preventive medicine which should be affiliated to the University of London. The want of money seemed fatal to the scheme; fortunately the Rockefeller Foundation with its customary princely generosity came to the rescue. It offered the British Government nearly £500,000, for the purchase of a site and for building and equipment, provided that the Government would see that expenses of upkeep were provided. This is now done in so far as the expenses are not met by students fees and the small amount derived from endowment. Thus it has become possible to build an imposing and extensive building in Keppel Street and Gower Street, close to the new University buildings. The Prince of Wales opened it in July 1929. There is a large Staff of Professors and other teachers in all branches of

Hygiene and Tropical Medicine. There are laboratories for ordinary education and for research, theatres, classrooms and everything that can be required for the purposes of this fine school. All this has flowed from a conversation between the Colonial Secretary and Manson.

SIR RONALD ROSS

Ronald Ross, scientist, poet, mathematician, novelist, water-colour painter and musician, was born on May 13, 1857, at Almora, in the Kumaon Hills, among the Himalayas, three days after the Indian Mutiny began. Many of the family had served in India. His father was General Sir Campbell Claye Grant Ross, K.C.B., a highly distinguished soldier and also an excellent water-colour artist. His mother, Miss Elderton, lived with her father at Effra House in Brixton; this had gardens, fields and a boat on the river Effra, which rises near the Crystal Palace and flows into the Thames at Vauxhall Bridge; it is now covered in. She was married in London in July 1836 and went with her husband to India. They had ten children, of whom Ronald was the eldest. In his *Memoirs,* from which I have taken most of my information, he gives an entertaining account of his ancestors.

Childhood and youth, passed in England, were happy years spent among those interested in the arts. He entered as a student at St. Bartholomew's Hospital: " But I must confess that the medical profession and all its associates and associations were little to my taste or inclination." When he should have been studying medicine, he was trying his hand at poems, stories and plays, composing music, painting or doing sculpture. As regards medicine he was idle, becoming qualified with difficulty and passing, low down on the list, into the Indian Medical Service.

He arrived in Madras in October 1881, subsequently moving to other places as ordered. Medical duties only occupied an hour or two a day; most of his time was given to writing poetry and studying mathematics. Before long he " began to recognize the futility of my mathematical efforts. I was only a self-taught amateur," so he devoted himself more vigorously than ever to writing novels and poetry. After seven years of this life, he came home on leave and, on April

25, 1889, married Miss Rosa Bloxam. He took a diploma in Public Health, attended classes in Bacteriology held by Professor Klein in London, and with his wife arrived back in Madras in September 1889. Next year he became Staff-Surgeon at Bangalore; this appointment was for three years; he continued his literary writings, spent much time with Greek and Latin poets, became depressed about mathematics, but took more interest in medicine. Long leave in Europe began in February 1894, the first part being spent on a delightful holiday in Switzerland, the rest in England. *Spirit of the Storm* was accepted by Methuen for publication. Two thousand copies were sold, the book was favourably reviewed and the author received £17 7s. 11d.

Ague or malaria is a disease known to have existed from Greek and Roman times, it has always been widespread in warm countries; it has killed many millions of people and has been the cause of ill-health to many more millions; large marshy districts are such hot-beds of the malady that they may be uninhabitable. It was supposed to be spread by an effluvium in the air from the marsh, hence the name malaria. Laveran had, in 1880, discovered a minute animal parasite, the malaria plasmodium, living in the red blood corpuscles of those who have the disease. This parasite belongs to the most elementary class of animals, the single-celled animals or Protozoa. It discharges spores into the blood; when it does so the patient has an attack of ague; the spores, which are asexual, enter other red blood cells, grow there, and the process is repeated. Not all the plasmodia form spores, for some, the sexual variety, assume a crescentic shape—they are then called crescents—these become spherical and full of melanin; they are called spheres or spherules and some of them become violently agitated and emit filaments which become loose and are the flagella. The cells, often called flagellate bodies, from which the flagella come, are now known to be the male sexual form of the parasite; the flagella are sperms. The female cells, also derived from the crescents, are round. The question was how do malarial parasites enter the man or animal—birds have malaria—affected with malaria. The principle of metaxeny or change of host was known; for example, the guinea worm which affects man passes part of its existence in the water flea, called cyclops. Laveran and others had suggested that malaria was conveyed to man by a mosquito.

When Ross arrived in England on leave in March 1894, he had failed to find Laveran's parasites in the blood of sufferers from malaria. He inquired of Professor Kanthack, the pathologist at St. Bartholomew's Hospital, who assured him that Laveran's discovery was sound and referred him to Manson, who showed him the parasites, whereupon he was convinced. Manson told him he thought that the question of how man gets malaria would be solved by studying mosquitos. This was natural, for Manson had shown that part of the existence of the Filiaria bancrofti, which causes chyluria and other diseases in man, is passed in a mosquito, being an example of metaxeny. Ross replied that Laveran had made the same suggestion, but he was immensely impressed with the argument and determined to test the hypothesis on his return to India. Manson attached importance to the fact that the flagella never appear till about ten minutes after the blood is drawn, suggesting that the process of their appearance occurs in the stomach of some suctorial insect.

During the winter 1894–5, Ross was writing two novels and also an essay on malaria, which won the Parkes Memorial Prize, in this he adduces arguments to show that the effluvium hypothesis for the cause of malaria is wrong, the chief being that, if it were true, the intensity of malaria should diminish inversely as the square of the distance from the marsh or other source, but this is not so.

Seldom does a poet tell the tale of his own scientific discovery; so it was, however, with Ronald Ross. I shall follow the story as recorded in his *Memoirs*.

He left England on March 1895, as he says, badly equipped for the fray, for he knew little about mosquitos or about the best way of staining malarial parasites. During the slow progress of the P. & O. boat *Ballarat,* he looked—without success —for malarial parasites in patients at the ports at which the ship touched; he spent much time with his microscope and in dissecting cockroaches; he was getting his hand in. Bombay was reached on April 21, Secunderabad, in Southern India, at midnight April 24–25. It was then the height of the hot weather, the ground was a desert, the wind terribly scorching and dry like that from the blast of a furnace.

Ross got to work at once and, within a few days, was able to find the parasites in the blood of 50 per cent of the cases of malaria examined. The mosquitos were a trouble; they would not bite the malaria patients on whom they were put to feed, or they died. Then the grubs of those that were bred died. He became nearly frenzied, but fortunately found out that by wetting the bed and mosquito curtains with water the creatures could be readily induced to bite. On May 13, 1895, his birthday, he for the first time found malarial parasites in the stomach of a mosquito which he had fed on a malaria patient. This excited him; next day more mosquitos were examined. In the blood of a man examined immediately after its withdrawal he found numbers of crescents (a stage in the life of the sexual parasite) but no spherules (a later stage of the same); in the same patient's blood kept two hours, there were mostly crescents and a few spherules. In a mosquito's stomach, half an hour after biting, nothing but spherules. This "seems to me to prove that the crescents change into spherules in the stomach of the mosquito as outside"; and suggests that they do so faster there than in controls of a patient's blood. Here was a step forward within three weeks of arrival at Secunderabad. "Talk of phagocytosis! I have seen things these last three days; I am dead beat now and the lids of my right eye are swollen and painful—at work from 7 a.m. to 7 p.m. with snatches at breakfast and tea," nevertheless, he continued his investigations. The spherules, which he usually calls spheres, were studied in the mosquito's stomach; by twenty minutes after the mosquito had had its feed of blood from a malarial patient, the pigment in them showed "an almost eruptive movement, as if flagella were about to burst forth in a moment, the spheres themselves were shaking"; in blood which had been in the mosquito's stomach half an hour he found "all the spherules bursting with excitement and exceedingly numerous" and flagellate organisms in every field; they were unmistakable "because they were being dragged about over the field generally or were quivering and being shaken as a dog does a rat." All the observations were repeated and controlled against direct examination of the patient's blood from the finger. The conclusion is reached that, very shortly after the crescents reach the mosquito's stomach, they are converted into spheres, some of which quickly show the above activity, flagella are then given off from them, the spheres from which they are given off may be seen as collapsed little bags containing pigment; these are more numerous the greater the time that has elapsed since the mosquito fed, which shows that they are not produced in the preparation of the specimen; the little bags are engulfed by leucocytes. Nearly half the spheres fail to throw out flagella, the movement of pigment in these gradually becomes slower and finally it collects to a heap at one side, then in two hours the bioplasm begins to swell up irregularly. (Subsequent investigation showed these spheres to be the females, those that emitted the flagella (sperms) being the males.) At this period of his study Ross thought that what were really females were simply parasites which had died. All this does not necessarily prove that the mosquito is the natural host which infects man with the parasite, but Ross urges that these metamorphoses proceed in the mosquito's stomach more rapidly than in controls of the patient's blood, which is strongly in favour of the mosquito being a natural host of the malarial parasite. Further he observes that quinine checks completely these changes in blood from the finger, but if the human being bitten by the mosquito has had quinine they are only delayed in the mosquito's stomach. In less than a month, during which the heat was intense, Ross had dissected 54 mosquitos, had made innumerable observations, and had arrived at the above conclusions, all the while doing his regimental duties.

About this time the Maharajah of Patiala wrote to the British Government asking that Ross should be sent to his country to investigate the fevers which abounded there. The Government could not give permission. Ross proposed that Manson should go, but nothing came of this.

It was suggested by Manson that the flagellated bodies work their way into the tissues of the mosquito, where they undergo unknown development, and when the creature dies, the human beings are infected by dead mosquitos either in drinking water or in dust. Ross put dead mosquitos, which had been kept alive for many days after biting a man who had malaria, into water which was given to healthy persons. One suffered from a slightly raised temperature but no malarial parasites were found in his blood, the others were unaffected. If

Manson's hypothesis about flagellate bodies was correct, they should increase in the mosquito as days passed by, but they diminished rapidly. (The reason for this was found later to be that being sperms they had entered the female spheres.) Therefore Manson's hypothesis had for two reasons to be put aside.

The cause of the rapid diminution in the number of flagella worried Ross. He studied them carefully and gives the following graphic description of one which he watched for three hours in the blood inside the stomach of a mosquito fed on a malarial patient.

He (the flagellum) wriggled round for twenty minutes . . . so that I could hardly follow him. Then he brought up against a phagocyte and remained so long that I thought the phagocyte had got hold of him. Not a bit, he was not killed or sucked in , but kept poking him in the ribs. . . . I was astonished, and so apparently was the phagocyte. He kept at this for about a quarter of an hour, and then went . . . straight at another phagocyte ! He pushed into this in several places with one end for a long time. . . . After 50 minutes, the beast seemed to be getting tired . . . . a third phacocyte came at him with mouth right open . . . the flagellum left his fallen foe and attacked the new one, holding on and shaking like a snake on a dog. In one minute the third phacocyte turned sharp round and ran off howling ! ! !

He concludes with " I shall dream of it. Good night. . . . I shall write a novel of it in the style of *The Three Musketeers*." Later on Ross was of opinion that what he saw was the male sperm attacking the female spores. What a pity he did not at that time grasp the significance of his observations.

Further investigations enabled him to verify completely all that he had seen up to now.

During August 1895, Ross followed another trail. In the stegomyia mosquitos with which he worked he found some little barley-shaped bodies, which were the psorosperms of unicellular parasites—coccidia and gregarines, which live in mosquitos, these psorosperms were in the Malpighian tubes which open into the pylorus, there were also in these tubes encysted gregarines, clearly the parents of the psorosperms. Was it possible, he said, that these bodies were another form of the malarial parasite ? Was it possible that free flagella developed into gregarines ? He found numbers of psorosperms discharged from the anus of the mosquito. Psorosperms could be found in mosquito grubs. " In short, I believe that psorosperms are meant for men as well as for re-infecting grubs." Men would be infected by psorosperms discharged from the mosquito's anus on to the skin of the patient on whom it alighted. This is more likely than that they infect drinking water, for then a simultaneous group of cases would be expected to occur among those who had drunk the same water. This is not so; malaria cases constantly come in driblets. Ross drank water in which were numbers of psorosperms, he did not get malaria, nor did many others who swallowed them. Another reason why it was suspected that the psorosperms hypothesis was wrong, was that it was contrary to all our knowledge that there should be two cycles—that of the malarial parasite and that of the gregarines —in the same creature, viz. the mosquito. Still, on the principle of trial by error, the hypothesis had to be investigated. In the Spring of 1896 he writes to Manson:

The psorosperms were given at all degrees of freshness and in large numbers, so it certainly looks, as it was to be suspected, that they are not the thing. But I will watch and pray and try a few more experiments . . . but the belief is growing upon me that the disease is communicated by the bite of a mosquito.

Manson wrote to say he did not think so.

Severe cholera broke out at Bangalore in Mysore, and Ross was transferred there on special sanitary duty in September 1895. He did not regret this interruption to his malaria studies, because it gave him an experience which was later invaluable when the mosquito-malaria theory, having been proved, was to be applied practically. He was given dictatorial powers, worked from 6.30 a.m. to near midnight, wrote his report on the cholera epidemic and, on his leaving in April 1897, the British Resident published an order highly praising all that Ross had done, which pleased him greatly.

In his *Memoirs* he speaks bitterly of the " humbugs " who opposed him in this cholera work, kindly of the enlightened who helped him, despairingly of officials who were so slow in their recognition of the value of the discovery of the cholera micro-organism. The following from his notebook " In Exile " refers to this period:

Twice have I driven thee hence,
Defeated, dreadful Guest—
O murderous Pestilence:
This time thou conquerest.

Loudly the people's cry
To thee in prayer swells;
I seek to purify
The deadly poisoned wells—

In vain. The languid child
Lies on his mother's knee;
The mother follows; wild
The people shriek to thee.

"Great," he cries, "is Sanitation—the greatest work, except discovery, I think, that a man can do. We must begin by being Cleaners."

We cry "God made us Kings,
Poets or Prophets here!"
The scornful Answer rings,
"First be My Scavenger."

When the cholera epidemic died down, he found a little leisure for malarial investigation. Mr. K. N. Appia, assistant surgeon to the hospital in Bangalore, courageously volunteered to be bitten by malaria-infested mosquitos. He was bitten by five, but remained absolutely free from malaria. This was disappointing: perhaps, says Ross, the proper species of mosquito had not been employed. He was distressed that he could not think of any explanation of the fact that only about half the crescents emit flagella. The already described "Adventures of a Flagellum" should, he says, have opened his eyes.

On 16th February, 1897, shortly before leaving Bangalore, I observed something which should certainly have revealed the truth to me in a flash. In the blood of a case of quartan malaria on that date, two parasites were lying close together, one emitting a number of struggling flagella, the other remaining a perfect sphere with one of the flagella moving slowly within it. . . . Of course only one sperm enters the female cell; but it did not occur to me that this one had entered the sphere—I thought it was trying to get out! I was so obsessed with Manson's hypothesis that these sperms were flagellated spores.

The honour of the discovery—nearly made by Ross—that the flagella were sperms which entered the female cells falls to W. G. MacCallum, who published his discovery in November 1897. Says Ross: "I have always felt disgraced as a man of science ever since."

He now reverted to the post of medical officer to his regiment, still at Secunderabad, and taking leave which was due to him,

joined his wife on March 27, 1897, at the delightful hill station
Ootacamund. Desperate attempts were made by Manson in
England, and by some of the authorities in India, to obtain
special leave for him to study malaria, but there was so much delay
that, at his own expense, during his leave, he went to a malarious
place, Kalhutti, near by, to investigate malaria. Unfortunately he
himself had a severe attack, parasites were found in his blood, he
made calculations that such enormous numbers of the infecting
agent must have been in the air or water, if infection had come
from either, that it would be easy to detect, but the examination
of stagnant water was negative. He convalesced slowly. Now
for the first time he observed and caught an Anopheles mosquito
full of blood from a human being, he also met with so many
Culex sylvestris mosquitos that he suspected they conveyed
malaria, but, as he found out later, Anopheles was the real
culprit. By this time he had become very suspicious that the
key to the problem lay in finding the particular mosquito which
transmitted malaria in man by biting as he surmised. He
had found other parasites besides gregarina in mosquitos.
Here was a difficult problem, an equation of two unknown
quantities, namely many species of mosquito, many kinds of
parasites, which mosquito and which parasite conveyed malaria.
There was only one method of solution: that of incessant trial
and exclusion. To this heavy labour, he now bent himself.
Considering the many observations that might have to be made,
he was very lucky to solve the problem as soon as he did.

After a rest—the heat was awful that summer in Secunderabad
—work began again in July. The punka was stopped because
it blew the mosquitos about, therefore crowds of flies tormented
him; "the screws of my microscope were rusted with sweat
from my forehead and hands." He found and bred Anopheles,
fed them on malarial patients, killed different ones at different
times so as to trace changes in them. On August 20, 1897—
afterwards always called mosquito day—he found in the stomach
of mosquito No. 37, which had been fed on the 16th, "a great
white expanse of cells." "The Angel of Fate fortunately laid
his hand on my head," so in spite of heat Ross continued to look
and observed that each cell had a circular outline with pigment
granules inside. These cells were certainly not part of the mosquito. Next day, mosquito 39 was examined, a day further

removed from the feeding : there were the cells again, only much larger ; they had grown in 24 hours. Therefore, as they contained pigment exactly like that in the crescents, they were almost certainly malarial parasites growing in the mosquito, and this was the stage of development after five days in the mosquito's stomach. " The thing was really done." (These white cells, called " zygotes," were shown later to be the female cells which had been fertilized by the sperms.) The night between examining No. 37 and No. 39 was spent in agony lest 39 should die, it being then the sole survivor of the batch. Notes being made in the scientific note-book, he wrote in it also the lines :

This day relenting God
    Hath placed within my hand
A wondrous thing ; and God
    Be praised. At his command,

Seeking His secret deeds
    With tears and toiling breath,
I find thy cunning seeds,
    O million-murdering Death.

I know this little thing
    A myriad men will save.
O Death, where is thy sting ?
    Thy victory, O Grave ?

The observations were confirmed on other mosquitos. Manson arranged for the publication of Ross's discovery in the *British Medical Journal*, December 18, 1897. Thirty-six years later a tablet was placed on the cottage at Secunderabad in which he had sweated in the heat. It has on it the following inscription :

To the memory of Sir Ronald Ross, and the discovery he made here on August 20, 1897, that the anopheles mosquito is the carrier of the malaria parasite.

To his intense disgust, malaria investigation was interrupted in September 1897 by his being transferred to Kherwara in Rajputana, where there was not any malaria. He, Manson, and others implored the authorities to give him leave; after months of delay he was accordingly appointed for special duty in research and arrived at Calcutta in February 1898. Here he found few cases of human malaria, so he turned his attention to that of pigeons, larks, crows and sparrows ; for malaria affects birds, the malaria parasite in them is similar to that of human malaria and is conveyed by mosquitos getting under the feathers and biting the bird. There were many difficulties, such as getting the right birds, the right mosquitos, finding birds with malarial parasites in their blood, keeping the mosquitos alive for a long time, which he did by feeding them over again. He worked enthusiastically, examining hundreds of mosquitos, and found that the zygotes by the sixth day after biting have passed through the mosquito's stomach wall, the number of them being proportionate to the number of parasites in the bird's blood. Then about a day later they discharge a number of elongated bodies which Ross called germinal rods, these a little later are found in the mosquito's blood, abdomen and thorax, they are abundant in the creature's salivary glands. "I am dead beat with excitement and work." On July 6, 1898, he writes of all this to Manson, saying :

In all probability it is these glands which secrete the stinging fluid which the mosquito injects into the bite. The germinal rods, lying, as they do, in the secreting cells of the gland, pass into the duct when these cells begin to perform their function, and are thus poured out in vast numbers under the skin of the man or bird. Arrived there, numbers of them are probably swept away by the circulation of the blood, in which they immediately begin to develop into malarial parasites, thus completing the cycle.

The problem started upon in March 1895 was solved.

The result was telegraphed to Manson who told the news to the British Medical Association held at Edinburgh at the end of the month. It "created quite a furore," and the Tropical Section passed a resolution of congratulation to Ross. Although much time had been compulsorily spent in harassing official work, he had in three years become a famous scientist. The pity of it is that he did not recognize that some crescents become females, others males, and that impregnation takes place in the mosquito's stomach, also that he was denied then the opportunity of completely working out the problem on human malaria.

Special leave had been given for research on malaria and kala-agar, consequently he went to Assam to study the last named, but nothing of importance came of this, and he returned to Calcutta in November. In December Dr. Daniels, sent out by the Royal Society, arrived to assist him in his malaria work ; he confirmed Ross's findings and left in February 1899. Some Italian observers extended Ross's results to human malaria and to mosquitos in Italy, a translation of their paper appeared in the *Lancet* of December 3 and 10, 1898. He was of opinion that his work was not properly referred to in this publication and that the authors had attempted to forestall his priority. This made him very angry; now, so long after, it would be a pity to quote what he wrote. In February 1899 Ross left India, taking his leave, and, at the end of it, retiring on pension; he arrived in England at the end of March.

The London School of Tropical Medicine had been founded. Liverpool had just decided also to have such a school and local merchants in that city had raised some money for the purpose; immediately after his arrival home Ross was invited to apply for the post of Lecturer on Tropical Medicine there, and was appointed on April 10. He felt disgusted with the salary—£250 a year, with a proportion of students' fees, in a few months it was raised to £300 a year, and three years later he became Professor with a salary of £600 a year. He went to Liverpool because he considered he would thereby get opportunities of studying the best way to eradicate malaria. Before settling down he visited Paris with Ray Lankester, met Laveran and Metchnikoff and showed his specimens in London at the Royal Society.

In the autumn vacation he and E. E. Austen, the authority on Diptera, travelled to Sierra Leone, free passages being given to them. Ross quickly found anopheles mosquitos containing human malaria parasites, he discovered that they bred in pools of water and therefore urged that the authorities should get rid of the pools in which these mosquitos breed. Directly he got back to Liverpool he brought out a pamphlet called *Instructions for the Prevention of Malarial Fever, for the use of Residents in Malarious Places*; this went through many editions. In 1902 he published *Malarial Fever, its Cause, Prevention and Treatment*; it was very popular, being translated into German and Greek. In several publications and at many meetings he urged that malaria should be attacked by destroying the breeding-places of mosquitos.

The Royal Society was asked, in 1900, to approach the Colonial Office on this matter. Michael Foster, its secretary, wrote a friendly letter to Ross asking him to name places where the experiment might be carried out. Ross, in his *Memoirs*, comments that an experiment was not desired, which would be like an experiment to prove that two and two make four, and that the Society were asking him to advise on a self-evident proposition. Not long after, with regard to the same matter, he was one of a deputation to the Colonial Secretary, Joseph Chamberlain. A sanitary commissioner was suggested. Ross comments: "I suppose he thought I had suggested a sanitary commissioner in order to find a job for myself." These are instances of Ross's unhappy way of taking offence when none was intended.

Fortunately Mr. Coats provided him with money to give, in West Africa, an object-lesson on mosquito reduction. He went with Dr. Logan Taylor, they drained pools and destroyed old tins and the such-like in which mosquitos breed. He returned in time to read a paper on malaria before the British Association. Lord Lister, in proposing a vote of thanks to him, said that the discovery "was due solely and simply to Major Ross" and, with regard to exterminating breeding places, "the results already obtained were an absolute proof of the efficacy of the means adopted." Ross writes: "I look upon these words as the red ribbon of my life."

In this year he obtained his F.R.S., and was invited to accept a post at the Lister Institute, and also to return to India; neither of these proposals came to anything. Next year (1901) he was awarded the Cameron Prize and journeyed to Ismailia, a hot-bed of malaria, where he found the mosquitos bred in sewage-pots and from thence flew into the open air up the ventilating shaft. A little kerosene on the surface of the contents of the sewage-pots eradicated malaria: in 1901 there were 1,990 cases, in 1902, 1,551, in 1903, 214, in 1906, 0. In the autumn of 1902 he received the Nobel Prize in Stockholm.

In 1906 he went to Greece to advise about malaria. While there the supposition that the decay of ancient Greece was due to malarial invasion entered his mind, it has since been supported by historians. In 1907 he visited Mauritius to advise upon the malaria there. Numbers of honours were conferred on him, he was made K.C.B. and K.C.M.G., banquets were given to him; he was a celebrated man.

After he left his official post in India he did no original work, saying he had lost heart for it, because of early opposition, and because of the attempts to deprive him of priority. "So the great Passion died." At Liverpool he gave much thought to malaria propaganda, a little to mathematics and to literature. He resigned his professorship there in 1912 and, coming to London, set up in practice at 18 Cavendish Square. Before beginning this he went on a malarial advisory tour, visiting Spain, Cyprus and Greece. On his return he became the editor of *Science Progress*. He entered wholeheartedly into a campaign for the payment of great discoveries by Parliament, and in the War, he, being in the Territorial Army, was employed chiefly in dealing with malaria. "My time at the War Office was nothing but pleasant to me." Subsequently he was made Honorary Consultant in Malaria to the Ministry of Pensions, but found leisure in 1920 to give a lecture on Science and Poetry before the Royal Institution.

A committee, with the Duchess of Portland as President, raised money to commemorate the twenty-fifth anniversary of the discovery that malaria is transmitted by the bite of a mosquito. The appeal was made in 1923; over 1,000 contributors came forward, among them were the Prince of Wales, fifteen tropical dependencies and eight rulers of states. A sufficient sum was obtained to found the Ross Institute, which was placed in a large house adapted for the purpose, facing Putney Heath. Ronald Ross was the first director. The cost was £25,000 and the running expenses from £8,000 to £10,000 a year. A fund of £15,513 was also raised to provide for Lady Ross; this gave her husband much happiness. The Institute contained two small wards, some research laboratories and a library; its object was, not to teach, but to foster research in tropical diseases and to act as a propaganda centre for information as to the prevention of malaria. It sent fourteen expeditions abroad to investigate malaria and to advise as to its extermination; it arranged lectures for laymen (engineers, tea planters, missionaries and others) who wished to be taught how to carry out antimalarial work; it published a little book, *Notes on the Prevention of Malaria,* many thousands of copies of which were given away; workers in its laboratories did research and, lastly, it was of great use as a kind of clearing-house of knowledge about malaria for the benefit of those whose business took them to malarious countries. All these activities and propaganda were exceedingly valuable; on the very day that I write this, there is a letter in the *Times* telling of the great fall, in recent years, in the deaths from malaria in Nigeria. The teacher at the head of the Ross Institute and the teacher at the head of the Tropical School (Manson) have reaped a great harvest. After the death of Ross the Institute was moved to and merged in the London School of Hygiene and Tropical Medicine.

As Director of the Institute, Ross went, in 1925, to Ceylon to advise about malarial prevention. He also visited Malaya and India early in 1926 and in Singapore he lectured on malarial prevention. The antimalarial work in Malaya had for many years been extensive and successful. Sir Malcolm Watson, who was in charge, showed Ross round. Afterwards he gave Watson a copy of his poems, with this inscription, " Sir Malcolm Watson, who proved that the piece on p. 77 was a damned lie." Turning to this page, Watson found a poem of which he prints the following part :

"THE ANNIVERSARY"
(AUGUST 20, 1917)

Now twenty years ago
  This day we found the thing;
With science and with skill
  We found; then came the sting—
What we with endless labour won
  The thick world scorned :
Not worth a word to-day—
  Not worth remembering.

And clapp'd our hands and thought
  Your teeming width would ring,
With our great victory—more
  Than battling hosts can bring.
Ah, well—men laugh'd,
  The years have pass'd;
The world is cold—
  Some million lives a year,
Not worth remembering !

. . . but when true
  Achievement comes—
A trifling doctor's matter—
  No consequence at all !

This anecdote is taken from Sir Malcolm Watson's fine eulogy of Ross in *Science Progress*, vol. 27, p. 377. Malaya was by no means the only place where Ross's teaching had borne fruit; for example, in 1914, Gorgas had written to him, "Your discovery that the mosquito transferred the malarial parasite to man has enabled us, at Panama, to hold in check this disease. . . . It was your discovery of this fact that enabled us to build the canal at the Isthmus of Panama."

Ross returned to England in time for the formal opening of the Ross Institute, on July 15, 1926, by the Prince of Wales, who said: "I can think of no single discovery in recent times which will earn the deep gratitude of so many thousands of human beings of all nationalities as the discovery made by Major Ross. . . . It is not too much to say that Sir Ronald Ross has made one third of the world inhabitable."

In 1927 he had severe paralysis of the left side; he slowly improved somewhat, but his activities were much impaired. He passed the time publishing or republishing some of his literary and mathematical works. His wife died in September 1931. After this he went to be nursed at the Ross Institute; he gradually became weaker and died there on September 16, 1932.

Four years previously he offered for sale his archives, chiefly concerned with his work on malaria. They formed a complete collection about this subject. Lady Houston bought it for £2,000, and the collection went to the Ross Institute. There is a bronze medallion of him in front of the General Hospital in Calcutta, near the site of the room in which he worked.

To many people Ross appeared as a critic and a fighter who both in his sayings and his writings was unnecessarily caustic. His great discovery was accepted by some and opposed by others; he did not stop to reflect that everything new always has been and always will be opposed by those who do not understand it, and should be severely criticized if we are to arrive at truth. The path of discovery is paved with the corpses of false discoveries killed by criticism. Darwin went quietly on, leaving his critics, for the most part, to be answered by others or to take care of themselves. Ross fought them fiercely. It is difficult to say which method ensures the quicker triumph of a new doctrine which is true. In private he was friendly; his memoirs are full of kindly appreciations of those with whom he worked, he goes out of his way to distinguish between his dislike of a man's opinions and his liking for the man. He gave his time freely to those who wanted advice.

The outstanding characteristics of Ross's make-up were his imagination, his vision and his sense of beauty. We have seen that he was not interested in medicine. He attacked the malarial problem because it appealed to the above characteristics and because its solution would benefit mankind.

He takes a place in the highest class of our minor poets. When Mr. Marsh published his first volume of Georgian Poetry, Ronald Ross was a chosen contributor because his poetry was eminent as such. Professor Lascelles Abercrombie, in an appreciation in *Science Progress* (vol. 27), writes:

Science gave him a profound æsthetic satisfaction, and art for him was but a transvaluation of scientific truth. When the poet in him saluted the Unknown Power it was in these noble lines:

> He is the Lord of Light;
> He is the Thing That Is;
> He sends the seeing sight;
> And the right mind is His.

The thing that Is—the seeing sight—the right mind; whatever was precious to the scientist was precious to the poet; scientist and poet only differed in expression. The result is something unique in our literature. . . . The remarkable thing in Ross was that he had mastered the technique of poetry as thoroughly as he had mastered the technique of science. . . . "In Exile" will surely stand as one of the masterpieces of modern poetry.

Osbert Sitwell speaks of the "great and unforgettable beauty" of Ross's poetry. Mr. John Masefield writes equally enthusiastically. He also wrote beautiful prose, witness some of the descriptions in his *Memoirs*. He could paint, he wrote music. For an account of his poetry, his novels and his mathematics, the reader should consult *Ronald Ross*, by R. L. Mégroz.

INDEX